Medical Enhancement and Posthumanity

The International Library of Ethics, Law and Technology

VOLUME 2

For other titles published in this series, go to
www.springer.com/series/7761

Bert Gordijn • Ruth Chadwick
Editors

Medical Enhancement and Posthumanity

Springer

Editors
Bert Gordijn
Ethics Institute
Dublin City University
Ireland
bert.Gordijn@dcu.ie

Ruth Chadwick
University of Cardiff
Cardiff Law School
Museum Avenue
Cardiff
United Kingdom CF10 3AT
chadwickr1@cardiff.ac.uk

ISBN 978-1-4020-8851-3 e-ISBN 978-1-4020-8852-0

Library of Congress Control Number: 2008933211

Printed on acid-free paper

9 8 7 6 5 4 3 2 1

springer.com

Contents

Part III Current Developments

Introduction

Bert Gordijn and Ruth Chadwick

> *We have given you, O Adam, no visage proper to yourself, nor endowment properly your own, in order that whatever place, whatever form, whatever gifts you may, with premeditation, select, these same you may have and possess through your own judgement and decision.*
>
> Giovanni Pico della Mirandola, Oration on the Dignity of Man (1486)

Since times immemorial the regulative idea of *restitutio ad integrum*, reinstatement of human wholeness or intactness, has dominated medicine. Currently, the idea of restoring the normal functions of the human body still plays a central role. However, another notion has recently entered the medical limelight as well. Beyond merely reinstating the original physical and mental states of the patients, physicians are currently increasingly envisaging the improvement of the traits of perfectly healthy persons. Thus, the *restitutio ad integrum* doctrine is gradually being forced to share its status in present-day medicine with the *transformatio ad optimum* idea, reshaping persons who are already in good physical shape to further improve certain characteristics. This phenomenon is commonly called “enhancement”.

Ideas about enhancing human traits with medical means emerged as far back as the 17th century (see Gordijn 2006). Prior to this, medicine, like the natural sciences and technology in general, played only a minor role in thinking about possibilities of improving the human condition. This situation changed in the 17th century. As achievements in science and technology mounted notions of constructability and controllability of the human body gradually emerged. Three scholars in particular were to advance influential optimistic views about improving human nature through further medical developments: Francis Bacon (1561–1626) in his *New Atlantis* (1627), René Descartes (1596–1650) in his *Discours de la méthode pour bien conduire sa raison et chercher la vérité dans les sciences* (1637) and the Marquis de Condorcet (1743–1794) in his optimistic work *Esquisse d’un tableau historique des progrès de l’esprit humain* (1795). These works touch upon central themes regularly to be found in writings of modern proponents of medical enhancement. These themes include extension of the maximum human lifespan and the improvement of physical and mental traits.

B. Gordijn, R. Chadwick (eds.) *Medical Enhancement and Posthumanity*,

However, there are two remarkable differences between the philosophical thinking about improving human beings with medical means that was prevalent in the 17th and 18th century and contemporary ideas about medical enhancement. The first difference concerns the extent in which medicine is being perceived as a particularly suitable means of ameliorating the human condition; the second regards the *de facto* power of medicine to change human physical and mental states.

(1) In the early days philosophical ideas about medical enhancement were firmly embedded in a more general sort of prevailing scientific optimism. It was widely accepted that human beings are able to craft their own ideal future, if only they make proper use of their intellect and organize and develop science in a methodically correct way. This basic optimistic thought was then set out in detail in three more specific ideas. The first idea was that of ruling over the living and inorganic environment surrounding us. Developments in the biology, chemistry, physics and the engineering sciences were thought to facilitate the endeavor of molding nature so as to flawlessly fit our human ends. The second idea was that of shaping a perfect society on the basis of historical, sociological or political scientific theories. The last idea was that of controlling and constructing the human body, as well as perfecting human nature, to be achieved by advances in medical science and technology.

At present, the naive sort of vigorous scientific buoyancy that was characteristic of the 17th and 18th century has vanished. Accordingly, the idea of attempting to control nature with scientific and technical means is regarded from a critical perspective by many. We have definitely lost our innocence after the Second World War revealed the terrible consequences of using nuclear arms. Weaponised nuclear technology may have contributed to the conclusion of the WWII, yet the human and environmental costs of deploying nuclear weapons in this fashion were immense. The threat of nuclear weapons was a deciding factor in the Cold War, and the use or misuse of nuclear technology remains a topic of enormous international concern to date. In addition, as the human population grew roughly fourfold in the 20th century ever increasing pressures on natural resources have deteriorated and depleted many resource bases, thus creating an increased potential for competition and conflict. Moreover, exploiting our environment we increasingly change its natural state. As vegetation and the animal kingdom cannot always successfully cope with these changes, species are now vanishing many times more quickly than by evolution and natural extinction. Furthermore, anthropogenic greenhouse gas emissions, from industry, transportation and agriculture, are contributing to global warming, a phenomenon that could have severe consequences for human kind. As a result of these and similar developments, enthusiasm regarding unbridled technological intervention in our environment in order to control nature has dwindled.

In addition, enthusiasm about shaping ideal societies has dulled significantly. More and more, it became clear that endeavors to radically improve our societies can have severe and uncontrollable downsides. The effects of 20th century attempts to change societies motivated by political ideologies such as Leninism, Stalinism, Maoism and Nazism have been unprecedented in terms of death and destruction. Dystopian and anti-utopian novels such as George Orwell's "1984", Yevgeny

Zamyatin's "We" and Aldous Huxley's "Brave New World" became part of the public consciousness. With the fall of the Soviet empire one of the last surviving "political utopias" had finally come to an end. In retrospect, many intellectuals in the West now seem to agree that most historical attempts to create "ideal societies" on the basis of certain historical, sociological or political theories have resulted in failures.

In contrast to the fading fervor for the ideas of creating ideal societies and technologically intervening in our natural environment so as to fit our ends, the idea of improving human nature with medical means is currently still triggering significant intellectual excitement. It is almost as if the disillusionment concerning dominating nature and shaping model societies has reinforced academic enthusiasm towards the idea of perfecting ourselves. Specific types of enhancements, such as cosmetic surgery, cosmetic dentistry, smart drugs and mood enhancers, seem to be counting on quite a lot of public support. Accordingly, many seem to believe that medicine may be instrumental in improving essential traits such as appearance; cognition and mood, provided certain medical research fields are appropriately promoted and financed. Thus, in contrast to the other two ideas of ruling over the living and inorganic environment surrounding us and shaping a perfect society, the idea of improving ourselves with medical means still seems to be viable and inspiring.

(2) From the moment the first ideas about medical enhancement emerged, the discipline of medicine was assigned enormous potential. However, in the 17th century medicine was *de facto* capable of very little. The general lack of medical knowledge and expertise meant that it was reduced to the alleviation of symptoms and moral support for patients. Initial enthusiasm surrounding the potential of medicine was therefore based chiefly on purely theoretical considerations and extrapolations. Today this has fundamentally changed. Enthusiasm is no longer reserved exclusively for theoretical considerations and hypothetical mind games. Contemporary euphoria is chiefly directed at real-life medical fields. Amongst the latter are fields that have already come up with clinical applications, such as cosmetic surgery, sports medicine, tissue engineering, psychopharmacology and bioelectronics. Moreover, developments at the preclinical stage are addressed. They include research fields like cloning, stem cell research, germ line genome modifications and interventions in the biological aging process. Last but not least, thoughts about medical enhancement are also inspired by developments which so far remain mainly theoretical, for example medical nanorobots and software resident intelligences. Be this as it may, the prospect of applying medical means in order to improve ourselves is currently much more realistic than it appeared two or three centuries ago.

Thus, medicine today has the public support as well as the scientific know-how and technological capability necessary to successfully realize the century old idea of *transformatio ad optimum*. More and more we will medically intervene in healthy persons in order to further improve certain characteristics. We have in fact already started to do so in many different medical fields. The best-known examples to date are anabolic steroids in sports, all manner of cosmetic surgical interventions and the use of Prozac, Ritalin and Viagra for non-therapeutic purposes.

Ultimately our striving to improve ourselves according to our own wishes might even result in a situation, where it is no longer appropriate to speak of a 'human being' at all. After all, interventions with the purpose of enhancement might bring about such radical changes that the result could only be regarded as a posthuman being, and no longer as a human being. Several contemporary authors argue that it is feasible and recommendable (or even morally required) that with medical help, we depart from our human existence, with all its innate weaknesses and imperfections. Various recent writings describe different scenarios of how this process could unfold.

In one example we will more and more apply bioelectronic and neural engineering systems in order to improve motorial, sensory and cognitive traits. This will result in an ever more symbiotic connection between the human biological system on the one hand and the various technical systems at work on the other. In fusing man and machine, human existence is ultimately surmounted and thus transferred into a posthuman mode of existence (Kaku 1997; Kurzweil 1999). In another example, humankind is reshaped with the help of germ line genome modifications. In contrast to so-called 'somatic gene therapy', in which only the genetic material of somatic cells is modified, germ line genome modifications can be passed on to the next generation. If they are performed consistently through successive generations, a genetically modified posthuman species might emerge (Silver 1997). A third example is 'uploading', a procedure that would involve transferring the contents of a biological human brain to a computer. This might be performed by first scanning the synaptic structure of a brain at a sufficient resolution by means of nanotechnology. This information would then be implemented in an electronic medium thereby bringing into existence a software resident intelligence. "Uploads" would not necessarily be disembodied. Not only might they have a virtual body, they might even use robot bodies in order to bodily inhabit physical reality (WTA 2007).

At present, all these "posthumanity scenarios" are still firmly in the realm of science fiction. However, this observation should not delay debates about the desirability of these scenarios. After all, space travel, IVF babies, radio, television, cell phones and the WWW were also science fiction only 100 years ago. Yet, they are very real phenomena today, influencing our lives in ways that we would never have imagined. It has turned out that our track record for predicting scientific and technological progress is not impressive.

It is a fact that we are increasingly using new medical technologies to change ourselves beyond therapy and in accordance with our own desires. Although at this early stage, it is impossible to predict exactly where this will lead us to, we will almost certainly enter new territory – not only in a medical sense, but also anthropologically, psychologically and politically. Against this backdrop, a well-researched and profound debate is essential. It is the only way in which solid concepts and ethical parameters necessary for a responsible future biomedical course may be developed. Therefore, this volume will focus on the topics of medical enhancement and posthumanity. Both topics are treated along the same general lines. The issues are first analyzed from an historical and a conceptual perspective. Against this backdrop then follow both a positive as well as a negative ethical assessment.

Authors well known for their favorable or critical views on enhancement and posthumanity try to make their strongest possible case. Finally, the issues of medical enhancement and posthumanity are discussed as and to the extent in which they appear in specific fields such as cosmetic surgery, biogerontology, germ line genome modifications, bioelectronics and NBIC converging technologies.

References

Bacon F (1627) The New Atlantis. In: Johnston A (1974) (ed) The Advancement of Learning and New Atlantis. Clarendon, Oxford: 1–212

Condorcet (1795) Esquisse d'un tableau historique des progrès de l'esprit humain. In: Pons A (1988) (ed) Esquisse d'un tableau historique des progrès de l'esprit humain suivi de Fragment sur l'Atlantide. Flammarion, Paris: 79–296

Descartes R (1637) Discours de la méthode pour bien conduire sa raison et chercher la vérité dans les sciences. In: Adam C, Tannery P (1897–1913) (eds) Oevres de Descartes (13 volumes), Léopold Cerf, Paris: vol 6

Gordijn B (2006) Medical Utopias. Ethical Reflections About Emerging Medical Technologies. Peeters, Leuven, Belium/Paris/Dudley/Massachusetts

Kaku M (1997) Visions. How Science will Revolutionize the 21st Century. Anchor Books/ Doubleday, New York

Kurzweil R (1999) The Age of Spiritual Machines. When Computers Exceed Human Intelligence. Viking, New York

Silver L M (1997) Remaking Eden. Cloning and Beyond in a Brave New World. Avon Books, New York

World Transhumanist Association (WTA) (2007) The Transhumanist FAQ (http://transhumanism.org, accessed 25 September 2007)

Part I
Medical Enhancement

Chapter 1
The History of Medical Enhancement: From *Restitutio ad Integrum* to *Transformatio ad Optimum*?[1]

Urban Wiesing

1.1 Introduction

The subject of medical enhancement has received growing attention over recent years predominantly due to the developments in the fields of biomedicine and to technological possibilities. This could lead erroneously to the assumption that the subject itself is new and that human beings are considering for the first time how they might improve themselves. This is not the case. The idea of human optimization and self-perfecting is not new. Human beings, as far as we can judge from the historical sources, have always been interested in creating or bettering themselves, and have always intervened in their own reproduction. The practical measures and theoretical concepts involved in enhancing human beings have, however, transformed considerably over the course of history. Presented below is an overview of the topic together with several important key conclusions, drawn from selected authors and related examples pertinent to the discussion.

1.2 Antiquity

In Antiquity, medicine was based on the idea of the healthy human organism as a well-ordered microcosm. If it's order, or the configuration of its individual components, became disturbed (if, for example, the 'good ratio between the humours' became imbalanced) this would then be the cause of disease. The task of the physician was, therefore, to reinstate the original order, the *eucrasy* of the human microcosm, and thus cure the disease, according to the concept of *restitutio ad integrum*. "What you should put first in all the practice of our art is how to make the patient well" (Page et al. 1959: 78). According to the theory of the four humours, eucrasia is a balance of the bodily liquids, with any possibility of enhancement neither presumed nor suggested. One could attempt to transform dyscrasia into eucrasia by

[1] The author thanks Johannes Brachtendorf, Ruth Chadwick, Bert Gordijn, Diane Kerns, Karl-Heinz Leven, Julia Peterson and Richard Toellner for their help.

B. Gordijn, R. Chadwick (eds.) *Medical Enhancement and Posthumanity*,

way of treatment, but eucrasia was itself not a condition that one could surpass; a *restitutio ad integrum* was a *restitutio ad optimum*.

This represents an understanding of medicine as an art, as a τέχνη (téchne). According to the theory of Aristotle (384–322 B.C.), which was considerably influential over a long period of time, techne, and thereby medicine as well, is a human activity that in a special way imitates nature. With nature as such being the model, art (or techné), following this model, will strive toward its inherent entelecheia. "[A]rt in general imitates the method of nature" (Butcher 1927: 117). For this reason, the range of active possibilities for the human being within the framework of an Aristotelian τέχνη is limited, and the direction of his or her activities is already preset by nature. "The human being, in his work and activities, places himself in the consequence of physical teleology: he brings about that which nature would bring about, nature's [...] immanent being as it ought to be" (Blumenberg 1981: 73). Appropriately understood then, achievement beyond the dictates of nature is not intellectually feasible, and this pertains as well to any alteration of the human being. The mimesis principle, according to Aristotle's definition of art (techné), has had a lasting effect upon European intellectual history.

In the religious and moral sense as well, the human being in the time of Antiquity could only strive toward self-improving from within a preset framework. According to the regulatory concept of 'becoming like a God' – όμοίωσις θεῷ (*homoiosis theo*) – a fundamental kindred of spirits exists between the human and the divine. The task of the soul is to maintain this kindred spirit during its lifetime on earth, that is, during its time away from God. If the soul is successful in this mission, it can reunite with the deity – its origins – once the human being it has been occupying dies. Plato (427–347 B.C.) adopted these teachings and developed them further. According to Plato, *homoiosis theo* can only be realized through philosophy, by recognizing the divine in ideas. In his view, a human being who has become similar to God is a just human being, because the gods themselves are just par excellence (Plato 1988: 352a–b). The *homoiosis theo* imposed upon people finds its expression in the development of the virtue of justice. Plato's image of human perfection thus included a moral component as well (Plato (1967; see Köing 1996). And philosophy, not biology, serves as the method by which humans are then capable of perfecting themselves. The limitations of *homoiosis theo* are twofold: firstly, the divine model cannot be augmented; secondly, the human being can only strive toward this image within his or her limited realm of possibilities, κατὰ τὸ δυνατόν, as far as this is possible (Platon 1946: 176a–b).

Within the further course of history, the idea of *homoiosis theo* assumed various philosophical and theological manifestations. Remarkably, the notion of human improvement associated with *homoiosis theo* remained firmly linked to the realization of moral virtues, just as it had been in the time of Plato and at the height of Christianity.

In classical antiquity, measures were known, e.g. infanticide, which would have been used to control the number as well as the quality of offspring. Several regulations of infanticide and references to it in the literature of classical antiquity indicate that infanticide was most probably performed in many societies of that time period.

Aristotle thus argues in *Politics*, "As to the exposure and rearing of children, let there be a law that no deformed child shall live" (Aristotle 1988: 7th Book, 1335b 19). Plato asserts this as well in the *Politeia*, in which he demands, in terms of selection of children after birth, the following, "Well, I suppose they'll take the children of good parents to crèche and hand them over to nurses (who live in a separate section of the community); and they'll find some suitable way of hiding away in some secret and secluded spot the children of worse parents and any handicapped children of good parents" (Plato 1988: V 460 c; see also 460a–b). Further, we find in Plato's *Politeia* the eugenic concepts for breeding: A state must make sure that "sex should preferably take place between men and women who are outstandingly good, and should occur as little as possible between men and women of a vastly inferior stamp. It also follows that the offspring of the first group should be brought up, while the offspring of the second group shouldn't. This is how to maximize the potential of our flock" (Plato 1988: V 459 d). The biological pursuits involved in improving the human being draw upon groups within a state and are implemented by means of breeding. They remained as such within the possibilities predetermined by nature itself.

1.3 The Middle Ages

During the Middle Ages, the idea of *restitutio ad integrum* was compatible with the dominant notion that God created the world and all the creatures in it according to His omniscient conceptions. Since the whole of creation was regarded as perfect – being, as it was, of divine origins – human beings, as the pinnacle of creation, were also regarded as fundamentally and naturally perfect, not in the sense of a perfection alone pertaining to God but in the sense of the form of the created human being. "All natural things were produced by the Divine art, and so may be called God's work of art. Now every artist intends to give to his work the best disposition; not absolutely the best, but the best as regards the proposed end. [...] Now the proximate end of the human body is the rational soul and its operations; [...] I say, therefore, that God fashioned the human body in that disposition which was best, as most suited to such a form and to such operations" (Aquinas 1948: quest. 91, 3). Medieval man viewed disease as a deviation from natural perfection. The fact that diseases could befall fundamentally perfect human beings was attributed to original sin and its repercussions: an erring of ways or possession by evil spirits. The process by which human beings might recover from their sufferings was equated with the resurrection of mankind on the Day of Judgement. According to Medieval precepts, earthly recovery to some extent pre-empted heavenly resurrection. *Restitutio ad optimum*, which means *restitutio* according to Gods plan, was, however, only possible in the life after death, and only through the mercy of God.

Any thought of human beings reaching beyond the preconceived plan of God in order to improve themselves did not occur, as nothing was capable of surpassing God's plan. It would have been unimaginable and would also have endangered the image of God if one wished to improve human beings beyond what was a condition pre-determined by God. This condition was optimal and binding, even when it could never be fully obtained in a person's lifetime due to original sin. One should not forget that the medieval efforts toward human self-improvement or perfecting are less concerned with the biological aspects; rather, these efforts were much more focused on the intellectual and spiritual side of human beings. By concentrating on the healing of the soul, one spent less time questioning the physical health of a person. The notion of *restitutio ad integrum*, therefore, contained not only medical but theological significance as well.

These are the ideas found, for example, in the work of St. Augustine (354–430). He described the notion of an "integrum" as "peace" (pax) and extended this peace to correspond with the integrity of the body, to the relationship between body and soul, between human beings with one another and between the human being and God. "The peace of body and soul is the ordered life and health of a living creature; peace between mortal man and God is an ordered obedience in the faith under an everlasting law" (Augustinus 1957–1972: Book XIX, Chapter XIII (p 175)). According to Augustine, this peace is a characteristic of the natural order, an optimum established in God's all encompassing design. The opposite of peace is turmoil, which is an unnatural condition expressing itself in the form of physical illness. Peace as the best of all conditions cannot, though, be completely found on earth due to the sins of "man." At best human beings will know peace as a *pax temporalis*. In order, though, to attain the most substantial form of earthly peace, God has made certain means available to human beings. In applying these means to acquire the peace, a *pax mortalium*, accorded to mortal men, human beings are paving the way for the eternal peace, or *pax immortalitatis*, to be found in a later life. For only in the resurrection can the absolute integrity of eternal peace be re-established for the just or good human being.

"God, then, the most wise creator and most just ordainer of all natures, who has set upon the earth as its greatest adornment the mortal human race, has bestowed on men certain good things that befit this life; to wit, temporal peace, so far as it can be enjoyed in the little span of a mortal life in terms of personal health and preservation and fellowship with one's kind, and all things necessary to safeguard or recover the peace (such as [...] light, speech, air to breathe and water to drink, and whatever befits the body, to feed or to cover it, to heal and adorn it); all this under the most just condition that every mortal who rightly uses such goods, that are designed to contribute to the peace of mortals, shall receive larger and better goods, that is the peace of immortality, and [...] an everlasting life spent in the enjoyment of God" (Augustinus 1957–1972: Book XIX, Chapter XIII (180–181)).

1.4 The Modern Age

The ideas concerning human beings and their possible alteration changed decidedly through the developments of modernity and the scientific revolution, which thus transformed the concept of *restitutio ad integrum* into *transformatio ad optimum*.

With the beginning of the Modern Age, a transformation took place regarding how one understood Nature, human beings and the possibility of human intervention; a creative self-confidence slowly emerged. The mimesis principle from Aristotle's concept of techne lost its strength while the creativity of human beings was discovered. Along with technical improvements, a "historical, and by no means obvious, link between achievement and self-confidence" (Blumenberg 1981: 58) developed. Beginning with Anatomy and Physiology, the concept of human and of the possibilities of intervention became transformed. Whereas the people of antiquity viewed themselves as a well-ordered microcosm, and medieval people as the pinnacle of God's creation, modern people saw themselves in many different ways, more like a machine, in a technical sense, and finally as the flawed result of chance evolutionary processes.

In the 16th century, Paracelsus (1493/94–1541) described the production of a small human being, a Homunculus, in his work "De Natura rerum" from 1537. Technical possibilities offered new means for Alchemy: "The propagation of all natural things is twofold: the first being that which is derived from nature without any art, the second that which is derived through what is art, namely through alchemy" (p 312). An artificially created human being could exist when human sperm was kept in a glass flask along with horse dung at a constant warm temperature, "until it becomes a living thing, and is moving and stirring" (p 317). This living being was to be nurtured over time under specific conditions so that Homunculi might develop. These "will become giants, dwarfs, and other types of great wondrous beings, who will become useful as mighty tools and instruments" (p 317). Due to their artificial origins, their abilities could also surpass human standards so that "with their strengths and deeds they will more resemble ghosts rather than human beings" (p 317–318).

Paracelsus' description of the creation of a Homunculus, Paracelsus (1928), a being similar to a human and conceived through alchemy, was read by later authors, especially during the time of the Enlightenment, as superstition. Alternatively, Rene Descartes (1596–1650), in the tradition of Iatromechanics, understood an organism as a machine that could be described completely through physical laws. Nature was no longer a well ordered cosmos but rather a well-functioning machine, for the most part. One had to proceed thus in the treatment of people. As such, the theoretically conceived possibilities were broadened by means of creative intervention in the structure of a machine.

As a consequence of the success accompanying the natural sciences, the idea prevailed that Nature can be influenced. Within this transformation of ideas concerning Nature, the means of approaching Nature, as well as the means for grappling with human nature, changed dramatically in the modern period. New methods, through observation and scientific experimentation, changed the approach to Nature. Nature was held to be an object that could be recognized simply through the methods of natural science. Nature was to be revealed through precise observation and experiment. The possibilities for intervention became in principle unlimited, with science, through its departure from religious and other traditional terms of reference, ridding itself of its own limitations, even when overriding these limitations was at this point merely theoretical. In turning away from the Aristotelian understanding of techne and the associated mimesis principle, a tendency developed "away from the dependency on the imitation of nature, while pushing forward from nature into the untrodden realm" (Blumenberg 1981: 83). The cosmos harbours within itself a multitude of possibilities, which stand fundamentally open to people and which through technology can be in effect realized. This theoretical notion became, at least for some authors, a reason for euphoria.

A striking example of a philosopher of the Enlightenment is the Marquis de Condorcet (1743–1794). His optimism with regard to progress extended as far as the possibility of influencing human nature. In his "Esquisse d'un tableau historique des progrès de l'esprit humain" from 1794, Condorcet proposed "that nature has set no terms for the perfection of human faculties; that the perfectibility of man is truly indefinite; and that the progress of this perfectibility, from now onwards independent of any power that might wish to halt it, has no other limit than the duration of the globe upon which nature has cast us" (Condorcet 1794: 4). He applied this historical-philosophical plan to all areas of human life in order to pose the question of whether this could pertain to the biological perfection of the human being. His answer is affirmative: "Organic perfectibility or deterioration amongst the various strains in the vegetable and animal kingdom can be regarded as one of the general laws of nature. This law also applies to the human race" (Condorcet 1794: 199). Condorcet focused especially on drastically increasing longevity and on the radical reduction of disease through progress in the sciences and the political application of scientific findings. Furthermore, he believed that newly acquired and improved moral and intellectual capabilities could then be inherited.

Medical practitioners are by rule more cautious with regard to the enhancement of human beings. The physician Christoph Wilhelm Hufeland (1762–1836), in his famous work "Die Kunst, das menschliche Leben zu verlängern" (The art of prolonging human life, 1796), does not see any possibility in "bringing about change to the grand scheme of nature" (Hufeland 1796: 55) but rather sees at best that the lifespan prescribed by nature could be lengthened through a healthy way of life and through "künstliche Mittel" (artificial means). Nature grants a certain amount of "Lebenskraft" or *vis vitalis* (vital power) to human beings. When this amount is consumed then each living creature will die. By being careful with the *vis vitalis* and taking certain pains in rejuvenating one's vitality by, for example, getting enough sleep, human beings may be able to lengthen their lifespan, but no more. This is also a point of view shared by Immanuel Kant (1724–1804) in his "Conflict between the Faculties" of 1798.

Long before the technical realization of human enhancement, literary authors took up the subject. Examples are mentioned here to serve as evidence of the transformation of theoretical conceptions. One of the most influential examples is the novel "Frankenstein or: The Modern Prometheus" by Mary Shelley (1797–1851), published in 1818. A scientist, Victor Frankenstein, creates a new human being with a method that he develops out of an almost self-destructive ambition. He accomplishes it not through breeding or through the creation of a machine, but out of body parts and through a new method, electricity. For all of this, the creator of the new human is exclusively thankful to science: "Some miracle might have produced it, yet the stages of discovery were distinct and probable. After days and nights of incredible labour and fatigue, I succeeded in discovering the cause of generation and life; nay more, I became myself capable of bestowing animation upon lifeless matter" (Shelley 1951: 45–46). Limitations within the scientific findings or with regard to the exertion of influence did not exist for Frankenstein, but rather the opposite: he praises himself, in the spirit of the Enlightenment and in the optimism felt for technology, as the means for bringing light into the darkness of the world. "Life and death appeared to me ideal bounds, which I should first break through, and pour a torrent of light into our dark world" (Shelley 1951: 47). The scientist Frankenstein is furthermore convinced that he is benefiting humankind with this attitude and with his creation. During the creation of his new human being, he is not befallen with any notion of skepticism concerning the results of his actions. "A new species would bless me as its creator and source; many happy and excellent natures would owe their being to me. No father could claim the gratitude of his child so completely as I should deserve this" (Shelley 1951: 47). But the catastrophic course of events that follows the invention is well known: The newly created being possesses a personality, desires love, warmth and security, but is an outcast among people who find his monstrous appearance too hideous. Out of revenge the monster kills the family and friends of his creator. Victor Frankenstein pursues his creation also out of revenge, and in doing so finds death.

1.5 Evolutionary Theory

The varying ideas from the modern period concerning nature and its influence on human self-awareness were once more surpassed through the theory of evolution from Charles Darwin (1809–1882). As a result of the theory, the human being becomes the product of chance in the course of evolution. This product is not perfect but rather, in all manners of speaking, deficient and predisposed to further deficiencies in relation to the evolutionary challenges. The boundaries demarking categories of species became accidental products of history, while new, even altered species could come into being. This knowledge was, on the one hand, a threat. The human being, his genus or a specific race could change for the worse, degenerate and even become extinct. The decadence of human beings und their societies were a topic often discussed, especially at the end of the 19th century. People believed themselves to be threatened with decline. On the other hand, the theory of evolution allowed for the possibility of improvement above all in connection with future scientific means. The characteristics, which placed humans in a specific genus, were no longer fixed and were therefore fundamentally flexible, open to our disposal. One could improve human beings – and not only a few believed that one must change human beings alone due to the supposed fact that civilization had become altered, was now anti-selective and therefore promoting degeneration. "The man-made – aesthetically as well as technically – with all its necessity presented itself to the randomness of natural formations" (Blumenberg 1981: 89).

1.6 Eugenics

When above all the field of molecular biology, and particularly genetics, is currently being associated with the bettering of human beings, then this is not being done, historically understood, for the first time. "The current revolution in molecular biology is not the first but the second large-scale attempt to modify the pattern of human heredity for the better. The eugenics movements of 1870–1950 came first" (Buchanan et al. 2000: 27–28; see Weingart et al. 1992).

The founder of eugenics, Francis Galton (1822–1911), a cousin of Charles Darwin, defined it in 1883 as the "science of improving stock, which is by no means confined to questions of judicious mating, but which, especially in the case of man, takes cognisance of all influences that tend in however remote a degree to give to the more suitable races or strains of blood a better chance of prevailing speedily over the less suitable than they otherwise would have had" (Galton 1973: 17). The Darwinian theory of evolution was the prerequisite for the eugenic movement.

Conceptually, eugenics is, in the contemporary world, understood negatively due above all to the eugenic politics under National Socialism. One should, however, not forget that in the first half of the 20th century there were many different eugenic movements, not only in Germany. Many civilised countries incorporated eugenic thought into their political agenda and, as an example of this, limited the immigration of particular population groups. There were more or less influential eugenic societies in many countries. Liberal and left-leaning political parties also argued from a eugenic point-of-view, not only the political parties tending toward the right. With its broad resonance as a social and political response to various issues, the eugenic movement of the 19th and 20th centuries was different from all previous but similar movements propagating eugenic thinking. Supporters of eugenics wanted to incorporate their utopian vision into the realm of politics (see Plötz 1911a, b).

The varying eugenic movements were striving toward different goals. Should one hinder "bad" offspring (negative eugenics) or should one encourage the propagation of people with a better genetic inheritance (positive eugenics)? The question of which measures should be implemented also brought on varying responses. Should one support only wished for propagation, should one encourage voluntary abstinence with regard to unwanted propagation, should one force the copulation of people with a "good" genetic structure and prevent by force unwanted propagation, or should people with a bad genetic make-up be eliminated?

Despite these differences there were some common views within the eugenic movements. They all follow, in broad terms, a biological approach. They assume that behaviour and the personal characteristics of human beings are overwhelmingly conditioned by hereditary and that the quality of the genetic make-up of the population in civilised countries is deteriorating due to unnatural conditions that impede selection.

As a response to this assumedly avoidable degeneration, the eugenic movement wanted to see a greater representation of certain types in the gene pool, types which were thought to be "better". In order to accomplish this, it is not only necessary but also legitimate to limit individual freedom. The eugenic movement has then stood in perpetual conflict with the protection of individual freedoms and human rights.

The eugenics movement has faced constant criticism and was accused of being a misguided science, not only after the moral catastrophe of National Socialism. In scientific terms, it has been doubted whether there is proof that the gene pool in civilised societies is deteriorating and that degeneration is now a threat (e.g. Raymond Pearl 1879–1940; (see further Pearl (1928a, b)). Accordingly, the fundamental question was raised concerning the criteria for determining what is good and desirable and what is bad and undesirable. Furthermore, eugenics has been criticised as non-scientific for applying valuations that do not pertain to science (e.g. Max Weber 1864–1920; see Weber 1911). A science is not capable of answering the moral question, to what end a gene pool should be manipulated. And in no lesser terms, eugenic measures have also been criticised from the perspective of humanism and individual rights (e.g. Friedrich Hertz 1898–1965; see further Hertz (1916–1918)).

The history of eugenics reached its political high point, and its moral low point, with National Socialism in Germany. Here we see clearly what it means to find the peculiarly horrific consequences of biological thought becoming part of a political agenda. Initially, "hereditarily defective" offspring were prevented through legally based forced sterilization; afterwards the separation of the races was controlled, then handicapped and mentally ill individuals were murdered and finally the Jews faced extermination. The presumably worst crimes of humanity were based on the absurd eugenic thought that one saves his own race through the extermination of another. Also, within the SS, a breeding program existed with the aim of creating a higher quality of racial offspring.

1.7 Eugenics After 1945

After National Socialism, the attempt to improve the quality of the gene pool of a particular group through forced measures, along with the acceptance of human rights' abuses, has been a taboo subject in the Western world. At the same time the eugenic intent in several immigration laws was not changed immediately after 1945, and particular elements from eugenic thought have been maintained, even when forced implementation is discussed only with great reserve. The CIBA Symposium in London of 1962 is described below in order to present in precise terms eugenic thought and a "modern" scientific identity.

Assembled together were 27 high-ranking scientists (among them six Nobel prize winners) who were addressing the threats of both over-population and atomic warfare; they considered their situation to be that of facing a challenge which was to be confronted by one means alone: "Most of the authors backed without qualification a scientific solution to the problems" (Wieser 1966: 10). One of the reasons for the inappropriate response to the scientifically-induced challenges discussed at the symposium was the quality of human beings themselves: "The challenge is man's obvious imperfection as a psychosocial being; both individually and collectively, he is sadly in need of improvement, yet clearly improvable" (Huxley 1963: 4).

Through science, especially through the theory of evolution, human beings find themselves in the peculiar situation that they alone have before their eyes the true history of the universe and they alone know the true path: "We are privileged to be living in a crucial moment in the cosmic story, the moment when the vast evolutionary process, in the small person of enquiring man, is becoming conscious of itself" (Huxley 1963: 1). On the one hand, science recognizes that the form of the human being is capable of being transformed; on the other hand, the human being (at least the smarter ones, in particular the participants of the symposium) perceives the crisis. Therefore, it is necessary to alter the human being.

This conclusion does not exclude eugenic measures: "Our present civilization is becoming dysgenic. To reverse this trend, we must use our genetical knowledge to the full [...]. Eventually, the prospect of radical eugenic improvement could become one of the mainsprings of man's evolutionary advance" (Huxley 1963: 21). The majority of scientists participating at the CIBA Symposium spoke in favour of eugenics. They discussed in particular the practical difficulties that arise in liberal and democratic societies. What limitations to personal freedom could be deemed acceptable? Could one attain the eugenic goals through education as well? Some of the participants were in favour of selective fertilization through sperm donations, as well as direct intervention in genetic material to enhance future offspring.

Although the CIBA Symposium was a small meeting of high-ranking scientists, it did present a poignant example of a self-immunising science and a paradigmatic style of argumentation. According to most of the participants of the meeting, science has contributed to the existence of a crisis because it has invented technology (medical and atomic) that is then causing the crisis. By way of evolutionary theory, scientists have recognized the crisis as a degenerative one, and have recognized the present make-up of human beings as being insufficient in abating the crisis. The scientists believe in the necessity of altering human beings, have proven the transformation of human beings in evolutionary theory, and are able to present the means for overcoming the crisis. According to this view, science is being impaired above all by traditional moral considerations – and those who do not realize this are, of course, not scientists, and therefore misguided.

Science as such becomes the final determining force; science alone is responsible not only for causing but also for eradicating the problems. The improvement of human beings through the means of biological applications becomes here a scientific necessity and can be advanced through scientific means in a goal-oriented manner. And in view of the level of difficulty of the problem, intervening in the rights of individuals is "the least of all evils" (Wieser 1966: 24).

Interestingly enough, the central opposing arguments at the conference were also pointed out: has it in any way been proven that genetic degeneration in civilized societies exists? Is there a crisis in the first place? And who produces the standards to evaluate this? Also, the cognitive theoretical difficulties, already long known, were mentioned: how can evolutionary theory, as well as other scientific theories, determine the goals that are to be followed? Would this not push scientific theory beyond its own limitations? (See discussion in Wolstenholme 1963: 274–298).

1.8 Medicine in the 21st Century

The eugenic theses presented at the CIBA Symposium are, in this form, no longer brought up today. But the challenges have since then become more acute and the technical possibilities through biomedical progress have gone through further expansion. This progress is advancing at a faster pace than ever before with the result of an "exponential acceleration of progress and growth" (Kurzweil 2005: 32). Never before have so many people collected, with the most complicated of technologies, so much knowledge about human beings and about possible interventions in the human body. In particular, the transformation of bio-medical inventions into a marketable product is occurring under a more stringent rationality and within a tempo never known to have existed before. This is historically significant: In times past, even in times of scientific progress, there has been "no proclaimed notion of a future determined by constant progress, and even more important, hardly a deliberate method worked out for its implementation, such as regards research, experimentation, means for risk-involving and unorthodox trials, a far-reaching exchange of information, etc." (Jonas 1985: 18). Constant progress has become a fundamental condition of life and work. This leads to the new historical situation that human beings must prepare themselves through the course of their lives for completely new technologies, since within one generation technical innovations will massively alter their lived-in world. It is understandable that this could lead initially to apprehension and fear in those who are affected.

Technical development, with its ever-growing and seemingly unlimited possibilities, has in turn had a stimulating effect on public euphoria. First, it appears technically possible in the near future to alter the human being for the – alleged – better through directed medical means, and not only for the sake of her descendents but rather during her own lifetime. While medicine and its possibilities were still severely limited up into the 20th century, many ideas concerning the altering of human beings are no longer simple illusions but have become seemingly possible in their technical implementation, in particular through the combination and convergence of technologies. While the medical dimensions of Utopia from the previous century were still theoretical speculations over a distant future, those dimensions of more recent utopias have become exact prognoses, drawn from concrete technologies as, for example, with regard to genetics or Man-Machine-Interfaces (for a summary, see Gordijn 2004). But the euphoria is by no means without its shadowy side. Along with the optimistic visions of the future we find horrific depictions of this same future as well. These were manifested already in the 20th century in the negative utopias of a totalitarian society, in which cloning technologies are implemented to control reproduction completely, as for example in Aldous Huxley's (1894–1963) *Brave New World*.

This increase in the range of medical activity has resulted in the intensive way in which the medical profession in the Western world tends to be closely involved in the lives of people – from the moment they are born until the moment they die. Many areas of daily life such as unusual behaviour, sexuality, aesthetic appearance or performance at school have become more and more "medicalized" for the first time in the history of humanity, placed under the responsibilities of medicine and described as medical issues. No longer is the priest or a family member responsible for certain problems, but rather the doctor or therapist. In addition, the achievements of modern medicine in many industrial countries are financed by insurance institutions and made accessible to the general population.

New to the present situation, from a historical perspective, is the emphasis placed on the methods from the biomedical fields. These methods are viewed as having the most potential for improving human beings. They are applied in many areas, not only in medicine, but also, for example, in pedagogy, through the use of pharmaceuticals to improve learning results. This can also be found in varying degrees, and for other aims, in sport or in the use of lifestyle drugs. Mainstream science hopes to generate the best possible success by way of biomedical methods, for example, in improving general capabilities in social behaviour, intelligence and concentration, to name only a few. Furthermore, one hopes to find improvement in specific qualities or attributes. The 'holistic' moral improvement of a human being through, for example, philosophy, or the training or the refining of moral behaviour, is currently hardly considered. Old methods such as spiritual or moral improvement through belief, meditation, and prayer or through the training of moral behaviour are seen as the goals of isolated, often religious-based groups. Medicine, within its possibilities, has more and more become an influential societal phenomenon. All of this – understood historically – is very new.

By the technical possibilities the aim of a *transformatio ad optimum* gets numerous facets, each raising different ethical questions: One can try to enhance, or even optimise, single partial capacities of a human being, several partial capacities or even the whole human being. And it has to be determined what the *optimum* of a human being is or whether there are several *optima* – an answer to this question is far from being trivial. Due to the variety of answers to be expected the *transformatio ad optimum* will become a *transformatio ad optima* and therefore in its practical realisation a *transformatio ad infinitum*.

Along with the known methods toward medical enhancement through pharmaceuticals or controlled reproduction, two technological approaches are above all making possible a new dimension in intervention: the direct intervention in the genetic material and the direct connection of the human being with a machine.

1.9 Modern Genetics

The possibilities of intervention through the technological developments in genetics have broadened dramatically when compared to "classical" eugenics. The possibilities of controlled reproduction, already discussed by Plato, are being well surpassed.

The interventions do not take place through selective mating, but rather through directly aimed intervention in the genetic material – which has already been successfully practiced in the animal world. Improving the human being cannot only happen intergenerationally through the process of heredity, but already in the lifespan of a human being, provided that gene therapy on humans is possible. When we, through directed intervention, manipulate the structure of the human being, we have come across, at least theoretically, something historically very new. Altering genetic material can also be understood as an intervention in perfectibility, in a perfecting of perfectibility.

The genetic paradigm can be found, moreover, moving in broad directions. Genetics became a leading science in the late 20th century. Other technologies are closely tied to genetics, such as tissue-engineering or stem cell technologies. Also in the field of pharmacology, one hopes for therapeutic breakthroughs through genetics.

An open eugenic discussion, such as that which occurred at the CIBA Symposium, has seldom taken place among leading scientists in Western countries. Current discussions concerning the use of genetics, as well as other medical technologies, are characterized above all by the ethical perspective of the individual. It is not a matter which concerns the improvement of the gene pool of a group of people, but rather how an individual, in the face of new technologies, or a couple, through questions referring to reproduction, might make the appropriate decision. An orientation based on grand political projects, which were meant to construct completely new societies in the 20th century through eugenic theories, is today no longer a topic of discussion. At the centre, at least officially, stands the individual. The desired biological alterations pertain to the individual; we allow the individual to answer largely for herself the moral questions concerning these alterations. That this course of action is not without dangers is perfectly clear. Could an individualistically styled practice in effect lead unnoticed to a new 'liberal' eugenics (Habermas 2001), or to 'back door eugenics' (Duster 1990)? Could people be put under pressure to make choices which pertain for the most part to matters of fashion?

1.10 Man-Machine-Interface

We know from older medical cultures that humans continually used prostheses to replace lost body parts, as for example, limbs or teeth. These could, however, only replace the function of the lost parts to a certain degree; seldom was the case that they could fully replace which was lost. This limitation is currently being overcome through technological development, and the improvement of human capabilities through prostheses and man-machine-interfaces has moved technically to the foreground. These are in part already to be found in clinical practice (e.g., Cochlea implants), but not yet so far as to improve human capabilities, rather to create a *restitutio ad integrum*. It is, however, technically close to becoming much more; not only in replacing certain functions, but in surpassing functionality, making the replacement better than the "natural" organ in the sense of *transformatio ad optimum*. When artificial organs establish a direct tie with the body and especially with the brain, then a threshold, in historical respects, has been crossed. Outer stimulus is not transformed through human sensory organs into information for the brain (e.g., "classical" hearing aids), but directly conducted to the central nervous system.

1.11 Science and Society in the 21st Century

The dramatic transformation occurring in the field of medicine in the 20th century has had an impact on how medicine is reflected upon, which is in many respects historically unprecedented. Discussion concerning medicine takes place openly at least in many countries and is a concern of governments. Bioethics has become institutionalised in the form of academic institutes, ethics boards, ethics committees, and others. The discussion over new technologies takes place at least partially before these technologies can be applied. Gene therapy is publicly debated with regard to its moral legitimacy before clinical application on humans.

Science, in a circular self-appointed involvement, determining moral and political questions as seen in the CIBA Symposium, is no longer accepted in democratic societies. The separation of the sciences and moral responsibility is widely recognized. Scientists do not decide what areas of possibility are legally admissible. Though an indirect influence of scientists does in fact occur, as they are usually predominant in ethics committees. But ethics committees are capable only of acting as advisory bodies. At least in democratic societies, the responsibility rests in the hands of lawmakers, with efforts made to involve the public. But the reach of the lawmakers with regard to technological development is dwindling. National regulation stands often helpless in the face of a global market. Therefore, there are efforts being made to establish international norms in regulating the new technical applications. This is also something historically new and sensible, since the techniques have been developed within structures involving a worldwide component. International compromises are, though, not easy to produce, for we must keep in mind that a distinguishing characteristic of modern societies – in particular in international communities – is pluralism, even in a moral respect. Not only technological possibilities, but also public reflections on these possibilities, as well as attempts to regulate them, are all now found in a completely new setting.

This pertains as well to the philosophical parameters. A norm, which is universally accepted as God-given with regard to the enhancement of human beings, cannot be determined in view of religious pluralism. At the same time, one can little hope for a binding natural philosophy, morally contrived for establishing the limitations for human enhancement. Unlike in the age of Aristotle, the limitation of what can be altered is difficult to establish through a binding, normative and substantive concept of Nature. The opposite proves to be the case. "For the technician, Nature could become more and more simply the substratum, whose given constitution blocks rather than facilitates the development of constructive ends" (Blumenberg 1981: 92). Something similar exists in terms of a binding anthropology that sets normative limitations in the improvement of human beings. Too many varying concepts exist with regard to the nature of humans, and one that could also be normatively binding would be impossible to implement. "The history of anthropology as a philosophical discipline can be written as the modern history of the liberation of people from the terms of reference of what they are to be" (Schmid 1999: 80). In so far as an all-encompassing God-given norm is concerned, as well as a normative, substantive and binding natural philosophy and a similarly regarded anthropology, we cannot expect direct solutions to moral questions. But on the other hand ideas about nature and anthropological assumptions unavoidably form the hidden background of the debate. The discussion on international standards will continue by way of a reflective and direct discussion of the moral question with reference to the consensus on human dignity and human rights (Lenk 2002).

1.12 Historia Magistra Vitae?

What use do we have for historical knowledge when we are facing contemporary moral decisions? Certainly a moral decision is not to be drawn from history. This pertains as well to the possibility of human enhancement. There is no historical legitimacy that can relieve us of our moral decision-making. But history is important in making a moral decision. It shows us the historical genesis of the current situation, and reveals to us the experiences made with previous attempts at improving human beings, the similarities in these attempts, and the differences as well, as compared to the modern ones. History can draw our attention to the great differences which have developed in terms of the image of human beings, the concepts of Nature and the respective prevailing moralities. Historical evidence can make us aware of crucial developments, can make us cautious, and can make us sensitive, realistic, and hence more prudent. In particular the history of eugenics is 'a cautionary tale', especially when we consider the history of National Socialism: "the magnitude of the evil waiting at this extreme terminus of the eugenics movement provides an enduring general caution for genetics in the foreseeable future" (Buchanan et al. 2000: 30). Along with other functions, one function at least of written history is wholly uncontested: "If we are to avoid the errors of the past, we must know what they were" (Buchanan et al. 2000: 28).

References

Aquinas St T (1948) Summa Theologica. Christian Classics, Westminster, London/Maryland

Aristotle (1988) The Politics. Everson S (ed) Cambridge University Press, Cambridge

Augustinus Saint (1957–1972) The City of God Against the Pagans. In seven volumes, Heinemann, London

Blumenberg H (1981) Nachahmung der Natur'. Zur Vorgeschichte der Idee des schöpferischen Menschen, in Wirklichkeiten in denen wir leben. Reclam, Stuttgart, Germany

Buchanan A et al. (2000) From Chance to Choice. University Press, Cambridge

Butcher S (1927) Aristotle's Theory of Poetry and Fine Art. Macmillan, London

Condorcet M (1794) Esquisse d'un tableau historique des progres de l'espirit humain. In: Barraclough J (trans & ed 1955) Sketch for a Historical Picture of the Progress of the Human Mind. Weidenfeld & Nicolson, London

Duster T (1990) Backdoor to Eugenics. Routledge, New York

Galton F (1973) Inquiries into Human Faculty and Its Development. Reprinted from the edition of 1907. AMS, London/New York
Gordijn B (2004) Medizinische Utopien. Eine ethische Betrachtung. Vandenhoeck & Ruprecht, Göttingen, Germany
Habermas J (2001) Die Zukunft der menschlichen Natur: auf dem Weg zu einer liberalen Eugenik? Suhrkamp, Frankfurt am Main, Germany
Hertz F (1916–1918) Rasse und Kultur. Eine Erwiderung und Klarstellung. In: Ploetz A (ed) Archiv fuer Rassen- und Gesellschaftsbiologie. BG Teubner Verlag, Leipzig, Germany/ Berlin
Hertz F (1925) Rasse und Kultur. Eine kritische Untersuchung der Rassentheorien. Alfred Kröner Verlag, Leipzig, Germany
Hufeland C (1796) Makrobiotik oder Die Kunst das menschliche Leben zu verlängern. Reclam, Leipzig, Germany
Huxley (1963) The future of man - evolutionary aspects. In: Wolsten holme (ed.) Man and his future. Ciba Foundation Volume, London
Jonas H (1985) Technik, Medizin und Ethik. Insel-Verlag, Frankfurt am Main, Germany
Kant I (1992) The Conflict of the Faculties. University of Nebraska Press, Lincoln, NE/ London
König H (1996) ὁμοίωσις θεῷ - Verähnlichung mit Gott. In: Hünermann P (ed) Gott – ein Fremder in unserem Haus? Herder, Freiburg, Germany/Basel, Switzerland/Wien
Kurzweil R (2005) Human 2.0. New Scientist, 24th September: 32–37
Lenk C (2002) Therapie und Enhancement: Ziele und Grenzen der modernen Medizin. LIT, Münster, Germany
Page T E et al (1959) (eds) Hippocrates. Withington E T (trans) University Press, Aberdeen, Scotland
Paracelsus (1537) De natura rerum. Bibliotheca Palatina, München, Germany
Paracelsus (Theophrast von Hohenheim) (1928) Medizinische, naturwissenschaftliche und philosophische Schriften. Sämtliche Werke Bd. XI, Oldenbourg, München, Germany/Berlin
Pearl R (1928a) Eugenics. In: Baur E et al (eds) Zeitschrift für induktive Abstammungs- und Vererbungslehre. Gebrueder Borntraeger Verlag, Leipzig, Germany
Pearl R (1928b) Eugenics. In: Nachtsheim H (ed) Verhandlungen des V. internationalen Kongresses für Vererbungswissenschaften. Gebrueder Borntraeger Verlag, Leipzig, Germany
Plato (1967) Phaedo. In: Cooper L (trans) Plato on the Trial and Death of Socrates. Euthyphro, Apology, Crito, Phaedo. Cornell University Press, Ithaca, NY
Plato (1988) Republic. Halliwell S (transl & comment) Aris & Phillips, Warminster, England
Platon (1946) Theaitet. Schwabe, Basel, Switzerland
Plötz A (1911a) Die Begriffe Rasse und Gesellschaft und einige damit zusammenhängende Probleme. In: Verhandlungen des Ersten Deutschen Soziologentages. Mohr Siebeck Verlag, Tübingen, Germany
Plötz A (1911b) Diskussion. In: Verhandlungen des Ersten Deutschen Soziologentages. Verlag Mohr Siebeck, Tübingen, Germany
Schmid W (1999; 5th corr edition) Philosophie der Lebenskunst. Eine Grundlegung. Suhrkamp, Frankfurt am Main, Germany
Shelley M (1951) Frankenstein. Dent, London
Weber M (1911) Diskussion. In: Verhandlungen des Ersten Deutschen Soziologentages. Verlag Mohr Siebeck, Tübingen, Germany
Weingart P, Kroll J, Bayertz K (1992) Rasse, Blut und Gene. Geschichte der Eugenik und Rassenhygiene in Deutschland. Suhrkamp, Frankfurt am Main, Germany
Wieser W (1966) Das umstrittene Experiment: Der Mensch. Verlag Kurt Desch, München, Germany
Wolstenholme G (1963) Man and his future. Ciba Foundation Volume, London

Chapter 2
Therapy, Enhancement and Improvement

Ruth Chadwick

2.1 Introduction

In the contemporary debates about human enhancement, the elaboration of the concept of enhancement has frequently been attempted via a distinction between therapy and enhancement, in the hope and expectation not only that it would enhance clear thinking but also so that it could be drawn upon for practical purposes (e.g., in resource allocation decisions). Although the therapy-enhancement distinction at first sight has a certain intuitive appeal, however, this has proved prone to disappear quite rapidly when the distinction is closely analysed.

The limitations of the distinction appear to be not only theoretical but also practical. It is likely that interventions deemed to count as enhancements may be brought about by using techniques that have originally been developed for therapeutic ends. To prevent uses of new developments that might be regarded as 'off-label', in other words, used for purposes not envisaged and possibly not approved, would be extraordinarily difficult if not impossible.

This chapter has two aims: first, to seek more clarity about the concept of enhancement. I shall examine attempts to distinguish therapy from enhancement, and shall argue that a more important focus for debate should be the relationship between 'enhancement' and 'improvement'. The second aim is to assess the extent to which it is possible to establish some general principles for the kind of enhancing interventions that are morally acceptable and desirable.

In pursuit of these aims the discussion will be divided into three parts: the first section examines the therapy-enhancement distinction. The second section is concerned with the moral issues and has two sub-sections; beginning with an examination of the thesis that enhancement is inevitable. If this is true, this is likely to affect how the moral issue is structured – is the usefulness of asking the moral question limited to 'how' rather than 'whether' enhancement should be effected? A second subsection attempts to move towards general principles.

B. Gordijn, R. Chadwick (eds.) *Medical Enhancement and Posthumanity*,

2.2 The Concept of Enhancement

In surveying the approaches to 'enhancement' in the literature I suggest that they can be allocated to four categories:

1. Enhancement understood in terms of using certain techniques, that have been developed for therapy, but in a way that goes 'beyond therapy' (the 'beyond therapy view') (President's Council on Bioethics 2003)
2. Enhancement understood quantitatively, as increasing or adding [to] a certain characteristic (the additionality view)
3. Enhancement understood qualitatively, as making the things to be enhanced better in some way (the improvement view)
4. Enhancement as an umbrella term for a number of particular potential changes e.g., extending the human life span (the umbrella view)

Now, one thing it is important to note straight away is a potential issue about (3), understanding enhancement in terms of a qualitative change. I have interpreted this in terms of improvement, but there is also another interpretation of qualitative change in which an x is changed to such an extent that it no longer counts as an x. This seems to be at stake in the debates about the human/posthuman distinction. There is also then a potentially complex relationship between (2) and (3), concerning the extent to which an additionality can be of such a degree that it becomes a qualitative change. I do not have the space to discuss this here in detail. At the individual level the issue of continuity of personal identity is clearly at stake: whether an intervention brings about an identity change will depend on the criterion of identity appealed to. At species level, analogously, the issue will turn on what counts as a species (e.g. a group whose members breed with each other) and on the criterion for species continuity.

2.2.1 *Beyond Therapy*

There are difficulties in trying to explain 'enhancement' as 'beyond therapy'. This is not just because it may be argued that some interventions which we want to count *as* enhancements may also be at least *partly* therapeutic, but also because what counts as therapeutic is itself a subject of considerable controversy. Prominent examples are the purported distinction between 'therapeutic' and reproductive cloning, and the discussion, particularly in the early days of assisted reproduction, as to whether IVF counted as a therapy. The distinction appealed to in both of these discussions has been therapy versus research; criteria appealed to in order to resolve this included therapeutic intentions, on the one hand; and outcomes or at least expected outcomes, on the other (Caplan 1992). It is difficult to support the view that intentions alone are sufficient, if there is no evidence base to suggest that a particular intervention is likely to have therapeutic benefit. But nor is it clear that therapeutic intention is a *necessary* condition of something counting as a therapeutic intervention. Experience with placebos shows the wide variety of types of intervention that can be therapeutic even if not intended.

But it is necessary to be careful here. There seem to be at least four different issues:

(a) Whether intervention x has or is intended to have a therapeutic *effect* in a particular case
(b) Whether intervention x counts as an instance of a [validated] therapy
(c) Whether intervention x is applied to a condition that falls within the proper scope of medicine. Here appeal may be made to the *nature* of the condition that is being treated or to its *cause*. The latter has come in for criticism from Norman Daniels for leading us to treat relevantly similar cases in dissimilar ways, so that, for example, whether or not interventions to alleviate shyness count as therapy or enhancement depend on what is understood to be the aetiology of the condition. But as Daniels also points out, this is constantly changing, as indeed one of the purported outcomes of the Human Genome Project is the greater precision with which disease conditions can be distinguished from each other. Why should we be more concerned with the cause of the condition than with the amount of suffering or discomfort that people experience (Daniels 2000)?
(d) The therapy-enhancement distinction takes place both with regard to the individual and to the species as a whole. For some, it is the latter application that is the more interesting of the two, as we debate the possibilities of creating posthumans. However, it is also important to discuss what it means to enhance an existing individual. If the therapy-enhancement distinction is to be useful it needs to be able to tell us both how to distinguish between therapeutic and enhancing uses of cosmetic surgery; and how to assess the options for the future of humanity as a whole. In some discussions the distinction between self/species enhancement is glossed over. Baylis and Roberts, for example, in their significant discussion of the inevitability thesis (Baylis & Robert 2004) at times appear to be discussing enhancement of humans as such; while at others they speak of enhancement in relation to 'the self':

> [T]he resulting alterations may be conservative (i.e., used to normalise the self). Liberal (i.e., used to liberate the self) or radical (used to fashion a self that effectively challenges others' conception of oneself) (Baylis & Robert 2004: p 2)

And yet it is precisely this last possibility that may be under threat from some enhancement projects, which is the source of one of the major objections to enhancement.

There are of course questions to consider about what *counts* as making a change (whether enhancing or not) at species level rather than at individual level. Suppose that there was agreement that introducing a third eye, e.g., at the back of the head, counted as an enhancing intervention in an individual. Would making this change in one person count as an enhancement of the species? If not, would a certain number or proportion need to be changed? While this is a difficult issue because of the contested boundaries of the concept of 'species', my submission is that (although it would not be appropriate to talk of all enhancement only in genetic terms), for an enhancement to count as an enhancement of the species it would have to be transmissible down the germ-line. In other words, species enhancement does require the introduction of a change at gene pool level. Otherwise the respect in which it makes sense to speak of enhancement of the species remains obscure.

To try to explain enhancement through making an opposition with therapy is far from a simple matter – and there is yet another complication, which is the issue of prevention. There is a view that preventive interventions can be enhancing: an example is a boost to the immune system to protect against infectious disease (Holm 1994). Is it possible, also, for a preventive intervention to be therapeutic: what would count as an example of such? Let us consider, as a possible candidate, preventive mastectomy in the case of a woman with a strong family history of breast cancer – what, if anything, makes this therapeutic? Since it is not known with certainty that the patient would have proceeded to develop breast cancer had she not had the preventive mastectomy, there are difficulties in saying that it is therapeutic in *that* sense although there might be therapeutic effects in terms of *reassurance* (cf. Eisinger 2007). Arguably, however, the main aim is to reduce risk status – so in what sense is that different from the enhancing immune system change? And yet intuitively (and quite independently of any aesthetic considerations) it seems counterintuitive to speak of a mastectomy as an enhancement. It seems that in order to understand the answer to these queries, we need more to the concept of enhancement than simply the 'beyond therapy' criterion.

2.2.1.1 Species-Normal Functioning

Norman Daniels introduces species-typical normal functioning as a way of distinguishing between therapy and enhancement, and this has the advantage that it can be used either in the individual or the species case. In the latter, if we have an idea of species-typical normal functioning it is possible to assess individuals as to how far short they fall of that ideal; and we can have an idea, with regard to the species, of normal life expectancy, for example. In the individual case, if an intervention restores a person to species-typical normal functioning it falls within the 'therapy' category; otherwise it counts as an enhancement. In the preventive mastectomy case the point would presumably be that the intervention restores the individual to the population level of risk (although that would not, of course, be zero risk). Although this does not rescue the therapy-enhancement distinction as the best way of understanding enhancement, at least partly because species-typical normal functioning is a shifting boundary, the latter may be useful in thinking about the moral issue.

2.2.2 *Enhancement: The Quantitative Approach (The Additionality View)*

As noted in the US President's Council report, the O.E.D. definition gives a quantitative interpretation of enhancement – to enhance x is to add to, exaggerate, or increase x in some respect. So on this criterion, to increase the range or degree of immune response would count as an enhancement. But how should the preventive mastectomy be assessed? Rather than an increase or an addition, it appears to be a (quantitative) *reduction* in at least two respects – both in the sense that a part of the body is removed, and in the sense that the risk of developing breast cancer is reduced. Any reduction in risk, however, is at the same time an *increase* in the probability of remaining free from disease.

What this example makes clear is that it is necessary to be specific as to the *respect* in which x is enhanced. While it may make sense to speak of enhancing x with regard to characteristic y, it is difficult if not impossible to speak of enhancing x *tout court*. Indeed to enhance x with respect to characteristic y may be at the expense of some other characteristic z. This is the 'no gains without compensating losses' argument discussed by Jonathan Glover: you cannot breed race horses that are also good cart horses (Glover 1977). There are trade-offs to be had. So whether or not a preventive mastectomy will count as therapy or enhancement, even on the quantitative approach, will be characteristic–specific. This too will be pertinent to any moral assessment.

2.2.3 Enhancement: The Qualitative Approach (Enhancement as Improvement)

Although the strict dictionary definition of enhancement is quantitative, however, many people appear to use it to make a qualitative judgment. Indeed the advertisement for one company offering breast surgery specifically draws a distinction between breast reduction and breast augmentation, but also between breast augmentation and breast enhancement. Breast enhancement, it seems, may be neither about reducing or increasing the size, but about changing the contours to bring about a more pleasing silhouette[1] (http://www.ebreastaug.com/breast-augmentation.html).

From a linguistic point of view the concepts of 'enhancement' and 'improvement' are distinguishable. Whereas to enhance, as indicated above, is to add to; to improve is to make better. The discussion in (2) above suggested that to enhance an x with respect to characteristic y is not necessarily to make x better overall. It is possible for breast enlargement to distort the proportions of the body, for example. Is there a case, however, for saying that to enhance an x with respect to characteristic y should be understood as introducing an improvement to x *with respect to that characteristic*?

The question seems to turn on what the criteria for improvement are. It cannot be explained in terms of 'bigger is better' *per se*, because that removes any distinction between the quantitative and the qualitative judgment. For an enhancement to

[1] (http://www.ebreastaug.com/breast-augmentation.html). Accessed on 19 October 2007.

count even as a characteristic-specific improvement it would be necessary to understand the background conditions obtaining, including the purposes or desires being served by the change introduced. So in order to assess whether any breast surgery is an improvement or not we need to know for what purposes it was carried out, and if those purposes are achieved, then it counts as an improvement and thus *on this definition*, an enhancement. If the intervention is sought in order to make the person more attractive, however, it is arguable that the judgment of success, or not, has to have regard to broader considerations than simply the breast alone, such as the new proportions of the body, by whom it is found attractive and so on.

There may be circumstances in which a characteristic-specific intervention can be introduced which meets a particular purpose without changing anything else. For example, suppose I need to increase my hearing range in order to do a particular job and this can be achieved by taking a pill that has no side effects. In that case this might appear to be an improvement and thus, on this definition, an enhancement with respect to the purpose – and moreover, as *ex hypothesi* everything else remains the same, an improvement overall.

It is necessary, however, to be very precise about the respect in which an improvement is introduced. In the hearing example, mentioned earlier, it is necessary to allow for the possibility that an improvement in the hearing range could be accompanied by a diminution of hearing discrimination. So the relevant characteristic cannot be 'hearing' but must be 'hearing range'. I submit, moreover, that to define enhancement in terms of improvement is also at least potentially misleading, in that it directs attention away from the need to ask what purposes are being served and complicates the issue of assessment of the intervention from a moral point of view. This is not necessarily decisive against the definition, however, provided that it is clear that to define enhancement as improvement does not preclude an adverse judgment on its desirability. Given this, the definition of enhancement as an improvement is quite uninformative, because it implies a provisional qualitative judgment which is open to revision, all things considered, whereas the quantitative definition allows us to settle the conceptual question separately.

2.2.4 Enhancement: The Umbrella View

It might be argued that it is not possible to find a definition of 'enhancement' that fits all cases that might attract the label 'enhancement': that the term is used to apply to a wide variety both of changes and techniques. Such interventions include lengthening the life span, making people taller, increasing cognitive powers or emotional sensibilities, and facilitating greater sporting prowess, among others. In addition, techniques of 'enhancement' could include cosmetic, genetic, pharmaceutical, prosthetic, for example.

This way of looking at the issue allows for the fact that some 'enhancements' may also be therapeutic; that they need not add anything (they can involve reduction); they may not constitute an improvement. Specific interventions would have to be assessed on a case-by-case basis – rather than a judgment on the acceptability or desirability of human enhancement overall.

The advantages of this way of looking at the issue would be that it would then be possible to avoid the difficult issues of disagreement when some individuals wish to make changes to themselves that they regard as enhancements but which seem to observers to be damaging (e.g. amputation). Whether or not it was an 'enhancement' would not be the issue; the specifics of the case would have to be considered in making an assessment. It remains the case, however, that there are debates to be had about whether enhancement *per se* is part of human nature.

A sense of enhancement is needed which does not prejudge the issue of acceptability and desirability. With this in mind the 'improvement' view is not helpful. The sense of enhancement, I argue, which is to be preferred is the additionality view, where an enhancement is an addition or exaggeration of a characteristic which may or may not constitute an improvement.

The fact that it is necessary to be able to deal with the possible counter example that some individuals regard the removal of a limb as an enhancement makes it even clearer that attention has to be given to the respect in which there is a claimed enhancement. If there is no respect in which something is added or exaggerated, then such an intervention would not count as an enhancement on this definition: to say otherwise would be a mistake.

2.3 The Moral Issue

A major reason why there has been so much discussion about the distinction between therapy and enhancement has been for the purposes of drawing lines over what is acceptable and what is not. Even though it may be necessary to assess interventions on a case-by-case basis, the therapy-enhancement distinction has served as a 'moral warning flag' (Daniels 2000), and there are issues about whether human enhancement is a desirable goal, over and above the issues surrounding the use of specific technologies.

2.3.1 The Inevitability Thesis

Baylis and Robert have argued, however, that enhancement is inevitable, and that this sets limits to the range of useful questions that can be asked. The inevitability thesis is a frequent guest at the feast when new technological possibilities are on the table. While it might appear that a simplistic technological imperative is implausible, and uninteresting if it simply means that someone somewhere will try it, there may be different explanations of why and in what way enhancement is thought to be inevitable, which have a bearing on the moral issue. Robert Sparrow, for example, in relation to nanotechnology, identifies three different strands of thought about inevitability, tracing inevitability to techno-optimism – development is self-evidently good; to an empirical claim about the impossibility of regulation; or to a resigned techno-pessimism based on contingent political circumstances, whereby regulation would in principle be possible but in fact is not. The first of these, Sparrow argues, may, in turn, depend on an innate human drive (Sparrow 2007).

This seems to be the position taken by Baylis and Robert. Surveying a number of objections to [genetic] enhancement, Baylis and Robert say:

There is no evidence as yet … that these arguments … or any other arguments, *however well developed*, will suffice to stop the refinement and use of genetic enhancement technologies. As it happens, contemporary Western democracies have no experience with permanently halting the development and use of any enhancement technologies on ethical grounds (Baylis & Robert 2004: 16).

And yet they are surprisingly willing to take the line that some proposals will prove impossible:

To be sure, not all of the envisioned genetic enhancements will come to pass. The complexities of organismal development are such that some of the genetic tinkering imagined and promoted by enhancement enthusiasts will prove to be impossible… What matters … is that *despite* the likely failure … there are some among us who will *inevitably attempt* to engineer the human genome for the purpose of improving *Homo sapiens* (Baylis & Robert 2004: 22).

Baylis and Robert do not put the purported inevitability down to a science-friendly social and political context, or to a kind of empirical slippery slope: their explanation of inevitability is rooted in what they present as an *avant-garde* portrayal of human nature. They posit a 'biosocial drive to pursue perfection' as an essential characteristic of humanness. They further suggest that the inevitability thesis is a key step in the ethical debate:

We maintain that accepting the inevitability of genetic enhancement technologies is an important and necessary step forward in the ethical debate about the development and use of such technologies. We need to change the lens through which we perceive, and therefore approach, the prospect of enhancing humans genetically. In recognising the futility of trying to stop these technologies, we can usefully direct our energies to a systematic analysis of the appropriate scope of their use (Baylis & Robert 2004: 25).

It is important to bear in mind the 'drive to perfection' argument as an important influence on the debate, which pushes towards an understanding of enhancement in terms of improvement, which I have suggested is a mistake. Indeed, the improvement view seems to be reflected in the account supported by Baylis and Robert, who by genetic enhancement technology understand "any technology that directly alters the expression of genes that are already present in humans, or that involves the addition of genes that have not previously appeared … for the purpose of human physical, intellectual, psychological, or moral improvement" (Baylis & Robert 2004).

Although the 'drive to perfection' argument plays a significant role in the debate, it is not supported by all pro-enhancers, such as John Harris (2007). The point I want to emphasise, however, is that it is something of a red herring in the debate, because it somehow implies that enhancement is connected with moving towards perfection or at least improvement, whereas my argument is that enhancement as a concept is distinct from improvement. In *assessing* any given enhancement it will be important to ask if it constitutes an improvement or not.

2.3.2 Towards Guiding Principles?

In assessing the extent to which enhancement is morally acceptable and/or desirable, it is important, as already indicated above, to distinguish different levels at which enhancement can take place. First, there is individual enhancement: individuals may seem out ways of enhancing particular characteristics, by any number of means – not only genetic but also dietary, surgical, through exercise or treatments emanating from new technologies such as nanotechnology. In another context, Abdallah Daar and Peter Singer have used the term 'boutique model' – and to use the term for this category of enhancement choice can be helpful as illustrating what is at stake (Daar & Singer 2005). In between this and the other end of the spectrum, the enhancement of the species, are enhancement questions that are specific to particular areas of life or practices, such as sport.

There are a wide variety of positions with regard to the moral import of the therapy-enhancement distinction. The following list builds on one devised by Baylis and Robert in their article:

- Enhancement is morally wrong in itself.
- Enhancement gives rise to concerns about equity.
- Enhancement is not a priority from a moral point of view.
- Both therapy and enhancement are morally permissible, other things being equal.
- Enhancement is morally required.

While I do not have the space to discuss all these positions in detail, clearly there are different issues relating to the individual and the species case. For present purposes I am going to assume that if individuals wish to enhance themselves, then other things being equal, that is morally acceptable. That is because the more difficult issues arise where other things are *not* equal, either because this has implications for others, or in cases where individuals are not choosing for themselves e.g., when decisions are made for future children. There are objections to this that go beyond lack of consent, to having one's dignity as a human being compromised by being designed by another (cf. Fukuyama 2003; Habermas 2003). Such arguments inform the view that enhancement is morally wrong in itself.

On the other hand there is an argument that there is a moral obligation to enhance. There might be at least two lines of thought here. One might be that enhancement could be a means of redress for certain existing social inequalities or other social ills. An example of the latter would be claims such as the argument that enhancement of IQ would lead to a reduction in the crime rate.[2] Whatever the truth of this specific claim, any such arguments have to be able to deal with the complexity of social phenomena in terms of chains of causal influence. To suggest that changing one thing will bring about a desired change might be unduly simplistic.

John Harris's argument for enhancement (Harris 2007), appears to be based on the ills of diseases and death, which, he argues, we have an obligation to postpone. He makes a distinction between those human ills we have an obligation to do something about by enhancement; and those we have not. There is no moral obligation for example, to make people more attractive. In so far as the argument rests on relief of the harms of disease and death, it might be argued that enhancement has in effect been reduced to therapeutic aims, which is an interesting reversal of the attempt to define enhancement by distinguishing it from therapy. Harris is unconcerned, however, by the possible effects that enhancement of the sort he favours might have on social inequalities.

My position is that enhancement is permissible under certain conditions. I want to consider two principles provisionally set out as follows:

P1. Morally permissible enhancements are those, which constitute an improvement, all things considered.
P2. Morally permissible enhancements are those which reduce, or at least do not increase, social inequalities.

Let us take an example of trying to use enhancement to reduce existing social inequalities, in accordance with P2. If it is the case that taller people have certain social advantages, people of below average height may seek to be made taller, sometimes through painful operations, in order to access social advantage. There are at least two problems with this. First, there is the obvious point that any apparent advantages may depend on the fact that not everyone can access them. Second, to go down this route may reinforce the social conditions that create the inequalities in the first place. This shows that the application of P2 is problematic. However, if it is the case that an enhancement is permissible if and only if both P1 and P2 are satisfied, that might make a difference. In terms of an overall assessment of the tallness case, it is far from clear that the enhancing intervention would constitute an improvement, either for the enhanced individuals themselves or for society.

To say that an enhancing intervention would have to constitute an improvement overall, however, would perhaps be too strong. In order to be *acceptable* perhaps it is sufficient that it does not make things worse – this is consistent with the position taken in relation to individual self-enhancers. This would apply, for example, where an enhancement introduced a characteristic-specific enhancement and left everything else the same. Improvement overall would be a necessary condition of desirability. In any case, where enhancement to the species beyond current capability is concerned, how do we know that it would be an improvement? Where do we look for criteria? There is a problem in that, we may be creating new sources of inequality

[2] Julian Savulescu, presentation at 'Genetics and Justice' conference, Oxford, 2 July 2007.

and it is difficult to know what the relevant criteria are for what would count as an improvement.

We can understand this best by looking at a particular practice or area of life – for example, the context of sport, which is one of the contexts in which much has been written about enhancement. I am here going beyond the individual choice of a sportsperson to pursue enhancement, to look at sport as an area of life with its own standards and purposes. The criteria for whether or not an enhancement counts as an improvement will clearly be different in sport from other contexts. Aristotle, in his doctrine of the mean, pointed out that the diet that is appropriate for an athlete is different from what would be suitable for other people:

If 10 pounds are too much for a particular person to eat and two too little, it does not follow that the trainer will order 6 pounds, for this is perhaps too much for the person who is to take it, or too little – too little for Milo, too much for the beginner in athletic exercises. The same is true of running and wrestling (Aristotle 1908: 1106a17).

The relevant *ends* in question are different. There is an issue not only about the ends of the individual but also about the point of sport in general. For the individual there might be different purposes involved in maximising performance – winning is an obvious possibility (which might be a means to other ends such as earning more money), but there are also others, such as pushing oneself to one's limits. When we talk about sport in general, however, there are further questions to answer. Is the point of sport primarily competition and winning? What about other elements, such as providing an opportunity for exercise of certain virtues (which will be different according to whether or not team-playing is involved); physical exercise; development of human potential; entertainment and so on (cf. Miah 2004). My point is that whether or not enhancement will count as an improvement is, first, relevant to the context of sport, and second, to the purposes for which sport is engaged in, both on an individual and a species-level. We might not agree on the good that is internal to the practice of sport, but at least it seems possible to understand the kinds of considerations that are involved in different models of sport.

When discussion turns to improving humans overall, however, it is a much more difficult issue, because it is not clear where to begin in looking for relevant purposes. Some appeal to a concept of human nature, but to do this can also lead in different directions. From a conservative point of view, trying to enhance human beings as such would be tampering with human nature, which is undesirable in itself and likely to create a new type of being, the posthuman. A liberal view on the other hand might attempt to argue that continually striving for self-improvement is an aspect of human nature which ought to be facilitated. But the question remains – in what direction? How is it possible to set criteria for what enhancements will count as an improvement or not without any agreement as to ends or purposes?

The provisional principles, then, do not do an entirely satisfactory job. In the absence of an agreement about what would count as an improvement, all things considered, it is difficult to use P2 for guidance on what enhancements would be desirable. It also appears that for establishing what enhancements are acceptable P1 and P2 are too strong. In their place I suggest:

P3. Morally permissible enhancements are those which constitute an improvement, all things considered, or which introduce a characteristic-specific enhancement that leaves other things equal.
P4. Morally permissible enhancements are those which reduce, or at least do not reinforce, existing social inequalities.

Some might want to argue that the fact that an enhancement does not meet the demands of P4 should not rule it out – a better view would be that it is not a priority from a moral point of view. My view, however, is that this would not do enough to point to the real harm that may result from the reinforcement of existing inequalities, as in the suffering that may ensue in the attempts of people to increase their height for perceived social advantage.

2.4 Conclusion

In sum, I have argued that the important issue is not the distinction between therapy and enhancement but the extent to which enhancement counts as an improvement, which will be dependent upon context and purposes. Improvement should not be included in the definition of enhancement. When we are talking about human enhancement overall this is a difficult matter in the light of lack of agreement over purposes.

Acknowledgements I am grateful to Bert Gordijn for comments on an earlier version, and to discussion at the annual conference of the European Society for Philosophy of Medicine and Health Care in Barcelona, 2005. The support of the Economic and Social Research Council (ESRC) is gratefully acknowledged. The work forms part of the programme of work conducted by the ESRC Centre for Economic and Social Aspects of Genomics (Cesagen).

References

Aristotle (1908) Nicomachean Ethics. Ross D (trans) Clarendon, Oxford
Baylis F, Robert J S (2004) The inevitability of genetic enhancement technologies. Bioethics 18(1): 1–26
Caplan A (1992) If I Were a Rich Man Could I Buy a Pancreas?: And Other Essays in Health Care. Indiana University Press, Bloomington, IN
Daar A, Singer P A (2005) Pharmacogenetics and geographical ancestry: implications for drug development and global health. Nature Reviews Genetics 6: 241–246
Daniels N (2000) Normal functioning and the treatment-enhancement distinction. Cambridge Quarterly of Healthcare Ethics 9: 309–322
Eisinger F (2007) Prophylactic mastectomy: ethical issues. British Medical Bulletin 81–82: 7–19
Fukuyama F (2003) Our Posthuman Future: Consequences of the Biotechnology Revolution. Picador, New York
Glover J (1977) Causing Death and Saving Lives. Penguin, Harmondsworth, London
Habermas J (2003) The Future of Human Nature. Beister H, Rehg W (trans) Polity, Cambridge

Harris J (2007) Enhancing Evolution: The Ethical Case for Making Better People. Columbia and Princeton University Presses, California

Holm S (1994) Genetic Engineering and the North-South Divide. In: Dyson A, Harris J (eds) Bioethics and Biotechnology. Routledge, London

Miah A (2004) Genetically Modified Athletes: Biomedical Ethics, Gene Doping and Sport. Routledge, London

Sparrow R (2007) Revolutionary and familiar, inevitable and precarious: rhetorical contradistinctions in enthusiasm for nanotechnology. Nanoethics 1: 57–68

[US] President's Council on Bioethics (2003) Beyond Therapy: A Report by the President's Council on Bioethics. President's Council on Bioethics, Washington, DC

Chapter 3
Medical Enhancement: A Destination of Technological, not Human, Betterment

S.J. Kevin FitzGerald

3.1 Introduction

With the rapid advance of scientific understanding and technological manipulation, many utopian prognostications have come into the public domain predicting the future of a new and improved humankind. One of the most far-reaching visions of a technological human future can be found in the reports from the NBIC conferences sponsored by the National Science Foundation, along with other organizations. A statement from their website explains the basic perspective of the conferences: "The convergence of nanoscience, biotechnology, information technology and cognitive science (NBIC) offers immense opportunities for the improvement of human abilities, social outcomes, the nation's productivity and its quality of life."[1]

As seen by the NBIC proponents, the scope of these opportunities is limited only by our imaginations. In the overview chapter from the 2003 report, the promise of an NBIC convergence is described in the following manner: "The twenty-first century could end in world peace, universal prosperity, and evolution to a higher level of compassion and accomplishment" (Roco & Bainbridge 2003: 6). This 2003 report goes on to discuss how this NBIC convergence will offer humankind much longer, disease-free, lives, with various opportunities for interfacing with machines and computers in order to extend one's abilities and capacities.[2]

One strategy these technological utopians have for grabbing attention is to proclaim how technology will take us "beyond" our human nature. In response to this proclamation, one can ask several questions. Can we go beyond? What kind of destination is this beyond? And if there is such a destination, should we go there? In addressing these questions it is critical to distinguish between going beyond our human physiological capabilities and going beyond our current abilities to treat disease and illness. Few, if any, argue against a continual effort to improve our ability

[1] http://www.infocastinc.com/nbic/nbichome.htm

[2] See Section C, "Improving Human Health and Physical Capabilities" (Roco & Bainbridge 2003: 179–275)

B. Gordijn, R. Chadwick (eds.) *Medical Enhancement and Posthumanity*,

to treat illness or care for those who are ill. Therefore, the issue to be addressed in this chapter is the alteration of the physiology of human beings in an effort to somehow make human beings better or more than they could be otherwise.

Before investigating this distinction between attempting to advance our health care capabilities and attempting to advance fundamental human physiological capabilities, it is legitimate to question whether or not the issue of going beyond human nature or human physiology should be addressed within the context of medicine and health care. After all, this context is usually defined with respect to returning someone to health, preventing disease, or at least minimizing illness and suffering. As is found on the United States National Library of Medicine's Medline Plus website: medicine is "the science and art dealing with the maintenance of health and the prevention, alleviation, or cure of disease"[3]; and health care is "the maintaining and restoration of health by the treatment and prevention of disease especially by trained and licensed professionals (as in medicine, dentistry, clinical psychology, and public health)."[4] Nowhere is there mention of improving, bettering, or going beyond health or human physiological capacity as they are generally construed within the health care professions.

Since "going beyond" is not usually cited as a part of health care, one could argue that an ethical evaluation of this idea is best done outside of the medical tradition. However, since the technological advances being suggested as the means for making us "better than well"[5] are oriented at altering human physiology, health care professionals will by necessity become involved. At the very least, they will be required to provide oversight for the procedures involved, and care for those harmed in any way by the physiological alterations that are attempted as a means for moving individuals beyond their normal capacities. Therefore, employing the lens of medicine and health care to evaluate the claims and goals of the technological utopians will give us at least a crucial, if not comprehensive, perspective on the purported benefits and goods of choosing to journey to the destination of human physiological enhancement.

One heuristic framework commonly employed within medical ethics to categorize and evaluate these multiplying technological possibilities that are to take us beyond our human nature is to distinguish between manipulations that would be considered therapeutic and those that would be considered more than or beyond mere therapy – in a word, "enhancements." The goal of a therapy is to prevent, minimize, or cure disease and illness, as stated above. The goal of an enhancement is…what? To go beyond therapy? In this chapter, it will be argued that although the NBIC goals – such as universal peace, prosperity, and compassion – are well worth pursuing, the means with which they intend to achieve these objectives, i.e. physiological enhancement, will be unsuitable. Instead, there are ample alternative means better suited to achieve these goals. This argument will focus primarily on three points.

---

[3] http://www2.merriam-webster.com/cgi-bin/mwmednlm?book=Medical&va=medicine

[4] http://www2.merriam-webster.com/cgi-bin/mwmednlm

[5] This phrase has been used by many authors. For example, see Elliott (2003).

The first point is that the therapy/enhancement distinction no longer provides a clear line of delineation among various proposals for physiological interventions. This lack of clarity is due primarily to the rapid expansion of biological information and manipulation. This rapid expansion is blurring the conceptual lines we have employed in order to distinguish health from disease, normal from abnormal, medical benefit from medical harm – and, hence, also therapy from enhancement since this distinction generally relies on these more basic distinctions.

The second point builds upon the first. Not only is the therapy/enhancement distinction inadequate due to its inapplicability to current advances in biotechnology and medicine, but this distinction also fails as a basis for any broad program of bettering or improving human nature or health. The concept of enhancement, as it is currently employed, is not practically applicable to the ends of large scale or global benefit that are often proposed as justification for pursuing enhancement in general.

In response to these first two points, the third point will be to argue for some directions and goals for biotechnology that will provide clear goods and benefits especially when applied on a broad or global scale.

3.2 The Problems of the Therapy/Enhancement Distinction

Though this distinction between therapy and enhancement is often used in discussions regarding the future of biotechnology and medicine, its application is also often qualified by the *caveat* that the boundaries between therapy and enhancement are currently neither precise nor accurate. The United States President's Council on Bioethics summarized this point well in their report, *Beyond Therapy* (PCB 2003: 14–15). Building upon their conclusion that the distinction between therapy and enhancement "is finally inadequate to the moral analysis," (PCB 2003: 14) the focus of the argument to be presented here will be on an aspect of this inadequacy particularly pertinent to the idea that one might employ the current advances in medicine to enhance people and make them better than well.

The critical problem with the current proposals for physiological enhancement is the confounding effect advances in biomedical research are having on the idea of the enhancement of health itself. If one is to enhance or improve upon something, one needs to know what is the norm or the average for that something to be. In the case of physiological enhancement, one must know what normal or average physiology is before one can make it better. However, advances in molecular biology, genetics, bioinformatics, and imaging technologies (the very technologies the physiological enhancers are often proposing to use) are all revealing unforeseen complexities, interchangeabilities, and interrelationships within our biological nature that undermine and unravel the norms and categories often employed in judging between illness and health, or physiological benefit and burden.

One of these norms that has been broadly applied to health, both culturally and historically, is the idea of balance or homeostasis. Illness and disease are seen as imbalances in our bodies.[6] This concept takes on new meaning and significance in the light of recent advances in areas such as genomics and bioinformatics. With the increasing ability to both decipher the genetic and epigenetic roots of disease, and then assess those roots for genomic variations within a given population through database analyses, many leaders in medical research are predicting the dawn of individualized medicine (for example, see Guttmacher & Collins 2002). If we can understand how a multitude of specific genetic and epigenetic variations function within certain genomic and environmental contexts, then we can predict with greater precision and accuracy the physiological consequences of such genetic variations and how they might respond to specific treatments. Hence, treatments will be able to be tailored more to a given individual's disease, genetic constitution, and environment. For example, since each individual's cancer is unique (though we do categorize them according to tissue source and general features to assist in diagnosis and prognosis), treatments will be formulated to tackle the specific abnormal genetic and epigenetic aspects of the tumor while minimizing harm to the specific genetic and epigenetic characteristics of the individual's normal cells and tissue.

While such an individualized treatment approach may work well to address specific genetic or epigenetic abnormalities using the healthy cells, tissues, and physiology of the individual as the norm, the same individualized approach is not as amenable to enhancing one's physiology to go beyond health. Any radical change made to healthy human cellular or physiological functioning would by definition be an abnormality or imbalance. In the era of individualized medicine, by what standard will a change be judged to be an improvement? Will there be some ideal standard, and, if so, what will it be? Who among us represents the perfectly healthy person or the perfect embodiment of a particular characteristic? Since our advancing genomic knowledge indicates how each of us are our own unique balance of molecular biology and environment, who will declare that a particular new alteration is good and healthy for all, or even for many?

In response to these questions, proponents of enhancement might argue that surely there are characteristics that most, if not all, would agree are worth trying to achieve – such as a longer life or greater intelligence than would be otherwise possible. Indeed, those enhancements might sound attractive in theory. However, neither is an easily delineated biological characteristic, especially with regard to a simple cause and effect predictability, and that lack of clarity does not even take into consideration the complexity or the interrelatedness of various human physiological, environmental, and behavioral attributes.

Regarding intelligence enhancement, going well beyond the normal range of intelligence (however one might measure or quantify intelligence) has long been associated with behavioral problems, especially in child development. Researchers

[6] Homeostatis is a concept used in medicine to refer to the proper equilibrium or balance among various elements of a system or organism. In ancient Greece, and later, illness was thought to be an imbalance in the four humours. For more on this see Kontopoulou and Marketos (2002: 124–125).

in psychology and child development are continuing to explore correlations between extreme intelligence and sociopathic or psychopathic behavior (see, for example, Salekin et al. 2004; Johansson & Kerr 2005). In addition, child development resources for parents with gifted children consistently cite both the advantages and disadvantages such children experience as they develop. One author of works on this issue of raising gifted children emphasizes that "the healthiest long term goal is not necessarily a child who gains fame, fortune, and a Nobel Prize, but one who becomes a comfortable adult and uses gifts productively."[7] It is intriguing that this author identifies the *healthiest* goal as one that could apply to any child, and is perhaps more easily attained by those children not considered to be especially gifted. From this perspective, one could easily conclude that the real enhancement might well be to biologically adjust those children who happen to be categorized as "gifted" to become biologically more average so that they might have a better chance of becoming happy, well-adjusted, productive adults.

In a similar manner, the target of altering the aging process by manipulating certain genes in order to extend the normal lifespan of human beings without incurring any detriments, individual or social, may well prove to be entirely deceptive. While it is the case that certain genes, such as those of the insulin growth factor receptor family, have been demonstrated to be linked to the aging process, direct manipulation of these genes will most likely only have a partial effect at best on the aging process, as it is also a complicated interrelationship among genetic, epigenetic, behavioral, and environmental factors (Geesaman 2006). In addition, even if the partial effect does extend a person's lifespan, it does not guarantee that the extension also provides for the capacity to engage in the kinds of activities one might desire for one's longer life. Again, proponents of enhancement might claim that further research will allow for a more complete understanding of these complexities and, hence, allow for the ability to manipulate each person's physiology to achieve a specific type of longer lifespan without any undesired side effects. However, we must investigate whether or not this assertion – that more research and more manipulation will always solve the problems that arise – does not in fact promise more than it can deliver, and may actually cause more problems than are remedied.

Two aspects of the current research on aging will help reveal the faulty foundations of this assertion. First, the vast majority of current medical research is focused on finding ways to help people live healthier longer. In other words, the goal is to help people avoid the diseases that often accompany older age and may significantly shorten or greatly diminish one's potential healthy lifespan (for example, see Perls 2006). The context of the research is not specifically to find ways to increase an individual's potential lifespan – though the promise of a longer, healthier life can easily be misconstrued as the promise of extending one's maximum lifespan beyond what one might otherwise expect even under the best of circumstances.

---

[7] Tolan S S, Helping your Highly Gifted Child, http://www.kidsource.com/kidsource/content/help.gift.html

At this point one might ask, "What difference does it make what the goal and context are as long as the medical intervention adds healthy years to one's life?" From the perspective of adding years of health to one's life – perhaps no difference. However, from the perspective of deciding whether or not this intervention is part of the usual medical, therapeutic project, or some utopian enhancement agenda – the goals and context are quite significant, though difficult to delineate biologically. One way to express this significance is to ask whether we are to consider aging to be normal or not?

Normal human aging results in certain physiological diminishments. When these diminishments become incapacitating or life threatening, medical professionals intervene to rectify, compensate for, or palliate these diminishments. In the end, though, we die. Since modern medicine has greatly increased the lifespan of many people who have consistent access to good health care, it is not easy to declare at what specific point biotechnology will take us beyond normal aging and into an enhanced state – short of the extreme prognostications of healthy life-spans in the hundreds of years or longer. Hence, even on this generic level of the issue, the therapy/enhancement distinction may not be helpful for all practical purposes.

If this inadequacy for practical purposes is not sufficient to cause us to avoid using this distinction between therapy and enhancement with regard to aging research and interventions, then this argument of inadequacy can be extended further by raising the second aspect of aging research that undermines claims for lifespan enhancement. As mentioned above, behavior is also an important component of aging. One's lifestyle choices can greatly affect one's lifespan. For years it has been known that spartanly restricting what and how much one eats and drinks can reduce the ravages of aging and result in a life that is longer than it might have been otherwise (Duff et al. 2006). The problem with this approach is that few people wish to undertake this strict dietary regimen even to achieve a longer life. Hence, the question arises: when people say that they want to live longer, are they instead actually desiring to indulge in certain unhealthy behaviors – such as overeating, avoiding exercise, and consuming excessive amounts of alcohol – and not have these behaviors cost them years of life or health? Is the goal to do what it takes to live longer, or to live one's full lifespan while still engaging in all the behaviors one desires to do, especially if what one desires to do will likely diminish one's health and shorten one's life? If the goal is indeed the latter (which the paucity of dietary ascetics indicates), then are we really discussing lifespan enhancements, or is this merely the age-old desire to have one's cake and eat it too?

In response to these criticisms of the use of a therapy/enhancement distinction to justify making people better than well, especially with regard to such goals as greater intelligence or lifespan, enhancement proponents might argue that a more focused and incremental approach to enhancement will best demonstrate its promises. A biologically isolated ability that has a more limited scope, and yet is still desirable to many, might be the best starting point for the enhancement project. For the sake of addressing this type of argument, the ability labeled "perfect" or "absolute" pitch will provide one possibility that fits these criteria. Recent research indicates that absolute pitch has both a genetic component and a relatively isolated neurological basis. Though proper training in childhood may be required for an individual to express this ability in full, brain scans reveal that a certain inherited developmental pattern may be necessary for one to possess the ability at all (Zatorre 2003). Therefore, research might actually isolate a relatively discrete genetic or physiological component that could be made available to all so that everyone might enjoy this ability.

From there, who knows? Perhaps civilization would experience a flourishing of music unparalleled in the history of humankind! Then again, civilization may instead discover just how imperfect and annoying our normal lives can be when it comes to the sounds we experience every day. One effect of having the ability to discern absolute pitch is to suffer from all the off-key and sour sounds of our world. Those who have this ability can pay a significant price. As with many things in life, knowledge of the perfect, or the vastly superior, brings with it the multitude experiences of frustrating imperfections. Since we will not be able to remove all imperfections from life, such as off-key sounds, one can rightly question the assertion that more precise or powerful abilities to perceive or know, such as absolute pitch, will indeed be experienced as an improvement or enhancement when compared to one's previous level of ability. In fact, one can easily imagine a situation where parents with absolute pitch desire to have children without the ability so that their children might enjoy rigorous musical training without having to suffer too much the noises of our off-key world. The parents, of course, would consider this intervention an enhancement of their children's lives – a result similar to the suggested parental conclusion stated previously concerning the enhancement of the gifted children by making them more average.

From the preceding examples and arguments, one can begin to see that there is a problem with the therapy/enhancement distinction. Not only is this distinction rendered inadequate by the current research that is indicating greater interrelatedness among the molecules and processes of human physiological balance, but also this distinction is blurred by the research on and experiences of individuals and their unique states of health and happiness, especially those individuals with heightened abilities who often reveal the true costs of having such abilities. It is one thing to attempt to use our new medical information and knowledge to return completely or partially a person's diseased tissues and organs to their normal levels of function. It is quite a different matter to use that same information and knowledge to attempt to improve or perfect the levels of functioning for which one's physiology is balanced, especially when targeted improvement will be nearly impossible to define or delineate in a precise manner for the thousands/millions/billions of targeted individuals who differ both according to their own complex physiological balance and their own complex expectations as to what the experience of any improvement will be. Hence, the claim that one will be able to tweak human physiology in some precise and significant manner to achieve a particular improvement (e.g. longer and diminishment-free life, greater intelligence, or even the neurological basis for absolute pitch) for the human species overall without any detriment to or dissatisfaction by anyone is not supported by the data or by human experience. Consider the Spartan diet and aging issue as a prime example of the choices people must constantly face in addressing health issues. Some few who greatly desire to increase their possibilities for a longer life embrace such dieting as a means to their desired end in spite of the sacrifices they must make in their eating habits. Most others, while perhaps still desiring at some level a longer life, decide not to make these dieting sacrifices – the cost is too great. Hence, though draped in futuristic and utopian terms, the enhancement proposals boil down to the usual choices regarding what people are willing to risk or sacrifice in order to obtain something else. Humankind remains without free lunches.

3.3 The Impracticality of Physiological Enhancement

Building upon this first point my argument – that the therapy/enhancement distinction is not an adequate basis for ethical evaluation or delineation of utopian enhancements – we now move to the second point. If we do attempt human physiological enhancement programs, we may well just waste time and resources without achieving any desired benefit.

Acknowledging these problems in delineating what would be a definitive enhancement – and, therefore, a clear benefit – for all or most human beings, proponents of enhancement could alter their pursuit of certain generic physiological enhancement targets and instead argue that each individual will be allowed to choose the physiological characteristics that individual desires to be enhanced. Such an approach avoids the difficulty of establishing broad standards of enhancement, and acknowledges the extent to which health – and, hence, any claim to enhance health – is a social or individual construct. A closer look at such an approach, though, reveals that it merely exchanges one serious set of problems for another.

The fundamental problem with this individualized approach to enhancement is connecting it to the often purported goal of technological utopians – sweeping, if not worldwide, benefit. If generic physiological enhancements are not possible,[8] then how will we proceed with large-scale enhancement projects? Who goes first? Who gets to decide what the particular enhancement will be for those who go first? Are we to physiologically engineer the strongest human being to be ten times stronger? Or the fastest human being to outrun a cheetah? What would be the justification for pursuing such enhancements when we already have machines and devices that allow us to do more than we might ever be able physiologically to engineer our bodies to do? If widespread benefit is the primary goal, then certainly much benefit could be achieved worldwide if useful machines and devices were

[8] It is critical at this juncture to repeat that the focus of this chapter is on physiological enhancements that supposedly will take human beings beyond current capacities for health or function. Hence, cosmetic changes that might be considered social or aesthetic enhancements, and that might be made widely available, are not within the purview of this analysis.

made available to all who have need of them. If longer, healthier lives are the goal, then imagine the number of people whose lives could be longer and healthier from the use of machines and devices they need to survive and thrive but do not have. Of course, proponents of physiological enhancements can always claim that their intent is for all to benefit from some biological alteration. However, if the goal is worldwide, or even widespread, benefit, then we must be rigorous in our assessment of how, where, and to whom to distribute our resources in order to achieve these widespread or worldwide benefits.

Many others have raised this issue of distributive justice both within health care and for societies in general.[9] Though the importance of this issue is almost impossible to overstate, eloquent works by others have already addressed this issue with more cogency and information than can be marshaled here. Consequently, while distributive justice in health care will be briefly addressed in the last section of this chapter, the focus in this section is on the claim that pursuing individualized physiological enhancement will lead to widespread or worldwide benefits.

The key feature that indicates the fundamental incongruity of this claim is the contradictory content of the terms individual, enhancement, widespread or worldwide, and benefit. As was explicated above, advances in individualized medicine reveal the difficulty one would have in determining a particular enhancement that would be, or even would be perceived as, beneficial to most or all. Hence, the retreat to a lesser or seemingly easier claim that each individual will get to choose his or her enhancement. The problem then arises in making this individualized approach available in such a manner that it would have worldwide benefit. How might such a worldwide benefit be achieved?

The most direct way to achieve a worldwide benefit would be to deliver an enhancement product or treatments that most, if not all, agree is beneficial. However this goal not only runs afoul of the problem of individual physiologies, but also of individual evaluations of what is beneficial. The complexities could be staggering. Do we really think that we can develop technologies that will, through physiological means, address the multitude of hopes and dreams individuals throughout the world have regarding what might make their lives or health better than well? The simple answer is no. However, one could still attempt to defend the pursuit of worldwide benefits through enhancement two ways: trickle-down and limited choice.

The trickle-down argument is used often to justify the pursuit of advances that initially will be available only to a few, due to expense or scarce resources, but are intended eventually for most if not all. The argument generally sets up along the lines of allowing initially limited access to a treatment or product that is costly and labor intensive in order to demonstrate the safety and efficacy of the advance. Then when this goal is accomplished, further developments can be pursued that will enable mass production and broad distribution of the advance. Regarding the

[9] If the reader wishes some examples of authors who eloquently raise this issue of distributive justice, especially with regard to health care, two powerful works are Farmer (2003) and Callahan (1998).

pursuit of physiological enhancements, this trickle-down approach would have two serious challenges – scalability and cost.

Again, as mentioned previously, any particular intervention that alters a physiological characteristic of one or a few individuals in such a way that the alteration is considered an improvement over the individuals' normal physiology, even if possible, is not likely to be applicable in the same manner to people in general. Hence, the particular intervention would face significant, if not insurmountable, technical challenges when it came time to scale up the technology for mass production. To get a sense of these challenges, one need only to review the difficulties faced by pharmaceutical companies in the production of a new drug, even drugs that will be used to treat serious diseases and can, therefore, entail significant side-effect risks. There are many examples of drugs that have cleared FDA testing protocols and gone to market, only to later be removed due to some patients experiencing dangerous side effects.[10] If this problem exists for interventions intended to treat devastating illnesses, how will companies justify even minor side effects for mass produced enhancement interventions that may actually be effective only in a small number of consumers?

If physiological enhancement interventions cannot be mass-produced, then a question of cost arises. How will specific interventions with limited applicability be developed in such a way as to make them broadly available? Will governments be required to fund both the research to create these individualized enhancements and the facilities to manufacture and distribute these treatments? If worldwide benefit is the goal, how will governments that cannot even meet the basic health care needs of their populations take on the extra burden of these individualized enhancement products? One could suggest that the wealthier nations cover the enhancement costs for those not able to do so. However, considering the abysmal track record we have for global health concerns currently, such as the devastating lack of sanitation and clean water that affects the health of billions of people, this suggestion for covering the cost of enhancements might readily be regarded as less achievable than the mass production of the individualized enhancement treatments themselves.[11]

Taking into consideration this past and current lack of success in bringing worldwide health care benefits to the millions and billions most in need, in spite of the fact that the treatments and technologies already exist, one can readily question the credibility of any utopian enhancement project – especially those that claim advancements that will deliver worldwide benefits of great magnitude such as the NBIC example at the beginning of this chapter. The problem is not just that these claims of benefit overreach, as has been explicated previously, but also that these claims actually reduce to the age-old human illusion of technological solutions to

---

[10] These side-effect problems can become lethal in certain patients resulting not only in the removal of the product from the market, but also significant injury claims and lawsuits. For example, see the FDA webpage regarding Merck's product Vioxx at http://www.fda.gov/cder/ drug/infopage/vioxx/vioxxQA.htm

[11] For a current assessment of the Millennium Development Goals with regard to global health care, see the World Health Organization website at http://www.who.int/mdg/en/

all our problems and desires. This problem was also identified by the President's Council on Bioethics in *Beyond Therapy*:

> These dreams have at bottom nothing to do with medicine, other than the fact that it is doctors who will wield the tools that may get them realized. They are, therefore, only accidentally dreams "beyond therapy." They are dreams, in principle and in limit, of human perfection (PCB 2003: 19).

To this statement one can also add that they are limitless dreams of what physiological perfection might be since even broadly desired generic goals of longer life or greater intelligence would require constant and unique tinkering of each person's physiology in order to meet any person's open-ended and changing targets of physiological perfection. The pursuit of these dreams of physiological perfection becomes all the more problematic when one takes into consideration an ethical obstacle to the fulfillment of the enhancement fantasy: that the most opportune time to begin this change in an individual will likely be early on in the development of the individual. With current technologies of genetic or cellular manipulation, such alterations are more likely to have an effect on the entire organism or target organ if done *in vitro* or *in utero* (especially if some genetic alteration must be done to enhance longevity or intelligence since one might need to get the alteration into as much of the body or brain as possible). Hence, the situation will be one where the dreams of the parent(s) are being physiologically embodied in the child well before the child has knowledge of them or the opportunity to choose whether or not it is worth the risks of pursuing these dreams of physiological enhancement. Though parents always have to make choices regarding what might benefit or harm their children, the uncertain and unclear benefits of physiological enhancement combined with the significant risks provide overwhelming reasons for not making such choices available.

Though often framed in terms of individual or parental choice, this pursuit of physiological enhancement or perfection will impact others well beyond the individual's or family's circle. This public impact raises yet another barrier to the enhancement quest – truth in advertising. Even if not successful for the initial fortunate, or unfortunate, individuals who experience an enhancement attempt, the idea of legitimately pursuing such a goal could be sold to the public.[12] Thinking this a potentially positive thing to do, others may be convinced to try and obtain physiological enhancements desired by or for them. Though the purported goal might be a successful enhancement, the proposals sold to the public would guarantee only the opportunity to attempt the enhancement. After all, as noted above, it would be practically impossible to guarantee a specific physiological outcome for each individual that would clearly and cleanly be assessed by all parties involved as sufficient and desirable. In addition, the personal experience of the enhancement might not live up to the individual's expectations, requiring either compensation or additional attempts.

[12] Such endeavors are already underway on a conceptual level. For example, see www.transhumanism.org

With such dynamics, it would appear that a program for physiological enhancements might be more likely to look like our current cosmetic enhancement market, and not some globally accessible program delivering benefits to most if not all. Such a situation would be likely to add to the disparities in health care – at least on the basis of the availability of opportunities for enhancement – already troubling our world. This result might then actually work against the purported goals of the pro-enhancement groups by leading to increased political tensions over these disparities, as well as greater division and discord within and between human communities regarding what is normal or healthy physiological functioning. Finally, even if profitable for those developing and selling enhancement technologies, one can question the appropriateness of involving public funds and health care resources in pursuing enhancement technologies since, once again, they are most likely to help only a few – and not necessarily those who are lured into purchasing these technologies for themselves or their offspring.

In spite of the objections raised above, proponents of physiological enhancement can and will respond that my negative assessment of their proposals unfairly takes hope away from all those who have the natural desire and the right to improve themselves. If these goals of improvement are indeed limited to desired increases in certain physiological functions, then I may, in fact, be dashing their hopes – but certainly not unfairly. My objections specifically point out the decidedly uncertain nature of any attempt at physiological enhancement – including delineating what an enhancement might be – and the certain costs of such attempts both to the individual attempting the enhancement and to global society in general. I am not stating that some attempt, at some point, with a given individual, might, in fact, lead to a specific increase in physiological functioning of some kind. That scenario may well occur. What will most likely not occur is any kind of broadly accessible and beneficial enhancement that fits the purported goals of the pro-enhancement groups, such as those stated by the NBIC conference. However, this conclusion does not mean that I disagree with their goals of universal peace, prosperity, and compassion – or that technologies such as nanotechnology, genomic medicine and medical imaging might not be of help in working toward these goals.

3.4 Real Hope for Human Enhancement

The third and final point to the argument of this chapter is that there is already ample opportunity at hand for global human enhancement. In fact, one easily finds support for goals such as universal peace, prosperity, and compassion. Though I have critiqued the means the proponents of human physiological enhancement wish to employ to reach these goals, the goals, themselves, are well worth pursuing. It is possible to work in a pragmatic fashion towards such ends. The key is to remain balanced in one's focus on the ideal ends. Using this approach, much enhancement of the human condition could be achieved – though none of it might involve increasing current levels of human physiological functioning.

As I have already mentioned, many have written on the need for those with abundant resources to address more effectively the extensive health care needs of the underserved.[13] In fact, many organizations, both public and private, are working hard to address this issue.[14] Here I wish to single out the issue of public funding of biomedical research. My main reason is that arguments concerning this funding often arise when proposals such as human enhancement come into the public sphere. This push for public funding is often due to the speculative and controversial nature of the research itself. Since funds are not as likely to come from private sources in the amounts required to pursue a broad research program, proponents of programs such as human physiological enhancement look to public sources of funding, such as the United States federal government and the European Union. The justification for obtaining this funding is tied to the claims of broad public benefit. In making this case, a false dichotomy can arise wherein the public is led to believe that the choice is either to support this cutting edge science with generous amounts of public monies, or to block or reject this scientific research because of fears that the science will do harm to our bodies or is simply too expensive. There are, in fact, many better options that fall between these two extremes.

It is the public's responsibility to choose among the options that best balance the efforts that need to be funded in order to achieve the goods the public desires. Too often the public is disenfranchised by claims that only the scientists and other experts can say what needs to be done in order to achieve goals such as world peace, prosperity, and well being. Though expert analysis and evaluation is certainly beneficial in the public assessment of research funding, the choice remains with the public. If the public does desire to enhance the human condition, then they should be informed that human physiological enhancement is by far not the only option, nor the best one.

To begin with, rejecting the use of public funds for genetic, cellular, and nanotechnology research into human physiological enhancement does not entail rejecting genetic, cellular, and nanotechnology research for other goals. Certainly the public can choose to employ cutting edge scientific techniques to pursue new and creative ways to treat the diseases that afflict people globally, or even to address the poverty and health care disparities that make so many more susceptible to disease. Such research may not increase the limits of human functioning, but it can certainly increase the physiological functioning of those ill who are currently not receiving care. This result will not only enhance the lives of those who will be treated, but will also enhance the lives of their families, friends, neighbors, and even those who developed, distributed, and treated these ill. Though no one may extend the human capacity for intelligence or lifespan through this process, certainly it will increase

[13] See Callahan (1998) and Farmer (2003).

[14] Such organizations range from local to international, and include private groups such as Doctors without Borders and the Catholic Charities, as well as public institutions such as USAID and the UN.

our global capacity for mutual care and concern – capacities that are very amenable to extensive enhancement.

Ultimately, research that is done which more directly targets the most pressing demands of global health and prosperity, taking each and all into consideration, has a much higher probability of moving us all toward our shared ideals of peace and compassion than the speculations regarding human physiological enhancement. If we truly are in pursuit of a world that is peaceful, prosperous, and compassionate – if that indeed is our destination – then the enhancements we desire are already within our grasp. We already know the way. What is before us now is to decide how we can best make use of rapidly advancing scientific and technological knowledge to serve the enhancement of human lives around the world.

3.5 Conclusion

In summary, though the human enhancement goals of technological utopians, such as the NBIC proponents, are greatly desirable – world peace, prosperity, and well being – one of their primary means for achieving these goals – human physiological enhancement – is seriously flawed conceptually, practically, and ethically. Pursuit of human physiological enhancement will not lead humankind to the world that is desired, but to a world where people are put into the service of technological enhancement. Such a world is not inevitable, nor is the only alternative a world without technological improvements. Technology can serve the pursuit of global human enhancement, as long as it is one part of a set of truly humane means that foster the health, peace, and prosperity of all humankind.

References

Callahan D (1998) False Hopes: Overcoming the Obstacles to a Sustainable, Affordable Medicine. Rutgers University Press, New Brunswick, NJ/New York

Duff G W et al. (2006) The future of living well to 100. The American Journal of Clinical Nutrition 83(suppl): 488S–490S

Elliott C (2003) Better Than Well: American Medicine Meets the American Dream. WW Norton, New York

Farmer P (2003) Pathologies of Power: Health, Human Rights, and the New War on the Poor. University of California Press, Berkeley, CA

Geesaman B J (2006) Genetics of aging: implications for drug discovery and development. The American Journal of Clinical Nutrition 83(suppl): 466S–469S

Guttmacher A E, Collins F S (2002) Genomic Medicine – A Primer. New England Journal of Medicine 347(19) Nov 7: 1519–1520

Johansson P, Kerr M (2005) Psychopathy and intelligence: a second look. Journal of Personality Disorders Aug 19(4): 357–369

Kontopoulou T D, Marketos S G (2002) Homeostasis: the ancient Greek origin of a modern scientific principle. Hormones 1(2): 124–125

Perls T T (2006) The different paths to 100. The American Journal of Clinical Nutrition 83(suppl): 484S–487S

Salekin R T, Neumann C S, Leistico A M, Zalot A A (2004) Psychopathy in youth and intelligence: an investigation of Cleckley's hypothesis. Journal of Clinical Child and Adolescent Psychology Dec 33(4): 731–742

The President's Council on Bioethics, PCB (2003) Beyond Therapy. Washington DC: 14–15

Roco M C, Bainbridge W S (2003) (eds) NBIC Convergence for Improving Human Performance. Nanotechnology, Biotechnology, Information Technology and Cognitive Science. KluwerPublishers, Dordrecht, The Netherlands/Boston, MA/London

Zatorre R J (2003) Absolute pitch: a model for understanding the influence of genes and development on neural and cognitive function. Nature Neuroscience 6: 692–695

Chapter 4
How to Defend Genetic Enhancement[1]

Nicholas Agar

4.1 Introduction

Science fiction novelists and Hollywood screenplay writers delight in presenting us with futures in which parents routinely genetically enhance their children. What should we make of these forecasts? Cautious commentators urge that we not overlook the technological challenges confronting those who would radically reshape us. They point out that many of the traits that we may wish to enhance are genetically multifactorial, meaning that the relationships between changes to genes and increases in intelligence, athletic ability, or resistance to disease may be immensely complex.[2] This chapter takes no stand on the issue of the technological viability of human enhancement, but instead addresses a moral question that must be answered as we await technological developments. What moral principles govern the use of technologies of enhancement? I defend a liberal answer to this question that would grant prospective parents the freedom to enhance some of their children's characteristics. The first move in this defence is to depart from the standard liberal text and refuse to view enhancement as an expression of procreative liberty. Instead, I position the genetic enhancement of children as an expression of the freedom to influence the direction their lives take. This move has the advantage of offering clear guidelines on how genetic enhancement is to be regulated.

4.2 Is Genetic Enhancement an Expression of Procreative Liberty?

We should open the liberal case for enhancement with an account of what it is for someone to be genetically enhanced. I propose to treat a genetic modification as an enhancement if it results in a child better than the norm for human beings in some

---

[1] I would like to thank Bert Gordijn and Ruth Chadwick for their comments on this paper.

[2] Pinker (2003) does a good job of presenting the scientific obstacles for genetic enhancers.

B. Gordijn, R. Chadwick (eds.) *Medical Enhancement and Posthumanity*,

significant respect. Liberals differ from the old polemicists about enhancement in giving a pluralist spin on what it means for someone to be better than the norm, with the consequence that what counts as an enhancement for one set of parents may not be similarly viewed by others.[3]

Some thinkers present our genetically enhanced descendents as members of a new species of posthumans, as if one-off genetic modification could make them as different from us as five million years of evolution has made us from chimpanzees (see for example Fukuyama 2002). Our definition of enhancement includes modifications that are altogether less spectacular than the posthuman label seems to imply – one might be genetically enhanced by having one's intelligence or athletic performance boosted from average to somewhat better than average. It seems odd to think of those genetically enhanced in this way as members of a new species when they could be no more intellectually or physically adept than many humans with unmodified genomes.

How might tomorrow's prospective parents go about genetically enhancing their children? While it is a mistake for a moral inquiry to rely on overly specific notions about future technological developments, the early embryonic stage in development is likely to be recognised as providing an ideal opportunity for genetic enhancement. Changes to the DNA of the small number of cells that comprise an early embryo are transmitted to every cell of the adult body, ensuring that genetic modifications whose purpose is to increase intelligence are expressed in brain tissue and that alternations made to enhance athletic performance find their way into muscles and lungs. Although there will probably be later opportunities for our descendents to genetically modify their children – or themselves – enhancement achieved by the genetic engineering of embryos raises the pertinent moral issues in their starkest forms and hence will be the focus of this discussion.

We need first to get clear about what kind of moral investigation we are undertaking. There is a legitimate moral question about risks associated with genetic enhancement. Those who attempt to genetically enhance their children's capacities in advance of major advances in our understanding of the human genome are much more likely to create suffering than super men or women. The issue addressed in this chapter is philosophically prior to that concerning risks associated with the various means by which human capacities might be enhanced. It concerns the very idea of genetic enhancement. We can bring this issue properly into focus by imagining that the technologies of genetic enhancement work perfectly. Such idealizations should not be seen as biasing debate in favour of enhancement. Indeed, they give opponents of genetic enhancement the opportunity to formulate objections whose force will not be diminished by any technological advance; we do not negate the objection that genetic enhancement is wrong in principle by making the tools of enhancement safer. We must be careful to not confuse technological idealizations with predictions. It is possible that genetic enhancement is defensible in principle but that the complexities of human biology mean that it will never be sufficiently safe to be morally acceptable.

[3] For useful histories of 20th century programs of enhancement see Kevles (1995) and Paul (1995). Agar (2004) is an exposition and defence of the liberal approach to enhancement.

The preceding paragraphs cannot pretend to clear up all of the conceptual ambiguities connected with genetic enhancement, however, they should at least permit us to explore the possibilities of a liberal defence of it.

A customary first move for liberals is to posit a freedom to enhance one's offspring as either a part of procreative liberty or a legitimate extension of it. In his seminal treatment of the notion, John Robertson defines procreative liberty as 'the freedom to decide whether or not to have offspring and to control the use of one's reproductive capacity' (Robertson 1994: 16). He presents procreative liberty as establishing a presumption in favour of free choices about whether and how one reproduces that may, on occasion, be overturned by conflicting moral considerations. Those who think that procreative liberty encompasses enhancement add the choice of what kinds of children to have to the list of more traditional expressions of the liberty.

The alleged connection with procreative liberty has certainly made a convenient target for opponents of enhancement who assume that if they can show that enhancement is neither encompassed by procreative freedom nor a legitimate extension of it then they will have undermined the liberal position (see for example Habermas 2003; O'Neill 2002; Sandel 2004).

Jürgen Habermas highlights one disadvantage of enlarging procreative liberty to encompass genetic enhancement (Habermas 2003). Robertson's view that procreative liberty establishes a *presumption* in favour of free procreative choices actually understates the liberal tradition in respect of our reproductive decisions. Liberals tend to deny the government and other authorities any role whatsoever in instructing individuals on the use of their reproductive capacities. This is a significantly stronger position than the view that there is a presumption in favour of free procreative choices that the state can occasionally override. The traditional liberal position gives rise to the genetic counsellor's norm of non-directiveness. A genetic counsellor can tell someone who carries the version of the huntingtin gene associated with the serious neurodegenerative disorder, Huntington disease, that there is a 50% chance that his child will inherit the gene (see Chadwick 1993). She can provide information about the medical realities of Huntington disease. But she is not supposed to furnish specifically moral advice; she is supposed to leave the couple to decide whether to have a child. The classification of enhancement as a procreative liberty pushes this tradition of non-directiveness beyond the point of decency. According to Habermas, once one commits oneself to a liberal approach to enhancement 'it virtually goes without saying that decisions regarding the genetic composition of children should not be submitted to any regulation by the state, but rather should be left to the parents' (Habermas 2003: 76). Habermas seems correct in finding this an unacceptable position. It may be plausible that a couple who leave a genetic counselling session informed that one of them carries a defective copy of the Huntington gene should be allowed to risk having a child with this condition. But it is much less plausible that they should be permitted to genetically modify their child's genome to ensure that, should he live long enough, he will suffer from Huntington disease, even if they endorse a view of the good life that celebrates living with the condition.

In this chapter I argue that although enhancement by genetic engineering affects the results of procreation, it is only incidentally procreative and as such should not be defended as an expression of procreative liberty. Realigning enhancement with a different basic freedom both permits proper defence of it, and enables us to properly distinguish between morally acceptable genetic enhancements and those that should be proscribed.

4.3 Why Genetic Enhancement Is (Usually) Not a Procreative Technique

To see that genetic enhancement is not protected by procreative liberty we need to establish procreative liberty's proper domain. I propose that we understand procreative liberty as protecting *intrinsically procreative techniques*, which we can understand as techniques that have the purpose of boosting the chance of procreating.

The suggestion that an intrinsically procreative technique has the purpose of boosting the likelihood of procreating prompts a further question. What should we count as procreating? Bringing someone into existence seems clearly necessary for procreating, but is it also sufficient? Some philosophers think so (see for example, Harris 2004). Others argue that there is more to procreating than creating. According to them procreation not only brings an individual into existence, it establishes a special kind of relationship between the procreator and procreated. John Robertson, for example, holds that the transmission of genes is essential to procreative relationships and therefore to procreation. He denies that a woman who gave birth to a clone of someone not genetically related to her would have procreated (Robertson 2003). I take no stand on this debate. The argument that most forms of genetic enhancement cannot be viewed as procreative techniques goes through regardless of whether a more or less restrictive account of procreation turns out to be true.

Some actions are not procreative simply because they do not result in procreation. If Robertson is correct, a woman's giving birth to a child cloned from a non-genetic relative falls into this category. Other measures should not be counted as procreative because, although linked with reproductive acts, their involvement does nothing to raise the likelihood of procreation; the chance of procreating is at least as high without their involvement.

Many uses of pre-implantation genetic diagnosis (PGD) are not procreative for this second reason. PGD is currently used by some people at risk of passing on serious genetic disorders to their children to avoid doing so. The first step in the procedure is to use IVF to create a collection of embryos. Cells taken from the embryos are then subjected to DNA analysis in search of the genetic variants associated with a disorder. Only embryos lacking these variants are introduced into the womb. One element of this procedure, the creation of embryos by IVF, is clearly procreative. But the next stage in the process should be viewed differently. The choice that practitioners of PGD make differs from the selection that is a standard part of IVF. Practitioners of IVF choose the embryos that they judge to be most viable, where viability is a measure of the likelihood that an embryo will make it through to birth. The form of selection that occurs in PGD is similarly procreative only if the genetic variant tested for makes miscarriage more likely. This seems not to be the case for many current motivations for PGD. For example, some people who carry a version of the Huntington gene linked with Huntington disease are currently using PGD to avoid having a child with the variant. The Huntington version of this gene typically has its ruinous effects only relatively late in life. Because there is no known relationship between different versions of this gene and the likelihood of accomplishing the transition from embryo to newborn this use of PGD must be described as non-procreative.

Defending the use of PGD to avoid having a child who carries the defective variant of the Huntington gene as an expression of procreative liberty is a mistake because it mischaracterizes the act. Of course, this does not mean that using PGD for this purpose cannot be defended. As I shall argue, recognising this technique as only incidentally procreative points us toward the correct way to defend it.

Most techniques that involve the modification of an embryo's DNA with the purpose of enhancing traits are, like most uses of PGD, improperly characterized as procreative because they do not increase the likelihood of procreation. I say 'most' because it is certainly possible to think of some cases of enhancement by genetic engineering that do have this aim. Some men are infertile because they have genetic material missing from their Y-chromosomes causing them to have very low sperm counts. One could imagine men suffering from this problem presenting themselves at a gene therapy clinic to have the Y chromosome DNA of the cells in their reproductive systems modified. Since the aim of this technique is to boost its recipients' fertility it might be defended by appeal to procreative liberty. Given that its aim is to elevate the fertility of men suffering from the problem to a level considered normal for males of the human species we should not describe it as enhancement. But suppose that the DNA of the cells of a man's reproductive system was altered so as to boost his fertility beyond levels typical for human males. The means that enabled this to occur would be both a procreative and an enhancement technology. It would be an enhancement technology by virtue of the fact that it boosts the functioning of a capacity beyond that considered normal for human beings, and a procreative technology by virtue of having the purpose of boosting the chances of having children.

Does the definition of a procreative technique leave any room to classify enhancements of intelligence or of athletic ability as procreative? Robertson imagines a couple trying to add weight to their request to boost their children's intelligence by protesting that they will not have children at all unless allowed to enhance them. He thinks that this argumentative manoeuvre might succeed in drawing the freedom to enhance within the orbit of procreative liberty (Robertson 1994: 166, 2003). But the couple's intransigence no sooner does this than would their claiming that they will only have children if permitted to film them in pornographic movies succeed in reclassifying a putative freedom to make child porn as a procreative liberty. It would be a mistake to see these parents' insistence as establishing a presumptive right to make child pornography as a procreative liberty even if we go on to say that this presumption is outweighed by considerations concerning the welfare of their children.

Perhaps the couple could argue that their particular procreative values make genetic enhancement a procreative technique. This argument would be presented in the context of pluralism about procreation according to which variation in values generates variation in what counts as procreation. This variation could come into play in describing the relationship between procreator and procreated that some theories make constitutive of procreation. The aspiring enhancers might argue that although most people succeed in procreating without enhancing, their particular procreative values prevent them from viewing unenhanced children as properly their own. They would therefore protest that a ban on the enhancement of a child's intelligence or athletic ability is tantamount to a ban on procreation.

There is no need to challenge the pluralist thesis about reproduction to show that this argument that enhancement is procreative does not succeed. We should certainly not allow people to invent whatever procreative values are required to bring a technology that happens to interest them within the orbit of procreative liberty. It is difficult to describe a coherent collection of procreative values that would deny that bringing an unenhanced child into existence is procreation while allowing that creating an enhanced child qualifies. The only plausible way to explain the disappointment felt by the aspiring genetic enhancers about their intellectually normal children is by pointing to their recognition that they have not only caused the existence of a normal child, but that this normal child is theirs. This disappointment might lead them to take steps to disown their unenhanced children. The option of disowning a child is available to any parent. Although it may go someway to devaluing, or perhaps even cancelling a procreative relationship, it does not make it the case that this relationship never existed, indeed it presupposes that it did. None of this should be taken to deny that there might be some future society of posthumans whose members would be incapable of viewing unenhanced children as properly their own. It seems unlikely, however, that such a claim is licensed by the procreative values of people here and now.

The enhancement of an embryo's intelligence by the manipulation of its DNA is incidentally procreative in much the same way as courtship. A romantic evening can involve procreative acts, but it doesn't have to. The same romantic goals might have been achieved by way of the gift of a box of chocolates and a shared bottle of pinot noir. Equally, parents could delay the act of enhancing their child's intelligence until sometime after its birth, thereby severing the connection between enhancement and reproduction. Exposing enhancement and courtship as non-procreative shows that they should not be defended by appeal to procreative liberty, but rather by appeal to different freedoms. In what follows I defend enhancement by locating it at the core of a basic freedom distinct from procreative liberty.

4.4 The Freedom to Influence the Direction of a Child's Life

It is time to unmask the freedom to genetically enhance one's child. I defend the claim that parents' freedom to influence the direction their children's lives will take encompasses choices about the modification of their embryonic DNA. Familiar expressions of this freedom do not involve the manipulation of genes. Rather they involve choices about which schools to send children to, how to feed them, who counts as a suitable after-school companion, whether children are to be given religions instruction, and if so of what type. Parents in liberal democracies make these choices in a variety of ways.

Other philosophers have defended genetic enhancement by comparing it with upbringing, tending to conclude that this establishes the freedom to enhance as a procreative freedom (see for example, Harris 1998: Chapter 7, Robertson 1994: Chapter 7).[4] However, it is better to think of this comparison as locating enhancement among core interests protected by the freedom to influence the direction of a child's life rather than among interests at the periphery of procreative liberty. In this section I present this reclassification as bringing two benefits – one more pragmatic and the other somewhat theoretical. The pragmatic benefit is the licence to properly regulate genetic enhancement and guidelines on how this should be carried out. The theoretical plus is that we can avoid the complex tangle of philosophical issues connected with the morality of bringing people into existence.

Remember that Habermas makes much of the liberal skepticism about a role for the state in citizens' procreative decisions. Liberals are considerably more tolerant of a role for the state in the raising of their children. Parents are required to meet minimum standards of education and nourishment and if these standards are not met then we think that the state should intervene. The freedom to direct a child's life comes into play only once these minimum standards are achieved. For example, parents are required to send their children to schools that provide instruction in basic mathematics, or to home-school them to this standard. Once this standard is met, parents who place particular value on mathematical skills can provide additional tuition. Parents must ensure that their children are adequately nourished. Their distinctive moral or religious commitments can guide them in precisely how they provide the requisite calories, minerals, and vitamins.

Not reaching minimum standards is not the only way parents can err in the raising of their children. Overbearing parents impose values in such a way that intrudes on their child's freedom to make her own choices about her life. Our children do not exist merely to execute our plans for them. Joel Feinberg has coined the expression 'the right to an open future' to describe the moral protection children have against parents' plans for them. He explains that any ideas that parents have about their children's future 'must retreat before the claims of children that they be permitted to reach maturity with as many open options, opportunities, and advantages as possible' (Feinberg 1980). Other writers favour analyses that protect children against overbearing parents at the same time as granting parental values somewhat wider latitude (see for example Ruddick 1999; Murray 1996; Archard 2003).

Traditional influences on the direction that a child's life takes are exercised in upbringing. The extension of the freedom that licenses this to genetic enhancement will fail if genes and upbringing make fundamentally different contributions to human development. Genetic determinists find such differences. According to them

[4] I also made this mistake – see Agar (2004: Chapter 6).

an organism's significant characteristics result mainly from the action of its genes, with environmental influences playing only a minor role. This view, now widely recognised as false, has been displaced by a view according to which organisms emerge from a complex interaction of genes and environment. The moral comparison of genetic engineering with upbringing does not depend on the assumption that genes and environment make identical contributions to the traits that we may seek to modify. Instead it specifies that when changes to genes and changes to diet or schooling have the same effects, we should evaluate them similarly. We should give different moral verdicts only when we find a difference in effects. Some traits are almost certainly more easily modifiable by genetic engineering, while others are more readily changed by structuring a child's environment.

Francis Fukuyama thinks that genetic modifications differ morally from innovations in upbringing because their consequences are of greater magnitude (Fukuyama 2002). According to Fukuyama genetic enhancements may change our descendents to such an extent that they lose their humanity. They will be posthumans. We might agree with Fukuyama that we should be more suspicious of radical changes to our immediate descendents than we are of more minor changes. But we should disagree with the suggestion that genetic enhancements are inherently of greater magnitude than environmental enhancements. The idea that they are depends implicitly on a determinist misconception of genes' developmental significance. Biologists keen to correct this misconception have introduced the concept of a *norm of reaction* to describe the range of different phenotypes produced by a gene across a range of environments. In describing the norm of reaction of plant genotype we might observe that it produces plants of a particular height in at a medium altitude while it produces considerably taller plants higher up.[5] Thinking in terms of a norm of reaction helps us to escape from the idea that the plant has a genetically preset height. What goes for plants may also be true of human beings. Imagine a yet-to-be-discovered dietary supplement that changes the uterine environment in such a way to dramatically increase a child's intelligence. This supplement changes a fetus's environment, but not its genes. To deny that such a supplement could exist is, in effect, to claim that human genotypes have very narrow norms of reaction. While this view conforms with the popular genetic determinist bias, it is without empirical support. Concerns about posthumanity, if indeed they are warranted, apply equally to genetic and environmental alterations.

Now we come to the theoretical advantage of separating enhancement choices from procreative choices. This move enables us to defer the solution of a vexing philosophical riddle concerning the morality of bringing people into existence.[6] There is a frequently expressed fear that reproductive cloning will harm those it brings into existence. Yet the fact that the purportedly harmful act is also an act of procreation makes it difficult to see how this could be the case. Had the decision been against reproductive cloning the clone would not have existed in some

[5] This example and discussion of norms of reaction comes from Sober (2000: 359).

[6] The locus classicus for philosophical discussion of such cases is Parfit (1984).

preferable state. He would not have existed at all. Philosophers have explored a variety of ways to explain why it might be immoral to create clones doomed to short, miserable existences (see for example, Parfit 1984; Buchanan et al. 2000). The separation of enhancement from procreative choices enables us to see how some attempts at enhancement can be straightforwardly harmful. Enhancement harms a child if she would have been better off brought into existence without her genetic modifications.[7] The modification of embryonic DNA can make someone worse off than they would otherwise have been in much the same way that misguided nutritional or educational choices do. It is true that this harm resulting from morally misguided genetic modifications may be more distant in time from the action that we identify as its cause than harms resulting from bad upbringing. But this should not affect our recognition of it as harmful. Similar points apply to benefits. If a pregnant woman's taking of folic acid supplements to promote the development of her baby's brain can be viewed as leaving his identity intact, and therefore benefiting him, then so should a genetic modification with similar consequences for cognition.

Of course, radical alternations to embryonic DNA may upset this moral compartmentalization. Suppose we are talking about a whole collection of enhancements that may jointly change the identity of the resulting individual. This radical enhancement cannot be straightforwardly viewed as beneficial or harmful. The interactionist approach to the development of human identities leads us to find no difference between major alterations to genes and radical changes to a fetus's environment. Both kinds of change are difficult to assess morally because they both substitute one individual for another.

I conclude my argument for the liberal approach to enhancement by considering a recent challenge due to Michael Sandel.

4.5 Michael Sandel on Why Genetically Enhancing Is Hyper Parenting

Michael Sandel has recently argued that genetic enhancement exemplifies an unhealthy attitude to one's offspring (Sandel 2004). He takes the lead of theologian William F. May, claiming that parents should balance two kinds of love for their children. The love of acceptance acknowledges that there is much about your child that is not up to you. For example, your child's genome is, depending on your religious commitments, either a chance recombination of parental genetic material or part of God's design. Accepting love both acknowledges and celebrates this independence from parental plans. Parents must do more than merely accept, however. The love of acceptance should be balanced with the love of transformation that seeks to actively to cultivate children's talents, rather than allowing them to go to waste. It is the love of transformation

[7] For a defence of such a view see McMahan (1998).

that directs parents to insist that their children take their insulin and persevere with the Japanese lessons that seem to have uncovered a gift for languages.

Sandel accuses parents who would genetically enhance their offspring of erring too much in the direction of transformation. If genetic enhancement is to be likened with environmental molding, Sandel insists that we pair it with the 'heavily managed, high-pressure childrearing' that he calls 'hyper parenting' (Sandel 2004: 58). Hyper parents acknowledge few limits to their efforts to transform their children into sports champions or academic superstars. Sandel thinks that genetic enhancers err in the same way.

Those with a propensity toward hyper parenting will almost certainly react with enthusiasm to the new degree of control afforded by the combination of genetic engineering and more traditional varieties of control. While our genes alone do not determine our characteristics, genes and environment together, do. In the era of genetic enhancement both forms of influence may be under parental control.

We can accept Sandel's warning about the dangers of hyper parenting while denying that genetic modification is inherently more controlling or transformative than the manner of influence that one exercises by selecting a child's diet, schooling, or religious training. There are a variety of ways in which parents can achieve the right balance between the loves of acceptance and transformation. One way is, as Sandel suggests, for them to limit their attempts at transformation to the manipulation of environmental influences, leaving the genetic makeup of their child to be fixed by nature or God. But they can also correctly balance the two loves of parenting with different mixtures of genetic and environmental acceptance and transformation.

Parents today have some control over an ever-widening spectrum of environmental influences on their children's development. Compare the experience of being pregnant in the rich world of the early 21st century with an era when pregnancy was a time when you could predict that you would have a child but did not view yourself as having much of a say on how this child would turn out. Now pregnant women are told that many things that they do shape their child. Mothers-to-be learn that their diets play a significant role in determining their children's food preferences by imparting flavour to the amniotic fluid. The wrong kind of maternal diet may lead to an unhealthy liking for junk food, or serious allergies. Women are told that stress during pregnancy may result in a more anxious child. Some chafe at the heavy burden that modern understanding of their special relationship with their child-to-be foists on them. Consider a possible future in which parents are able to back-pedal in their exercise of some of the more onerous varieties of environmental influence. These parents might reject the suggestion that they are being too accepting by pointing out that they achieve an appropriate degree of transformation by manipulating some genetic influences. The genetic enhancements they have purchased might allow a pregnant woman to consume both pre and postprandial gins and tonic and excuse her from a diet rich in omega 3.

Merely exchanging one influence for another might seem of dubious value to those worried about the overall quantity of control exercised by parents. Yet there may often be reasons to prefer the manipulation of genetic influences to more traditional varieties of control. Philosophers have distinguished between general-purpose abilities and those more tightly focused at specific tasks (Agar 1995; Buchanan et al. 2000). General-purpose abilities equip one for a wide variety of endeavours. Intelligence is an obvious example. One can use one's intellect to design computer software, play bridge, or hunt wild pigs. The ability to play a devastating no-trumps bridge hand is an obvious case of special-purpose ability. It is of great value in certain trick-taking card games but of little use elsewhere.

Manipulating general-purpose and special-purpose abilities achieves different transformative ends. The enhancement of general-purpose abilities is inherently less directive than is the enhancement of special-purpose abilities. Given that general-purpose enhancement improves prospects associated with a wide variety of ways of life, a child who has been modified in this way may end up pursuing a life plan radically opposed to the values that motivated their parents' enhancement of him. This means that the cultivation of general-purpose means is more representative of the love of acceptance than is the cultivation of abilities directed at specific ways of life. When parents enhance a child's general-purpose ability, they accept that the skill that they have awarded their child may be used in many ways. Although this more accepting form of enhancement can be achieved by environmental measures, there is reason to suspect that genetic influences will be, on the whole, more accepting. The linkages between specific upbringings and particular life-plans are well understood, or at least better understood than the connections between specific combinations of DNA and particular life plans. A further reason for finding environmental influences more discriminatory is simply that they operate closer in time to the child's acquisition of his or her own values.

Consider an example that illustrates why genetic enhancements may be in general less directive, and hence more accepting, than environmental enhancements motivated by the same or similar values. Suppose a couple is keen to have a child who has religious faith. They have at their disposal some of the more traditional environmental means of directing their child toward a life of faith – regular attendance at places of worship and frequent readings from holy books. They may also be empowered to manipulate genetic influences on religiosity. Dean Hamer has recently argued for a link between the gene VMAT2 and a trait labelled self-transcendence (Hamer 2004). He follows the psychologist Robert Cloninger in defining self-transcendence as people's 'capacity to reach out beyond themselves – to see everything as part of one great totality' (Hamer 2004: 10). There is, Hamer thinks, a correlation between different versions of VMAT2 and different degrees of self-transcendence which in turn influences one's propensity for religious or spiritual belief. Suppose that Hamer is right about VMAT2. We can imagine that parents who subscribe to a religious creed permissive of human genetic modification may want to select their child's version of VMAT2. The most religiously ambitious parents will seek to combine this form of genetic modification with the appropriate religious environmental inputs. Such a combination seems overly transformative. However, the purpose of comparing their transformative properties is best served by considering genetic and environmental strategies pursued in isolation.

Consider parents who select their child's version of VMAT2 but put little effort into religiously organizing her environment. This form of religious direction seems more accepting than its developmental counterpart, which involves instruction in the tenets of a particular religion and participation in its rituals but no attempt to manipulate embryonic DNA. Traditional environmental forms of religious influence are oriented toward specific religious or spiritual creeds. This is not the case with the selection of a child's version of VMAT2. For example, a Southern Baptist who seeks to pass on her religion to her child but limits herself to modifying his copy of VMAT2 is liable to find that her child has become a devoted Hare Krishna. Introducing the version of VMAT2 linked with high levels of self-transcendence is, after all, as much an enhancement for Hare Krishnas as it is for Baptists. This is not so for schooling in the specific tenets of Baptist belief. Although parents who restrict themselves to these more traditional forms of religious influence may find that their children have become Hare Krishnas after all, this spiritual conversion will have occurred in spite of their religious training, not because of it.

The fact that some forms of genetic enhancement are more accepting than their environmental counterparts does not permit us to ignore the threat posed by parents who seek to combine the two forms of manipulation. There are likely to be combinations of genetic manipulation and religious instruction against which it would be near impossible to rebel and hence which involve too much transformation and too little acceptance. How frequently would one need to convince oneself of the soundness of The Argument from Evil to resist the plans of someone who has not only manipulated your copy of VMAT2 and any other genes shown to influence spirituality, but has also saturated your childhood environment with religious homilies and imagery? Transferring genetic enhancement out of the domain of procreative liberty and into the domain of the liberty to exercise some control over the direction a child's life clears the way for the genetic manipulation of religious influences to be legally regulated. Officers of the law should be present in the facilities in which embryos are engineered on a similar basis to their occasional entry into family homes. Of course this is not to say that it will be easy to work out when to involve the state. The choice about when child welfare provisions should be enforced in the case of parents' genetic choices may be as fraught as decisions about when threats to children's welfare warrant police entry into a home. Other forms of regulation may be less heavy-handed. While some parents are either neglectful or overbearing to an extent that demands intervention by the state, others err in either direction in such a way that is best responded to with cautionary words by fellow parents or relatives.

4.6 Concluding Remarks

My purpose in this chapter has been to show how liberals should argue for genetic enhancement and to argue that they can make a rationally persuasive case. Genetic enhancement is only rarely a procreative technique and hence is not to be defended as an expression of procreative liberty. Recognising the genetic enhancement of children as an expression of the freedom to influence the direction their lives take not only shows how enhancement can be defended, it also shows how it is to be regulated.

References

Agar N (1995) Designing babies: morally permissible ways to modify the human genome. Bioethics 9: 1–15

Agar N (2004) Liberal Eugenics: In Defence of Human Enhancement. Blackwell, Oxford

Archard D (2003) Children, Family and the State. Ashgate, Aldershot, England

Buchanan A, Brock D, Daniels N, Wikler D (2000) From Chance to Choice: Genetics and Justice. Cambridge University Press, Cambridge

Chadwick R (1993) What counts as success in genetic counselling? Journal of Medical Ethics19: 43–46

Feinberg J (1980) The Child's Right to an Open Future. In: Aiken W, LaFollette H (eds) Whose Child? Children's Rights, Parental Authority, and State Power. Rowman & Littlefield, Totowa, NJ: 124–153

Fukuyama F (2002) Our Posthuman Future: Consequences of the Biotechnology Revolution. Farrar, Straus & Giroux, New York

Habermas J (2003) The Future of Human Nature. Polity, Cambridge

Hamer D (2004) The God Gene: How Faith Is Hardwired into Our Genes. Doubleday, New York

Harris J (1998) Clones, Genes, and Immortality: Ethics and the Genetic Revolution. Oxford University Press, Oxford

Harris J (2004) On Cloning. Routledge, London

Kevles D (1995) In the Name of Eugenics: Genetics and the Uses of Human Heredity. University of California Press, Berkeley, CA

McMahan J (1998) Wrongful Life: Paradoxes in the Morality of Causing People to Exist. In: Coleman J, Morris C (eds) Rational Commitment and Social Justice: Essays for Gregory Kavka. Cambridge University Press, New York

Murray T (1996) The Worth of a Child. University of California Press, Berkeley, CA

O'Neill O (2002) Autonomy and Trust in Bioethics. Cambridge University Press, Cambridge

Parfit D (1984) Reasons and Persons. University Press Oxford, Oxford

Paul D (1995) Controlling Human Heredity: 1865 to the Present. Humanities Press, New Jersey

Pinker S (2003) Session 3: Human Nature and Its Future: Address to Council on Bioethics http://www.bioethics.gov/transcripts/march03/session3.html

Robertson J (1994) Children of Choice: Freedom and the New Reproductive Technologies. Princeton University Press, Princeton, NJ

Robertson J (2003) Procreative liberty in the era of genomics. American Journal of Law and Medicine 29: 439–87

Ruddick W (1999) Parenthood: Three Concepts and a Principle. In: Houlgate L (ed) Morals, Marriage, and Parenthood: An Introduction to Family Ethics. Wadsworth, Belmont, CA

Sandel M (2004) The case against perfection. The Atlantic Monthly 293(3): 51–62

Sober E (2000) The Meaning of Genetic Causation. In: Buchanan A, Brock D, Daniels N, Wikler D (eds) From Chance to Choice: Genetics and Justice. Cambridge University Press, Cambridge: 347–370

Part II
Posthumanity

Chapter 5
A Critical History of Posthumanism

Andy Miah

5.1 Introduction

A meaningful discussion about the history of posthumanism first requires distinguishing the concept from a range of related concepts with which its history is intertwined. Thus, one must first recognise that a historical analysis of posthumanism is not synonymous with the history of medical enhancements. Indeed, discussions about posthumanism are not necessarily about enhancements and, even when they are, they do not always involve the advocacy of enhancement freedoms. To this extent, there is no single form of posthumanism that we can identify that portrays a unified history of the term. Moreover, theories of posthumanism do not wholly reveal the moral import of enhancement ambitions. Additionally, the history of posthumanism is not synonymous with the history of technology and neither are theoretical contributions to this literature found exclusively within philosophical inquiries into technology. Certainly, technological change has become central to contemporary articulations of posthumanity. Indeed, the term implies an emergent leap from some present status of being human, to a future characterization as *after* humanity. In this sense, one must suppose that this is necessarily technological subject matter. However, I will endeavour to present a more diverse view of the history of posthumanism, which relies on the range of literatures and biopolitical spheres that have contributed to shaping concerns about the future of humanity.

From this interpretation of posthumanism, it will be possible to more fully appreciate the growing prominence of this term, as it is employed in often oppositional ways to argue for or against the use of human enhancements. The connections across disciplines is critical to build into our theoretical appreciation of posthumanism, so that we come to terms with the breadth and depth of its implications. For instance, posthumanism speaks to such issues as animal ethics by interrogating the significance of *species boundaries*, a concept that has shaped a series of moral commitments to both animals and humans. Such discussions are prominent in discussions about hybrid embryos, for instance, and the broader debates about transgenics. Each of these topics can be viewed from the perspective of posthumanism and a number of emerging philosophical stances can be characterized as posthumanist responses to such prospects.

B. Gordijn, R. Chadwick (eds.) *Medical Enhancement and Posthumanity*,

Developing a broad understanding of posthumanism also enables us to offer insights into how debates about human enhancement have been characterized by specific value laden terminology, such as the language of cyborgs, automata, robots and various scenarios that allude to the creation of Frankenstein's monster. Posthumanism connects debates about the ethics of, say, embracing the prospect of synthetic biology, by drawing on the cultural texts that enrich our philosophical discussions. As such, posthumanism has also transgressed disciplinary boundaries in its endeavour to reflect on humanity's distinct and special place in the world. In this fashion, a crucial premise of posthumanism is its critical stance towards the idea that humans are a superior species in the natural order. In this sense, the 'post' of posthumanism need not imply moving beyond humanness in some biological or evolutionary manner. Rather, the starting point should be an attempt to understand what has been omitted from an anthropocentric worldview.

Within this essay, I investigate how the concept of posthumanism has been developed, assumed, implied and appropriated in a range of (contemporary) philosophical and cultural contexts. In so doing, I explain the various analytic and continental traditions that have defined and theorised posthumanism, but which rarely speak to each other. Of particular importance is how one might read the history of philosophy from the perspective of posthumanism and how such an interpretation should inform the specificity of current debates about this term, particularly within bioethics. In so doing, I suggest that the history of posthumanism is partially a history of disagreements about the value of human (medical) metamorphoses. Yet, this history is also an inquiry into the social conditions within which the need for *justifying* self-modification (through technology) has become a necessary and crucial characteristic of contemporary socio-political processes.

First, I begin with an account of various attempts to characterise posthumanism, most notably by Francis Fukuyama who, in 2002, proposed that 'our posthuman future' would involve the inevitable commercialization of biotechnological innovations that could lead to worrisome human enhancements. The significance of Fukyuama's intervention is major, insofar as his language would come to shape lay-understandings of posthumanism as a future state of affairs where the traditional human might no longer be valued. He portrayed that this inevitable commercialization would replace humans with a new kind of being and, in turn, people of our current status would become devalued and potentially have their fundamental rights violated. I will go on to argue that this is not at all apparent when one examines the concept in depth. Nevertheless, Fukuyama's posthuman imaginations have become constitutive of a new chapter of posthumanism's history, which has been made meaningful by its repeated presence in media and political discourses.

Second, I examine how the concept of posthumanism has been constructed within a range of cultural and critical theories. This analysis lends support to the claim that posthumanity implies something more nuanced than merely moving beyond the human subject. These recent political and cultural stories of posthumanism are subsequently informed by considering the broader history of philosophical ideas that surround posthumanism; the third section of this essay. In this final section, I consider how visions of posthumanity are visible in a number of literary and philosophical texts, which are underpinned by unambiguous moral narratives that warn about biological transgressions such as human enhancements.

5.1.1 The Politics of Posthumanism

Fukuyama's *Our Posthuman Future* (2002) was published alongside Greg Stock's *Redesigning Humans* (2002), at a time when Fukuyama was a member of the United States President's Council on Bioethics, itself concerned considerably with the prospects of human enhancement (US President's Council on Bioethics 2003). During this year, the two authors undertook a combative lecture tour, which embodied the parameters of posthuman positioning: the polarisation of the *bioconservative* (Fukuyama) and *technoprogressive* (Stock) perspectives. Fukuyama's analysis of a future where human biotechnological enhancement is rife invokes the concept of posthumanism to frame and define this future. However, on closer inspection, the concept of posthumanism is advanced as a *negative* case rather than a positive one. Thus, Fukuyama explains that posthumanism is the *absence* of humanism, the transgression of crucial moral boundaries, rather than telling us what posthumanism might involve that is additional to and different from just being human. He explains this absence by appealing to the idea that there is an essence to humans that can be corrupted by too much technology, calling this essence *Factor X*. This Factor X – which is elaborated by Fukuyama as a kind of human dignity – would be compromised by a permissive, commercial environment within which medical enhancements would emerge.

Yet, rather than theorise posthumanism, Fukuyama uses the concept as a signifier to warn about a future of human enhancements. In his view, there are insurmountable challenges associated with the prospect of becoming posthuman, principally because the commercialisation of life will diminish the value of being human. To support his view, one can look at contemporary discussions in the medical sphere that suggest such prospects. For instance, one might extrapolate from stem cell research to a situation where organs are mass produced and are designed to be better than their originals. It is not difficult to foresee a commercial market for such technology, even if the initial consumers would be those in need of organ transplants. Alternatively, one might look to the recent moral imperative arising from stem cell research that involves storing cells from the umbilical cord. Today, parents are confronted with the choice to pay the significant sum that is required in order to safe guard against a prospective blood related condition their child might have. This obviously valuable technology is, nevertheless, available in many countries *only* as a private endeavour and the costs are substantial thus far. This type of commercialization over biological products represents the first stages towards the corruption of Factor X, on Fukuyama's terms.

In this context, Fukuyama's posthumanism is an observation from the perspective of political economy rather than moral philosophy. He indicates that the politics of biotechnology – or biopolitics, as they are often described – are such that, where human enhancements are allowed, this will weaken the moral force of human rights by the claims of chimeric, cybernetic or transgenic species, or over disputes about the ownership of DNA. He envisages a situation where what is, today, regarded as a normal level of health, might be seen as grotesquely inadequate from the perspective of a super-enhanced human and this will translate into social pressure to become enhanced.

Fukuyama's (2002) apocalyptic tone – which began as a re-working of his *End of History* argument (Fukuyama 1999) – is later reinforced by his article in *Foreign Policy* (2004), where he announces that *trans*humanism is the 'world's most dangerous idea'. This intervention accentuates the rich confusion over whether the concepts of post- and trans- humanism differ and I would suggest that Fukuyama is actually interested in *neither* of them. Rather, he is concerned about medical *enhancements* generally and the politics of groups who argue on their behalf specifically. It is evident that he considers the ethics of biotechnology as inextricable from this broader political economy of scientific research. Indeed, Fukuyama is concerned that a commercial model of biotechnology will overwhelm an ethical foundation to society that is based on humanitarian concerns and that this will, in turn, corrupt his *Factor X*, ushering in a posthuman future:

> Human nature shapes and constrains the possible kinds of political regimes, so a technology powerful enough to reshape what we are will have possibly malign consequences for liberal democracy and the nature of politics itself (2002: 7).

For Fukuyama, this prospect of biopolitical transcendence is alarming and is critical to understanding the recent history of posthumanism, since such a history is located within the broader politics of health care and trends within technological governance. Fukuyama's posthuman nightmare is nothing less than the destabilisation of established political boundaries and processes through the debasement of human dignity, the fundamental concept that informs all major international and domestic instruments of human rights protection. Thus, Fukuyama's posthumanism begins with an analysis of political history and a projection of its future within a permissive, biotechnological world. Further evidence of this is found in Fukuyama and Furger (2007), which draws attention to the politicization of bioethics and how it has shaped the political terms by which the debate about a posthuman future has developed. For instance, when considering 'embryo politics' the authors note that: 'there are several deeply held alternative views on this issue, over which it is not likely that there will be consensus any time in the near future' (p 45). Their provocative title *Beyond Bioethics*, is further evidence of the perceived limits of ethics within this debate about the future.

In sum, Fukuyama (2002) argues that a fixed, if inarticulate, conceptualisation of the human is crucial to the organisation of society and this is why debates about posthumanism are so controversial. Yet, his argument is only ever a thesis on the commercial character of human enhancements, rather than the morality of posthumanism. At most, it re-asserts the fundamental values of humanism, rather than establishes why it is that the prospect of enhancements should be considered as indicative of our posthuman status. Characterising posthumanism as the absence of

Factor X will not suffice. Thus, for Fukuyama, the concept of posthumanism is invoked and imagined rather than characterised by his analysis. His use of the word posthumanism is expected to do the work of establishing what is immoral about human enhancement. While this is not sufficient from a philosophical perspective, Fukuyama's contribution to the history of posthumanism has been to constitute the terms through which posthumanism is imagined and discussed within contemporary political spheres.

Other recent theories on posthumanism utilise the concept to characterise an emerging technological culture, but in doing so they also do not adequately distinguish posthumanism from other concepts. For example, Pepperell (1995/2003) discusses posthumanism as a form of *anti*-humanism, which is re-enlightened by modern science. On his view, posthumanism is also characterised by an absence, but it is the absence of humanist naïveté that interests him:

> Humans have imagined for a long time that the ability to develop and control technology was one of the defining characteristics of our condition, something that assured us of our superiority over other animals and our unique status in the world. Ironically, this sense of superiority and uniqueness is being challenged by the very technologies we are now seeking to create, and it seems the balance of dominance between human and machine is slowly shifting (Pepperell 1995/2003: 3).

Yet, this articulation of posthumanism is not straightforward to accept either. Pepperell's plausible notion of posthumanism as 'the end of…that long-held belief in the infallibility of human power and the arrogant belief in our superiority and uniqueness' (p 171) is later diminished when he appears comfortable to discuss posthumanism as if it were a temporal, progressive concept – i.e. humanity moves from transhumanism to posthumanism – and largely about using technology to achieve even greater productivity or functionality (Pepperell 2005). This move towards something more like transhumanism betrays Pepperell's vision of the history of posthumanism.

These two examples of how posthumanism has been positioned within political science and the philosophy of medicine or bioethics are indicative of the multiple meanings and expectations that are inscribed onto the concept. They indicate why there are conflicting histories to posthumanism that each deserve attention. Fukuyama (2002) uses posthumanism to constitute what people should consider as the immorality of human enhancement. He achieves this by invoking the idea that the posthuman future will make today's humans redundant. In contrast, Pepperell's posthumanism offers scope to embrace human enhancement, albeit in a way that rejects traditional technological determinism. He indicates that, we should not be tempted to utilize technology to replicate morally dubious values about preferable modes of existence, but stretch our imaginations to consider what other obligations we might have by being able to undertake such transformations. Other recent visions of posthumanity – such as Stock (2002) – can more easily be characterised as transhuman and much of what I argue here claims that there is both common and distinct ground between these concepts. Nevertheless, the history of posthumanism should *not* be seen as the same as the history of transhumanism (Bostrom 2005) and the reason for this is revealed when examining their conceptual trajectory within the literature, as well as the mobilization of advocates and critics that surround each concept. While one might identify that their common ground is an emphasis on technology, theorists from each tradition have made quite different value claims associated with the relationship between technology and humanity. Moreover, authors from each tradition arrive at a concern over medical ethics from quite different points of origin. To elaborate further on this, the next section of this chapter examines other visions of posthumanism, which have emerged within critical theory and cultural studies, rather than philosophy or bioethics. Indeed, the literature that has appeared to speak more explicitly to theorising posthumanism has come from studies in English literature, cultural studies, and communications.

5.2 Posthumanism in Cultural Theory

5.2.1 Posthuman Bodies

The origins of what might be termed *cultural posthumanism* are revealed within Halberstam and Livingstone's *Posthuman Bodies* (1995). The various essays within this book look to a range of texts such as film to advance an understanding of posthumanism that is informed by cultural manifestations of moral perspectives on technology.[1] Halberstam and Livingstone (1995) outline that their objective is to address challenges to 'the coherence of the human body' and in doing so, their authors engage with the posthuman idea that there is no coherence to being human and, perhaps, no basis on which to appeal to the idea of a human essence or a common form of human dignity. Also, the posthuman discussed within the book refers not to 'some subsequent development state' to humanity, but its 'collapses into *sub-*, *inter-*, *trans-*, *pre-*, *anti-*' (p viii). In their view 'posthuman bodies are the causes and effects of postmodern relations of power and pleasure, virtuality and reality, sex and its consequences' (p 3). Moreover, they emphasise that,

> The posthuman does not necessitate the obsolescence of the human; it does not represent an evolution or devolution of the human. Rather it participates in re-distributions of difference and identity (p 10).

Their approach to posthumanism is less apocalyptic than Fukuyama's and provides further explanation for why it is necessary to tell the combined histories of philosophical and cultural posthumanism, in order to offer a comprehensive analysis of its past. For, it would appear that there are quite different expectations and imaginations about this imminent posthuman condition.

Neil Badmington (2000, 2001, 2003) has also pioneered cultural posthumanism. His work explains how posthumanist interventions are a critical 'working-through

[1] Consider, for example, the genre of 'Body Horror,' which describes the integrity of human subject corrupted and its boundaries breached (Clarke 2002).

of humanist discourses' (2003: 22). His view bears close resemblance to Elaine Graham's (2002a) posthumanism, which draws on narratives from within literature to study Otherness as it is manifested within culture. Graham's posthumanism is constituted by studies of the 'interplay between the world of scientific, bioethical theorizing and the world of the cultural imagination – myth science fiction, popular culture and religion' (Graham 2002b). She discusses various 'representations' of the post/human, considering aliens and monsters to wonder how influential these images have been as frames for constituting moral discourses about scientific and technological change. Her findings have considerable importance to discussions that take place within bioethics. For example, it is widely recognised that the range of metaphors that have been used to describe genetic technology has limited the progress of research in this area. Thus, its public depiction as the 'holy grail' of science allowing humanity to 'Play God' and discover the 'book of life' in a way that is alleged to correspond with Mary Shelley's (1818) representation of 'Dr Frankenstein' all seem to have had a pejorative effect on the development of genetics. As such, the contribution of Graham's inquiry to our history of posthumanism is in revealing the narrowness of language that is used to characterize science and to show that these limitations restrict our capacity to come to terms with the more diverse implications of technological development. In short, genetics might also be neither the holy grail, the book of life or playing God, but without a more diverse range of metaphors, we are condemned to repeat these expectations of science. As Jon Turney notes, the continual referral to Frankenstein's monser 'tends to polarise a debate which we urgently need to take forward to a point where other answers, more complex than yes or no, are possible' (1998: 220).

5.2.2 *Cyborg Rights and Wrongs*

One of the most celebrated cultural posthumanists is N. Katherine Hayles. Her defining text for this area of inquiry, 'How We Became Posthuman' (1999), discusses the implications of translating bodies into information via digital technology, a project which occurs at a time when such authors as Hans Moravec discuss the prospects of brain downloads onto computers. One might think of everyday technologies that allude to this transformation. For instance, the digitization of social relationships through the Internet or the shift of commercial transactions to entirely digital monetary exchanges, are each examples of an increasing shift towards the digitization of various aspects of our lives. Hayles' posthumanism draws from Hassan (1977) who invites the suggestion – rather like Foucault – that the era of Man[2] is approaching some form of end point.

[2] The word 'sic' is not appropriate here, since the implication is both of a gendered claim and a claim about humanity generally.

Hayles explains how the body's boundaries have been compromised and that our current era is characterised by a desire to erase the burden of the body by reconstituting it as information or non-matter. This perspective draws attention to the development of legal instruments that emerged during the latter part of the 20th century, which endeavoured to broaden the respect and recognition of certain ways of being human. Thus, legal acts to protect disability, ethnicity and gender rights reflect a frustration over narrow preconceptions of what counts as morally relevant life that deserves protection via civil law. Where, in the past, certain modes of being were treated as 'invalid' or less morally relevant to take into account, today, these variations are celebrated. For Hayles, posthumanism is characterised by a (desired) loss of subjectivity that is based on bodies losing their boundaries. To this extent, the origins of Hayles' posthumanism are also visible in Donna Haraway's biopolitics. Haraway's work in fashioning the contemporary use of the term *cyborg* is a crucial component of how posthumanism has developed in the last 20 years. Her 'Manifesto for Cyborg's (1985) has become a central document to appeals on behalf of posthumanity. Yet, in later work, Haraway indicates that her cyborg must be read, first, as a feminist project located in a desire to reconstitute identity politics, particularly as it concerns assumptions about gender norms. This reading of Haraway allows one to explain how her ideas have become central tenets for some posthumanist scholars, as it advances the notion of a post-gender world where being a cyborg is preferable to being a goddess.

While there is little doubt that Haraway's work has been influential in recent expectations of posthumanism, there are numerous reasons to believe that this presents an ambiguous fortune for Haraway. Indeed, Haraway expresses considerable concern that her ideas have been appropriated by a particular vein of posthumanists that expresses biological transgressions as a utopian break with evolution. In an interview with Haraway (Gane & Haraway 2006), she expresses her disdain for the future-talk of such authors as Hans Moravec whose work embodies a notion of posthumanism that is located in the prospect of radical futures rather than sociocultural reform. For Haraway, this interpretation of posthumanism is at odds with the work she had intended for her post-gender, cyborgian world – she is more interested to understand 'how we became posthumanist' (Haraway, in Haraway & Gane 2006: 140) rather than 'posthuman'. Haraway's posthumanism, if there is one, interrogates the human, rather than celebrates the prospect of human enhancement. Her post-cyborg concept of 'companion species' is offered to engage with the prospect that humans might live among other, non-human entities, but rather than discuss this in the context of aliens or new life forms, she considers how domestic pets have become companion species. In sum, Haraway's claims about cyborgs were *not* based on an interest to enhance humanity, but intended to disrupt uniform ideas about what it means to be human and the social and political entitlements this might imply. In this sense, cultural posthumanists are considerably different from philosophical posthumanists. Haraway and Hayles each emphasise the dis-integration of the liberal humanist subject as the core characteristic of posthumanism. Moreover, they suggest that this change in subjectivity leads humanity towards a situation where it treats seriously claims about the moral status of artificial life.

We will see later how these ideas correspond with parallel debates taking place within analytic philosophy, but it is useful to note that these authors draw on key philosophical authors within the area of human enhancement and posthumanism. For instance, Hayles' use of Hans Moravec (1988) is also informed by Marvin Minsky (1985) and even Alan Turing (1950). Indeed, Turing's classic 'imitation game', which proposes a test to discern whether a machine is intelligent has infiltrated cultural spaces in various ways. For instance, the 1997 chess contest between IBM's Deep Blue and Grandmaster Garry Kasparov – machines vs human – was re-written through the documentary film 'Game Over' (Jayanti 2003) to explore assumptions about the relationship between the two. During this movie (and the contest itself, where the human lost to the machine) one is confronted with the demise of the human and the tragedy that this implies. This is embodied in the moment where, at the close of the contest, the IBM team and Kasparov enter the stage where the tournament was set and the crowd expresses its disapproval of the result by failing to congratulate the IBM programmers. Here, the age old narrative of the human as hero and machine as villain is replicated in full force.

The overlaps between philosophical and cultural posthumanisms are accompanied by crucial differences. For while philosophers have rejoiced at the prospect of understanding what it *doesn't* mean to be human by seeking to replicate or recreate it using science, cultural critics have often drawn attention to how literature has shaped our *evaluation* of this aspiration. There are other instances of cultural posthumanisms that also contribute to this history of the concept. For instance, in 2002, the journal *Configurations* published an entire volume on the term, which was shortly followed in 2003, by another full volume in the journal *Cultural Critique*. Here, the authors' immediate context is the cyborgology of Chris Gray (2002), Donna Haraway (1985) and, by then, an emerging number of artists whose work engaged matters of the body, such as Australian performance artist Stelarc (Smith 2005) or the French performance artist Orlan (O'Bryan 2005) each of whom have undergone surgical interventions for their work.

Taken together, these contributions to the recent history of posthumanism are crucial to explaining why views on the morality of human enhancements have become polarised. Unlike transhumanism – cultural posthumanists makes no direct claim made about the *ethics* of emerging technologies, though our ethical culture might find itself under considerable scrutiny by such authors (Zylinska 2005). Unlike transhumanists, cultural posthumanists have observed and developed theories of change and have positioned technology in relation to this change. In short, human subjectivity and embodiment have become the focal point for these analyses of change, rather than the prospect of human enhancement or species transgressions. However, there is a latent ethical stance that is often present within these analyses that might be characterised as a general concern that emergent technologies further frustrate the achievement of social justice, which is perhaps the common ground between culture and philosophy.

5.3 Philosophical Posthumanism

Thus far, I have located the history of posthumanism within a series of political and cultural shifts. From these offerings, it is now useful to examine their philosophical underpinning. As was mentioned earlier, Fukuyama's reliance on the instrumentalisation of such phrases as human dignity indicates the philosophical challenge from posthumanism: whether society can accommodate an expanding circle of moral concern to include the pursuit of medical enhancements. The emerging and varied perspectives on cyborgism (Haraway 1985; Gray 1997, 2002), posthumanism (Hayles 1999; Fukuyama 2002) and transhumanism (Bostrom 2005) seek to critique humanism as a guiding normative framework, though they go about this in different ways. Each of them resonates with a 21st century fetish for imagining the consequences of technological advancement, which stems from a 19th and 20th century post-Enlightenment skepticism over claims that technological development constitutes progress. For example, Hayles' (1999) thesis rejects the sanctity of stable biological distinctions, such as species categories. Alternatively, Gray (1997) articulates a 'cyborg bill of rights' to argue on behalf of broadening our narrow conception of humanness. These analyses are also inextricable from other cultural critiques, such as that of Furedi (2005a, b) and Beck (1992, 1999).[3] Indeed, Furedi (2006) contextualises his culture and politics of fear within an attempt to reconstitute the values of humanism. He notes that,

> Instead of celebrating man's attempt to transform nature, history and civilisation have been recast as a story of environmental destruction. From this standpoint the application of reason, knowledge and science are dismissed as problems because they help intensify the destructive capacity of the human species. 'Humans are, literally, a species out of control', notes a misanthropic contribution. From this perspective humanism itself is the problem.

To this extent, Furedi's perspective can be construed as posthuman, as his thesis on the politics of fear is implied by the various discourses on the dangers of biological modification. Moreover, his *Therapy Culture* (2004) offers specific connections to Fukuyama's analysis via its analysis of lifestyle medical care and the more general interest in personhood and vulnerability that concerns the main stay of bioethics. This section moves from these recent thinkers to further historical analyses of philosophical thought on posthumanism.

5.3.1 *Locating the Human*

Stories about the transformation of biology and the rise of machines are often imbued with narratives of fear and uncertainty, which intend to reveal the insecurity of humanity that arises from the prospect of having to share (control of) the world

[3] Beck's risk society is bound up with scientific and technological innovation.

with the living machine, or the cyborg. Such alien beings are frequently represented as a threat to humanity, calling into question their identity and powers of domination. Literary examples abound on this topic, including Hans Christian Anderson's fairytale story, *The Nightingale* (1844), Mary Shelley's (1818) *Frankenstein*, and more recently, Isaac Asimov's robot stories. Within each of these examples is a recurring narrative about how the new being creates a problem for the humans around it. Anderson's *Nightingale* tells the story of a mechanical nightingale that charms a Chinese Emperor far more than his *real* nightingale, even though the real bird had been a companion to the Emperor for many years. The mechanical bird's greater beauty and more pleasant song results in the real nightingale being banished and fleeing from the Emperor's side. A year later, the artificial bird breaks down and cannot be repaired and the Emperor begins to die. Hearing of the news, the banished nightingale returns and the Emperor returns to good health once again. The story symbolises the conviction that it is biological life that endures and that matters, rather than machines. The narrative is a part of a recurrent moral discourse on technology that asserts that being alive or natural is good and that being mechanical or artificial is bad.

Other texts convey a similar narrative. In Shelley's *Frankenstein*, the monster is a human creation that is part biological and part mechanical (through its reanimation). Despite its human form, the resulting being is grotesque and alien to the human world, within which it soon becomes monstrous and violent. Importantly, the monster of Frankenstein becomes terrible only when it is rejected from human society. As such, the text reveals an ambiguity about this creation – its monstrosity is not a product of its creation, but a consequence of its lack of acceptance by other humans who fail to embrace it. On this point, Mazlish (1993: 44) argues that the story provokes the following warning about the future of the human species:

> [I]f humans insist on their separateness and superiority in regard to machines (as well as other animals), viewing them as a threatening new "species" rather than as a part of their own creation, will they, indeed, bring about the very state of alienation that they fear.

These stories of automata, cyborgs, and robots all pose the same question: how do humans differ from non-humans, or more simply, what does it mean to be human? To this extent, they should be construed as integral parts of posthumanism's history. They also intimate at the inadequacy or interference of artifice in the reordering of nature.[4] More recent examples include Kafka's *Metamorphosis* (1948) and Atwood's *Oryx and Crake* (2005).

---

[4] Moreover, to confirm the links between the cultural and philosophical, Clarke (2002) discusses these ideas in the context of *The Fly* indicating the crucial component of telephony as an anarchic intermediary of natural processes. In his analysis, the posthuman is both a non-essential claim, but also a position taken on the relationship between biology and information where 'The metamorphic spectacles unleashed by the variants of *The Fly* are posthuman transformations brought about precisely by fantastic adaptation of modern communicative technology' (p 174).

5.3.2 *The Critique of Humanism*

These observations from literature of moral concern about the extension of human control over nature must be seen in the context of the post-Enlightenment period. The Industrial revolution provoked a significant development in writing about the relationship between humans and other entities. The discourse reflects a scientific concern for automata and the Romantic revulsion against the mechanical Newtonian worldview. It illustrates the range of curiosities, embodied in scientific inquiry and legends about the creation of life from inanimate material.

During these post-Enlightenment years, one perceives the works of philosophers and scientists with a far more sophisticated uncertainty about the *ends of science* than had existed before and, to reiterate, the enduring challenge of posthumanism is to wrestle with this issue. This period of 'isms' (Transcendentalism, Idealism, Existentialism, Nihilism, Realism, Pragmatism, Socialism, Communism, Liberalism) included such icons of western history as Charles Darwin, Karl Marx, and Schopenhauer. The presence of machines in everyday life made the distinction between humans and non-living entities more acute, particularly during the late 19th century and early 20th century, where machines would be far more confrontational to a worker's life than ever before and, increasingly, within the family home.

The machine became an object of human interest, a means to an end, accentuating the role of the human being as a tool user. Tools were used to extend personal power and freedom, at the same time as subjecting individuals to its impersonal organisation (Mazlish 1993). Tools became the mediator between humanity and the environment; an artificial skin separating humans from other animals. The division of labour transformed the human into mere body parts and reduced a worker's relationship with other into functional, economic value. From here, it was a small conceptual step towards the computer revolution (and our return to Turing and Hayles). The computer reflects the current articulation of machinic automation, extending human faculties as well as replacing humans and making them more machine-like, physically and cognitively.

Darwin's biological humanism allowed the human to be reduced to a level of mechanics, a view that pervades contemporary understandings about being human. The classification of species and the survival of the fittest hypothesis reduced the complexity of life to neat and tidy relationships. However, these barriers between animals and humans have now begun to collapse, identifying the difference between them as being one of degree, rather than of kind. Indeed, in Darwin's view, the most fundamental difference between humans and animals is that humans possess a developed sense of morality, or conscience, and religion. From here, the debate about whether humans are comprised mainly by genetic, inherited qualities, or whether humans are more socially determined – the nature versus nurture debate – begins to ensue.

The move from modern to postmodern articulations of the human condition also plays an important role in explaining the history of posthumanism, as it is articulated in contemporary ethics. The underlying narratives of such classic texts as

Huxley's (1932/1990) *Brave New World* or George Orwell's *1984* (1940/1983) recur frequently within contemporary discussions about the genetic revolution. The ideas within these works continue to characterise technological change in terms of warning and alarm, reminding of how easily the use of technology can lead to disaster. This period of redefining the human condition as distinct from other entities is not limited to any specific technology. It encompasses biotechnologies, but also includes such innovations as artificial intelligence, life extension and genetic or nanotechnological engineering. Yet, the symbiosis of the organic and machinic takes place in its most extreme form through the merging of humans with medical technology, allowing the transplantation of limbs, and the re-constructing of life, which utilises technology and biology.

It is in this vast historical context of conceptualising the human where we find a range of posthumanisms that challenge the idea that humanness is a fixed concept, but where also questions about humanist ideology arise. Moreover, it is these applications that have constituted the political rise of posthumanism, as a challenge to established medical ethical principles. Thus, one might characterise posthumanism as a crisis of delimiting the proper role of medicine in an era of enhancement and lifestyle treatments. To this extent, it is useful to further examine how such principles came to be; to understand the foundation on which a humanistic ethics has been developed. Indeed, this inquiry alludes to some of the broader philosophical origins to posthumanism and will allow greater clarity on how bioethics is challenged by posthumanism.

5.3.3 Identifying Our Ethical Other

Since the drafting of the Nuremberg Code after the Second World War and later the Helsinki Declaration (World Medical Association 2000), human biological integrity has become a subject of moral protectionism through the notion of individual human rights. Recall again that such conceptual assumptions are crucial to Fukuyama's *Factor X*. This is not to say that what one aims to protect by the observation of human rights is a new kind of moral concern. Indeed, wherever one finds codes of ethics or morality throughout history, there is evidence of an interest to protect some form of human vulnerability. Yet, insofar as this period established standardized ethical limits to the conduct of medicine, it is a useful moment from which to gaze upon the challenge these codes face from posthumanism.

The ethical principles of autonomy, beneficence, non-maleficience, and justice underpin modern, western medicine and any research involving human subjects. As such, an initial attempt to define what is uniquely valuable about being human is found in discussions about *dignity* and *rights*, which in turn give rise to discussions about *humanness* and *personhood*. In the past, philosophers have attempted to define humanness by distinguishing it from other kinds of entity, such as animals, machines, automata and even God. This reveals some of the most important contributions to the contemporary debate about posthumanim. As I mentioned earlier, distinguishing the *Other* or, as Rorty (1989) and Singer (1981) both characterise the dilemma: what should be within our circle of moral concern, is one of its central tenets.

A number of philosophical approaches of this kind are useful to mention, though I will not exhaust the entirety of philosophical history here. For example, Michel de Montaigne's (1533–1592) ideas about being human arise out of a frustration for understanding the place of humans in the natural order. Montaigne endeavours to explain humanness by contrasting the *differences between humans* and the *differences between humans and animals*. Arguing that beasts are more natural than humans and that there is greater difference among humans than between humans and animals, Montaigne claims that humans should aspire to be more like non-human animals rather than to mark themselves of as distinct and/or superior to them.

Subsequently, Rene Descartes (1596–1650) develops a philosophical approach to understanding the human being, which rephrases the question in the context of animal intelligence. Descartes foregrounds the instinctive volitions of animals, rather than whether or not they possess a soul to consider how they are different from humans. By characterising animal actions as *perfect* – rather like an automaton – Descartes concludes that they, unlike humans, do not have free will or the ability to determine actions. Whereas animals are perfect, humans have the ability to *chose imperfection* and make mistakes, represented by the story of the Garden of Eden. Additionally, humans must strive for perfection through reason and, from here, Descartes concludes that the method through which humans reason is rational doubt. Again, these concepts of *choice* and *perfection* are both central points of contestation within the literature on posthumanism, though as I have also mentioned, their content is not prescribed. Thus, it would be mistaken to characterise posthuman thought as the pursuit of human perfection or the limitless valuing of personal freedom. Rather, one can depict this literature as the site where competing views on these terms are played out.[5]

Distinguishing humans from animals is not the only way that philosophers have attempted to characterise what it means to be human. Philosophers have sought to distinguish between humans and non-living entities or automata and one can observe how this way of understanding humanness contributes to discussions about new technology. Mythical and fantastical ideas about human/machine hybrids are present from stories of Icarus' wings, to Chinese, Greek, and Arabic text that are rich in the subject of automata (Mazlish 1993). Indeed, a further characteristic of posthumanism appears to be an interest in the conflation of fact and fiction, as a rich aspect of these discussions rather than a confusing influence.[6] It plays an important role within the ethical consideration of new technologies. The ability to conceptualise the abstract being, the automata, the cyborg, or the genetically engineered human, is a useful way of approaching a clearer understanding of what constitutes the human

[5] Again, the Fukuyama and Stock counter positions are useful examples here. It is the staging of this conflict rather than the substantive differences of opinion that I suggest is characteristic of posthumanism.

[6] Indeed, Ansell Pearson (1997a) seems useful here in his characterisation of Stelarc as Lyotard's experimenter.

and what might be desirable circumstances for the future of human societies. Again, if one examines more contemporary debates on posthumanism, attempting to understand the role of fiction within this moral landscape is important.

5.3.4 The Philosophy of Technology

In offering this historical explanation, one might ask further how the history of posthumanism is distinct from the history of philosophical inquiries into technology. As far back as Aristotle, whose notion of 'form' located technology within the world as an instrument of humanity, philosophers have endeavoured to make sense of technology's transformative potential. Aristotle's ideas have informed other philosophers of technology, from Jacques Ellul (1964) to Martin Heidegger (1977).[7] While these authors never use the term posthumanism, their ideas on technology and nature are integral to contemporary theories of posthumanism.[8] For instance, Heidegger's concept of *enframing* offers a critical view of technology, which treats it as a *process* rather than an *artifact*. Indeed, Heidegger famously notes that the 'essence of technology is by no means anything technological' (1977: 4, 13) and his notion of enframing describes how technology is a process of revealing specific modes of being. Often considered to be a pessimistic view on technology, Heidegger's concern was that technology is perpetually an assault on nature since it always involves its alteration through destruction.[9] This struggle over how technology corrupts nature is visible in contemporary notions of posthumanism and is, as I suggest, the version of posthumanism that is a critique of *humanism*.

Thus, posthumanists treat technology as an ideology that enframes our utilisation of it, rather than an artifact that merely enables new kinds of functionality.[10] This is why one should not conflate the history of technology with the history of posthumanism, because only part of the posthumanist ideal seems connected to artifacts and our use of them. Instead, posthumanists have treated technology as an ideology, a particular kind of instrumental attitude that shapes the world. One might even question whether historical inquiries into nature (and how it is distinct from

---

[7] Again, an indication of how the cultural and the philosophical have a common history is evident from Foucault's admission of Heidegger's positive influence on his own analyses of culture, including its medicalisation (Rayner 2001).

[8] It is inconsequential that each of these authors thought of technology as pessimistically deterministic, as I have already argued that posthumanism does not establish a clear evaluative stance to accept technology.

[9] In this way, one is also drawn to the etymology of the word 'techne', which has its Greek root in the notion of 'art'. While it is not possible to consider in great depth the practice of posthuman art, such performers as the French artist Orlan and Australian artist Stelarc seem to be useful examples here. Moreover, Heidegger has often addressed the similarities between these two concepts of art and technology.

[10] Again, transhumanism seems more interested in where humanity might go in a world where it has those faculties.

artifice) are part of the posthuman concern. Thus, while Mill's *On Nature* appeals as an attempt to disrupt the assumed design of nature as an appeal to human agency, posthumanism seems critically shaped by a commitment to *transformation*, which itself might be characterised as an essentialist view on humanity (and nature).[11]

From this perspective, one might also include Nietzsche's *Übermensch* within our category of posthumanist thinking. Again, this is one way in which the history of posthumanism is only partially connected to the history of transhumanism. So described, Nietzsche applies in the sense that he was interested in various forms of 'becoming' (Roodt 2002) and transcendence rather than biological change specifically. Thus, when Nietzsche characterises the human state as provisional or, as the 'as yet undetermined animal', he beckons at an ideological transformation.[12] Further support for this view is evident if one characterises Nietzsche's *Übermensch* as a political philosophy. Indeed, Ansell Pearson (1997b) notes that to construe Nietzsche's ideas as limited solely to biological transformations would be inadequate. However, rather than claim that his arguments could not be applied to such changes, he is more concerned that such a focal point of application would be to the neglect of Nietzsche's much broader expectation for becoming.

Thus, while Ansell Pearson notes that 'Nietzsche informs us that he writes for a species that does not yet exist' (1997b: 17), he also indicates that Nietzsche had a much more profound becoming in mind than might be expressed simply by, say, human enhancements. Ansell Pearson's point is that we *cannot assume* that the changing of mere biology is always accompanied by a radical 'transvaluation of values'. This reinforces the suggestion that posthumanism constitutes a general claim about overcoming, which is located within the sphere of the biological. Perhaps it is, as Ansell Pearson describes through Deleuze and Guattari (1988), the recognition of biology's 'originary' function as inherently technical and where, today, we encounter the shift in matter – symbiosis rather than hybridity – as a 'desiring-machine'.[13] So conceived, Ansell Pearson reviews Stelarc's work – and

[11] Again, I stress that posthumanism is characterised by the tension between plural and essentialist views. Nevertheless, the philosophical perspectives I mention are affected by posthuman claims about the malleability of nature. Crucially, these authors describe a Newtonian mechanistic world view that is, as I suggest, extended by posthumanism through the employment of biological metaphors.

[12] This interpretation is increasingly relevant as technology progresses to make possible modification of cognitive capacities, such as the faculty of memory. In this sense, Nietzsche's view that the human capacity to act out memory as a distinguishing characteristic of humanness becomes all the more poignant as this acting out extends to erasing out or merely modifying.

[13] This is why I would consider Lewis' (2003: 51) question 'how much time in your day are you not on the telephone, at the computer, watching T.V., listening to the radio, in the care, on the train, in a climate controlled environment?' to be dubious. The point it aims to make about the newness of technological culture neglects the fact that a human is always a technological-being-in-the-world. In contrast, I concur with his observation that 'a central task in a post-human politics of Prozac is to challenge the hegemonic regime of bioscientific (and increasingly administrative) psychiatry and their pharmaceutical supporters. Crucially, to a large extent, Lewis is articulating a valuable cultural studies of ethics that should be seen in the context of Zylinska's (2005) 'ethics of cultural studies'.

more broadly the interface of art and science – as the 'site of a symbiotic complex which involves new mutant potentialities, preceding need and functioning beyond the pleasure principle.' Thus, Stelarc – either through his suspensions or extra ear – does not become a machine through his performance; he *is* a 'becoming machine', literally an evolving and unfinished entity. This characterization of posthumanism avoids the claim that emerging technological changes must be seen as a break from evolutionary processes. Indeed, this view seems consistent with Fuss' articulation of Nietzsche's all too human when she notes that 'the only way to reach the human may be to overreach it, to exceed the boundaries that fundamentally delimit and define the human' (Fuss 1996: 4). So understood, posthumanism is a critical practice of understanding the kind of overreaching that seems characteristic of humanity.

5.3.5 An Ethics of Undecidability

To conclude, other continental philosophers provide additional historical context to the development of posthumanism*s*. As I mentioned at the outset, the preoccupation with Otherness is characteristic of posthumanism's distinct history. The various areas of inquiry discussed here establish and negotiate boundaries of posthuman concern, whether they are moral, political or cultural. From here, one can infer from other authors, such as Emmanuel Levinas (1969), to explain how posthumanism consists of a plethora of moral imperatives to confront various kinds of changes. Indeed, one might describe the recent revival of posthumanism – evident by this book and various other recent analyses I have mentioned – as a moral imperative to attend to the collapse of social responsibility that is presented by catastrophic human change. Levinas conceives of this problematic by invoking the concept of the *face*. This term explains that a condition of human existence is being required to stand in opposition to an Other, in a form of ethical encounter. He indicates that 'my being in the world requires justification' just because the extension of my being (the body as technology) involves an unavoidable violence towards the Other. Exemplars of this encounter within medical ethics are various. For instance, it could include the use of genetic selection, which would require selecting one embryo over another. However, it also extends to other spheres of biological responsibility, such as questions of kinship that are implied via such diverse areas of social policy as immigration to organ transplants. Indeed, it is this breadth of concern which reveals the all encompassing content of posthumanism. Levinas conceives of the Other as the source of 'both my reason and my obligation'. The ethical imperative we encounter by considering this Other is explained by Derrida (1999) who draws attention to the intrigue of undecidability:

> [T]here would be no decision, in the strong sense of the word, in ethics, in politics, no decision, and thus no responsibility, without the experience of some undecidability. If you don't experience some undecidability, then the decision would simply be the application of a programme, the consequence of a premiss or of a matrix. So a decision has to go through some impossibility in order for it to be a decision. If we knew what to do, if I knew in terms

> of knowledge what I have to do before the decision, then the decision would not be a decision. It would simply be the application of a rule, the consequence of a premiss, and there would be no problem, there would be no decision. Ethics and politics, therefore, start with undecidability (1999: 66).

Thus, histories of posthumanism consist in an ongoing undecidability over the value of transgressing boundaries, in some cases as they relate to biological change. For Derrida, considerations of posthumanity are, unavoidably, questions about the future. It 'relates to what is to come, to that which will occur in ways that are not appropriable, unforeseen and therefore urgent, before anticipation (Derrida 1994: 31). In this sense, responding to the potential Other of the posthuman has become 'a thought of pressing need' as it is a process through which self characterisation or the 'performative character of morality' is played out. Posthumanism is the theoretical consideration of the ongoing re-definition of an 'ethics of bodies that matter' (Zylinska 2005).

I have not offered a view on whether these various philosophical perspectives are in agreement about the value of biological modification and the cultures to which it might give rise. Rather, I have aimed to elaborate on works that have clearly shaped contemporary theoretical views of posthumanism that re-construct humanism in an era of biotechnological change. Yet, it would be wrong to characterise this history as one of stalemate between technophobe and technophile. Indeed, some recent contributions to the question set by Derrida are visible within bioethics. For instance, Parens (2005) attempts to distinguish the different value systems of those who argue on behalf of medical enhancements and those who argue against by describing the former as operating from a 'creative' framework and the latter existing within a 'gratitude' framework. Parens' careful analysis seems consistent with Derrida's concern for ethical judgement to be hospitable so as to avoid a stalemate between seemingly oppositional view points. While I do not conclude from this that Parens is advocating a posthumanist view, his analysis arises at a moment where posthumanism is constituted by an intrigue over what might become of this seemingly impossible struggle between competing value systems.

5.4 Conclusion

Within this chapter, I have endeavoured to outline the origins of contemporary discussions about posthumanism. In doing so, I have distinguished between the political, cultural and philosophical contributions to this developing theoretical viewpoint. While it is fatuous to claim that these distinctions are wholly separate, identifying the different questions they have asked is crucial to explaining the emergence of polarised views about the ethics of medical enhancements. Indeed, the consequences of this challenging situation – typified by the debate about the federal funding of stem cell research in the USA – is reflected in Fukuyama's recent contribution, *Beyond Bioethics* (Fukuyama & Furger 2007). Here, one is struck by the need to locate ethical debates about medical enhancements within a broader social and political framework.[14]

In conclusion, the history of posthumanism has no obvious beginning, middle or end point in philosophical thought. Indeed, the current stage of theoretical interventions on this topic seems comparable to where postmodernism was located in the early 1990s. Indeed, this analogy extends to the potential divisiveness of the concept within and across disciplines. Nevertheless, the history of philosophy is scattered with specific moments of appeals to posthuman idea(l)s. So understood, posthumanism is as much a particular reading of the history of philosophy, as it is an attempt to rework philosophical views about what it means to be human, within the context of emerging technologies. Appeals to posthumanism as a series of philosophical concerns about biology compels it towards the pursuit of novelty and originality, which explains why it is inherently future oriented. One might add further to its usefulness as a concept by taking into account Virilio's (1977, 1995) claims about the acceleration of society, which, again, is an identifiable characteristic of the social discourses surrounding many emerging technologies. In this sense, the novelty of posthumanism should be understood as the rapid emergence of new ethical dilemmas and its capacity to develop a new sociology of ethics, rather than the newness of ethical theory that it might provoke.[15]

To its advantage, authors from across disciplinary boundaries have theorised posthumanism, which suggests its capacity to become a relevant and distinct philosophical paradigm. Yet, despite the proliferation of various views on posthumanism, many of them remain obscured in some of the crucial, policy-oriented debates about the legitimacy of medical enhancements. As such, I am inclined to conclude that we are still becoming posthuman, in the sense that these disconnected perspectives have yet to be written into its historical development, where, for instance, posthumanism is understood as a critique of humanism.

Nevertheless, despite acknowledging the overlap between the philosophical and cultural approaches to posthumanism, one might attempt to distinguish them in quite simple terms. Thus, cultural theorists are concerned about narratives of Otherness and their capacity to be politically divisive. On this view, the appeal of the posthuman is in the destabilisation of humanist values – such as the aspiration of perfectibility or the value of controlling nature.[16] In contrast, while philosophers of posthumanism often seem to share this view, they are also often engaged in a broader project that aims, nevertheless, to continue the Enlightenment ideal of *aspiring* to bring about progress through the employment of technology (as knowledge). This project has found its most visible articulation within the concept of

---

[14] Further evidence of this need is the recent trends towards *empirical ethics*, where various authors have called upon the need to underpin ethical research with social scientific and science communication investigations (Haimes 2002; Miah 2005).

[15] However, one might legitimately discuss, for instance, Sherwin's (1998) *relational autonomy* as one such new ethical response to such changes.

[16] Indeed, I would conceive of the animal rights movement as a pre-cursor to a posthuman philosophy, since it similarly is concerned with the circle of moral concern and the relevance of locating such concern outside of species boundaries.

transhumanism, which has become an organised movement and an aspiring philosophical perspective in its own right (see the *World Transhumanist Association* website).

Alternatively put, cultural posthumanists appear unified in their interest to provide a voice for marginal communities. In contrast, philosophical posthumanism makes a similar attempt for, as yet, *non-existent* communities who are expected to be marginal – such as the genetically modified or transgenic human. Indeed, perhaps it is the increasing proximity of these possible communities that constitutes their emergent common ground. For example, the world has already witnessed the utilisation of xenotransplantation, which has provoked concerns about the crossing of species boundaries. Cultural posthumanism foregrounds the political process over and above the value of individual agency and, in this domain, it differs from the priorities of philosophical posthumanisms. Also, cultural posthumanisms are more inclined to treat prosthetic devices as supportive to illness, rather than to espouse their potential to eventually surpass the normal range of human functioning and enhance humanity. Moreover, such authors are significantly less enthralled by the promise of technology, compared with philosophers in this area.

It would be misleading to portray cultural posthumanists as the more pessimistic authors on the prospects of medical enhancements. Yet, it is rare that one reads a posthuman philosopher who writes in the following manner: 'my dream is a version of the posthuman that embraces the possibilities of information technologies without being seduced by fantasies of unlimited power and disembodied immortality' (Hayles 1999: 5). Thus, cultural posthumanists seem much less willing to accept that technological development is indicative of a 'linear model of the development of the human, from the "natural man" to the "posthuman cybernetic organism" (Zylinska 2005: 149).[17] Rather, cultural posthumanism involves a commitment to engaging with the 'multiplicities of life' (*ibid*). On this view, posthumanism is the study of the collapse of ontological boundaries, of which one central, but not isolated element, is the study of how moral landscapes might be transformed by this occurrence. Indeed, such a perspective seems adequately summarised by Wallace (2005) who invokes the notion of the 'posthuman humanist' (p 102) to draw attention to the interest of scholars, such as Haraway, in the relationships between varies kinds of beings – 'humans, animals and machines' (*ibid*).

Nevertheless, in both the philosophical and cultural analyses, posthumanism emerges as a *visionary stance*, which also explains why it has invited suspicion by less enthusiastic academics. As was noted earlier, critics – who often do not distinguish between post- or trans- human authors – have been concerned about future-oriented views that seemed to neglect socio-political concerns about both the implementation of technology within society and the prospective replacement of the human with something else. The remnants of these concerns are still visible within most recent critiques of trans/post humanism, such as Zylinska (2005). This, more nuanced view is also expressed by such philosophers as Ansell Pearson (1997b)

[17] A claim that I expect would be disputed by many leading transhumanists but which, I would suggest, is often assumed of transhumanist thought.

who argues that, 'the transhuman condition is not about the transcendence of the human being, but concerns its non-teleological becoming in an immanent process of "anthropological deregulation"' (p 163). Nevertheless, while it would be tempting to characterise philosophical posthumanism as essentialist and cultural posthumanism as pluralist, this would be too quick a judgement.

As I have suggested, these various articulations of posthumanism have often been conflated and this chapter attempts to clarify the differences between theoretical work on this subject. Their semantic differences become crucial when attempting to articulate the history of the concepts, because their definition and use have become constitutive of the ethical landscape.[18] Earlier, I mentioned that cultural and philosophical posthumanism are distinct in relation to enhancements because they arrive at medical ethics from different points of origin and with different interests. This is neatly surmised by the earlier disjunction between the rise of *cultural studies in ethics* (Haimes 2002; Miah 2005) and Zylinska's (2005) recent call for an *ethics of cultural studies*. More broadly, one might characterise this through such cultural analyses as Foucault's (1974/2004) interest in medicalisation versus Jonsen and Toulmin's (1988) casuistry and the subsequent development of narrative ethics (Lindemann 1997; Chambers 1999).

I have argued that the history of posthumanism is often written from within cultural texts through which moral narratives emerge and become the subject of political concern.[19] Indeed, this is perhaps the main space where one finds common ground between the philosophical and the critical theory approach to posthumanism. For, all authors who speak about post- or trans- humanisms (or humanism more generally), discuss some crucial texts where ideas about the future of humanity emerge. Indeed, when studying these texts, one becomes aware of how technology is often the scapegoat for ideological bad practice. It seems relevant that both approaches to posthumanism have become particularly interested in cognitive modifications and understanding the mind's capacities. Even within Gray's (2002) cyborgology, his tribute to Turing's (1950) work is crucial. This prioritising of biology as information, rather than matter, is appealing to both digital theorists and post genomic understandings of nature.

There are areas of interest that I have not considered in much depth here, though they further challenge the claim that posthumanism is a subject located solely in high technology. For instance, more must also be said about the shift 'from chance to choice' (Buchanan et al. 2000) that also seems to characterise contemporary versions of posthumanism, where the possibility of radical biological change is afforded by new scientific discoveries. Again, in this context, posthumanism is best understood as the interplay of competing responses to these new encounters with moral dilemmas, rather

[18] Again, we can recall the narratives of *Frankenstein* or *Brave New World* as having become part of the common language of framing high technological futures.

[19] A further example would be the emergence of the Ron's Angels website in 1999, which purported to auction ova and sperm, thus allowing bidders to purchase the genes of their offspring. In this case, there is little evidence that the company was anything more than a media spectacle. Alternatively, the telephone tooth implant that made the cover of Time magazine and which was developed by design provocateurs James Auger and Jimmy Loizeau at the Royal College of Art are constitutive of the moral debate about technology's limits.

than simply a limitless embrace of such change. While there are undoubtedly scholars of post- and transhumanism who would hold value in such choices, it is mistaken to characterise this enthusiasm as a lack of concern for social responsibility.

Also, I have not discussed the development of 'magic' as a form of technological knowledge (Stivers 2001), or other modes of body modification, which have different transformative cultural meanings, such as tattoo, scarification or body piercing (Fisher 2002). It is crucial to inquire into how these practices and rituals of metamorphosis are different from, say, cosmetic surgery or the interest to extend life, both in terms of the ethical stance from medical regulation and as a claim about what would constitute posthumanity. It is a common misconception that posthumanism is grounded solely within technological change, yet these examples suggest that there is more to the transformative notion of posthumanity than is revealed by emerging technology.

Thus, an historical analysis of posthumanity cannot be grounded solely in technological transformation. Rather, it must be more broadly described as part of a set of interconnected discourses and philosophical claims surrounding concepts of mind, body, nature and artifice. It must take into account the historiography of concepts that have emerged and the cultural, political and media instantiations through which moral claims about a shift of humanisms can be asserted. Surrounding these debates has been the continual fluctuation of technological change specifically, but *change* more generally. At various points in time, the subject of that change has differed and contemporary posthumanism involves a change in kind to the boundary (and integrity) of nature and artifice.

In sum, the philosophical project of posthumanism can be marked by a set of boundaries and our cultural relationship to them. To this extent, posthumanism is a philosophical stance about what might be termed a *perpetual becoming*. It also describes a cultural stance on the embeddedness of change within social processes. Posthumanism is indicative of a struggle of perspectives, perhaps analogous to the struggle of humanity's shedding of its biological limitations. It exhibits moments of concern about the fragility of biological decision making, which might be more broadly conceived as a postmodern anxiety. Yet, while posthumanism is struggling to be accepted, it is not a distinct perspective. It is the detritus of perspectives.

References

Ansell Pearson K (1997a) Life Becoming Body: On the 'Meaning' of Post Human Evolution. Cultural Values 1, no 2: 219–40

Ansell Pearson K (1997b) Viroid Life: Perspectives on Nietzsche and the Transhuman Condition. Routledge, London

Atwood M (2003) Oryx and Crake. Bloomsbury, London

Badmington N (2000) (ed) Posthumanism. Palgrave, New York

Badmington N (2001) Pod Almighty! Or, Humanism, Posthumanism, and the Strange Case of Invasion of the Body Snatchers. Textual Practice 15, no 1: 5–22

Badmington N (2003) Theorizing Posthumanism. Cultural Critique 53, Winter: 11–27

Beck U (1992) Risk Society: Towards a New Modernity. Sage, London

Beck U (1999) World Risk Society. Polity, Cambridge

Bostrom N (2005) A History of Transhumanist Thought. Journal of Evolution and Technology 14(1): http://jetpress.org/volume14/bostrom.html
Buchanan A, Brock D W, Daniels N, Wikler D (2000) From Chance to Choice: Genetics & Justice. Cambridge University Press, Cambridge
Chambers T (1999) The Fiction of Bioethics: Cases as Literary Texts. Routledge, New York
Clarke B (2002) Mediating the Fly: Posthuman Metamorphosis in the 1950s. Configurations 10: 169–91
Deleuze G, Guattari F (1988) A Thousand Plateaus. Massumi B (trnas). Athlone, London
Derrida J (1999) Hospitality, Justice and Responsibility: A Dialogue with Jacques Derrida. In: Kearney R, Dooley M (eds) Questioning Ethics: Contemporary Debates in Philosophy. Routledge, London/New York
Ellul J (1964) The Technological Society. Vintage Books, New York
Fisher J A (2002) Tattooing the Body, Marking Culture. Body & Society 8, no 4: 91–107
Foucault M (1974/2004) The Crisis of Medicine or the Crisis of Antimedicine? Foucault Studies 1: 5–19
Fukuyama F (1999) Second Thoughts: The Last Man in a Bottle. The National Interest Summer: 1–18.
Fukuyama F (2002) Our Posthuman Future: Consequences of the Biotechnology Revolution. Profile Books, London
Fukuyama F (2004) Transhumanism: The World's Most Dangerous Ideas. Foreign Policy, no Sept/Oct: 42–43
Fukuyama F, Furger F (2007) Beyond Bioethics: A Proposal for Modernizing the Regulation of Human Biotechnologies. Paul H. Nitze School of Advanced International Studies, Washington DC
Furedi F (2004) Therapy Culture: Captivating Vulnerability in an Uncertain Age. Routledge, New York
Furedi F (2005a) Culture of Fear: Risk-Taking and the Morality of Low Expectation. Continuum, London
Furedi F (2005b) Politics of Fear: Beyond Left and Right. Continuum, London
Furedi F (2006) The Legacy of Humanism. In: Cummings D (ed) Debating Humanism. Imprint Academic, London
Fuss D (1996) Introduction: Human, All Too Human. Routledge, London/New York
Gane N, Haraway D (2006) When We Have Never Been Human, What Is to Be Done: Interview with Donna Haraway. Theory, Culture and Society 23(7–8): 135–158
Graham E L (2002a) Representations of the Post/Human. Manchester University Press, Manchester, UK
Graham E L (2002b) The Politics of the Post/Human. Paper presented at the Presented 3 September 2003 at Yale University, Technology and Ethics Working Research Group, Yale Interdisciplinary Bioethics Program, New Haven, CT/New York
Gray C H (1997) The Ethics and Politics of Cyborg Embodiment: Citizenship as a Hypervalue. Cultural Values 1, no 2: 252–58
Gray C H (2002) Cyborg Citizen: Politics in the Posthuman Age. Routledge, London
Haimes E (2002) What Can the Social Sciences Contribute to the Study of Ethics? Theoretical, Empirical and Substantive Considerations. Bioethics 16, no 2: 89–113
Halberstam J, Livingstone I (1995) (eds) Posthuman Bodies. Indiana University Press, Bloomington, IN
Haraway D A (1985) Manifesto for Cyborgs: Science, Technology, & Socialist Feminism in the 1980s. Socialist Review 80: 65–108
Haraway D (2006) The Companion Species Manifesto. Prickly Paradigm, Chicago, IL
Hassan I (1977) Prometheus as Performer: Toward a Posthumanist Culture. In: Beramou M, Caramello C (eds) Performance in Postmodern Culture. Coda Books, Madison, WI
Hayles N K (1999) How We Became Posthuman: Virtual Bodies in Cybernetics, Literature, and Informatics. University of Chicago Press, London
Heidegger M (1977) The Question Concerning Technology and Other Essays. Lovitt W (trans). Harper & Ro, London

Huxley A (1932/94) Brave New World. Flamingo, London
Jayanti V (2003) Game Over: Kasparov and the Machine. 84mins, Canada/UK
Jonsen A R, Toulmin S (1988) The Abuse of Casuistry: A History of Moral Reasoning. University of California Press, Berkeley, CA
Kafka F (1948/1992) The Metamorphosis. In: Klieman L, Lewis S (eds) Philosophy: An Introduction Through Literature. Paragon House, St Paul, MN: 147–74
Levinas E (1969) Totality and Infinity: An Essay on Exteriority (trans Lingis A). Duquesne University Press, Pittsburgh, PA
Lindemann N H (1997) (ed) Stories and Their Limits: Approaches to Narrative Bioethics. Routledge, New York
Mazlish B (1993) The Fourth Discontinuity. Yale University Press, London
Miah A (2005) Genetics, Cyberspace and Bioethics: Why Not a Public Engagement with Ethics? Public Understanding of Science 14, no 4: 409–21
Mill J S (1969) Three Essays on Religion: Nature, the Utility of Religion, Theism. Prometheus Books, Amherst, MA/New York
Minsky M (1985) The Society of Mind. Simon & Shuster, New York
Moravec H (1988) Mind Children: The Future of Robot and Human Intelligence. Harvard University Press, London
Nietzsche F (1891/1961) Thus Spoke Zarathustra. Penguin Classics, London
O'Bryan C J (2005) Carnal Art: Orlan's Refacing. University of Minnesota Press, Minnesota
Orwell G (1949/83) 1984. The New American Library, New York
Parens E (2005) Authenticity and Ambivalence: Towards Understanding the Enhancement Debate. The Hastings Report 35, no 3: 34–41
Pepperell R (1995/2003) The Posthuman Condition: Consciousness Beyond the Brain. 3rd edition, Intellect Books, Bristol, UK
Rayner T (2001) Biopower and Technology: Foucault and Heidegger's Way of Thinking. Contretemps: An Online Journal of Philosophy: 142–156
Roodt V (2002) The Loss of the Human: Nietzsche and Arendt on the Predicament of Morality. Ethical Perspectives 9, 1: 31–47
Rorty R Contingency (1989) Irony and Solidarity. Cambridge University Press, Cambridge
Shelley M (1818/1994) Frankenstein. Penguin, London
Sherwin S (1998) A Relational Approach to Autonomy in Health Care. In: Sherwin S (ed) The Politics of Women's Health: Exploring Agency and Autonomy. Temple University Press, Philadelphia, PA
Singer P (1981) The Expanding Circle: Ethics and Sociobiology. Oxford University Press, Oxford
Smith M (2005) (ed) Stelarc: The Monograph. The MIT Press, Cambridge
Stivers R (2001) Technology as Magic: The Triumph of the Irrational. Continuum, New York
Stock G (1993) Metaman: The Merging of Humans and Machines into a Global Superorganism. Simon & Schuster, London
Stock G (2002) Redesigning Humans: Choosing Our Children's Genes. Profile Books, London
Turing A (1950) Computing Machinery and Intelligence. Mind: A Quarterly Journal of Psychology and Philosophy LIX, October no 236
Turney J (1998) Frankenstein's Footsteps: Science, Genetics and Popular Culture. Yale University Press, New Haven, CT/London
The U.S. President's Council on Bioethics (2003). Beyond Therapy: Biotechnology and the Pursuit of Happiness, Washington DC
Virilio P (1977) Speed and Politics: An Essay on Dromology. Semiotext(e), New York
Virilio P (1995) Speed and Information: Cyberspace Alarm! CTHEORY Article a030: http://www.ctheory.net/articles.aspx?id = 72
World Medical Association (2000) The World Medical Association Declaration of Helsinki: Ethical Principles for Medical Research Involving Human Subjects: http://www.wma.net/e/policy/b3.htm
Zylinska J (2005) The Ethics of Cultural Studies. Continuum, London

Chapter 6
Posthumanity, Transhumanism and Human Nature

Dieter Birnbacher

6.1 Introduction

"Posthumanity" has established itself as a label for a form of human existence radically transformed by the most advanced medical techniques and by the use of neuro, bio and nano and other technologies for human enhancement. In itself, "posthumanity" is a value-neutral term that neither implies nor excludes any specific attitude one might assume towards the prospect of a "posthuman" future. Nonetheless, the concept is bound up with a fairly fundamental controversy about values. It has done much to lay open the split in attitudes in our culture between those who welcome "posthumanity" as a positive vision appropriate to guide our strategies in scientific research, technology and medicine, and those who think that the dangers inherent in this vision so much outweigh its promise that we should resist the temptation to "improve" the human race by means of science and technology. "Transhumanists" like Nick Bostrom (cf. 2003, 2005) define themselves by taking a decidedly positive view of the prospect of a "posthuman" future, whereas "bioconservatives" like Leon Kass (cf. 1997) are more sceptical of this prospect and tend to warn us not to invest too much, mentally and economically, in what is seen as a threat rather than as a paradise. Semantically, the terms "transhumanism" and "posthumanity" are closely connected. "Transhumanism" can be defined as a movement that wants us to get on the way to "posthumanity" by going *beyond* humanity in its present form. Transhumanists want us to enter upon a process that will ultimately lead to "posthumanity" by attempting, now and in the near future, to transcend certain limits inherent in the human condition as we know it.

It should be borne in mind, however, that the terms "transhumanist" and "bioconservative" describe ideal types rather than concrete realities. There is a broad range of positions between the extremes, and it will be no less hard to find a "bioconservative" opposed to literally *any* attempt to improve the human condition by medical and non-medical techniques than to find a "transhumanist" in favour of literally all such attempts. As it is usually the case with polar opposites, most people can be expected to adopt some kind of intermediate position. Even many of those who unreservedly welcome the advent of neurobionics for non-medical purposes, for example, will probably have doubts about the desirability of reproductive cloning or

B. Gordijn, R. Chadwick (eds.) *Medical Enhancement and Posthumanity*,

about attempts to extend the average life-span to more than 100 years. And many of those who are opposed to cloning as a technological extension of human reproductive options will welcome other and more hopeful medical advances, for example in the field of the prevention of cancer and other crippling diseases.

6.2 "Posthumanity" and "Transhumanism" – Conceptual Puzzles

There are two reasons why it seems more appropriate to understand "posthumanity" and "transhumanism" as slogans rather than as well-defined concepts. One is the fact that both expressions are inherently paradoxical if taken literally. The other is that both expressions, even if taken with a grain of salt, are partly misleading. They might be misunderstood as suggesting that changing the natural "outfit" of man by means of science and technology amounts to a change of human nature. This suggestion, however, seems doubtful at best. I will discuss both puzzles in turn.

The first puzzle is that taken literally, "posthumanity" and "transhumanism" are inherently paradoxical. "Posthumanity", for one might be thought to be a state of existence in which the human species has so far moved beyond its biological limits that it constitutes an entirely "new" species. Or it might be thought even to ascend to a higher level in the ontological hierarchy and to become what Samuel Alexander called "finite gods" (Alexander 1927: 346), a category of superhumans related to humans in a way similar to how humans are related to non-human animals now. However, with possibly only a few exceptions, those who make use of these expressions do not really think that posthumanity will no longer consist of human beings but of beings of a different biological species. Julian Huxley, who is believed to have been the first to use the word "transhumanism" in an essay of 1957, explicitly denied a species change. "Transhumanism", as he conceived it, was to be a process of perpetual self-transcendence, but one which leaves the biological nature of man unchanged. The improvements he envisioned were primarily improvements in the social and physical environment of man rather than improvements of man himself or of human nature. "New possibilities of and for his human nature" should be realised, but man should remain what he has been (Huxley 1957: 17).

Though much more radical in their vision of man's future, today's "transhumanists" seem to share Huxley's belief that the kind of self-transcendence to which the improvement of the human race is expected to lead up to will not transcend the limits of the biological species. Though the beings at the end of the road will possess powers and abilities that from the vantage point of the present cannot be called other than "superhuman", these beings will still be humans. They will be humans just as Nietzsche imagined his *Übermensch* to be human. With his vision of "superman", Nietzsche gave expression to his very personal ideal of perfect autonomy and unfettered artistic creativity. With "posthumanity", transhumanists express their vision of a form of human existence in which certain restrictions inherent in the human condition have been overcome. In both cases, the changes are thought to be effected primarily by changes in the human being itself rather than in its physical and social environment. And in both cases, the higher level of existence envisioned is characterised not by a transmutation of man into a different kind of being but by the development of powers he possesses in virtue of his specific nature.

But though a minority, we certainly cannot completely ignore those who talk of a possible species change in the sequel of further technological advance. In the present debate about human self-transcendence, talk of a possible species change can be found at both opposites of the controversy, and with opposite values attached to it.

On the bioconservative side, talk of the "abolishment" of man, as in C. S. Lewis' diatribe against technological civilisation (Lewis 1943) is primarily a rhetorical device adding emphasis to the normative claim that modern technology and modern medicine, however sincerely motivated by the desire to improve the human lot, endanger the very essence of man. "Essence" refers, in this context, to what the respective author sees as most valuable in man: respect for tradition, spirituality, the ability to find some overarching value in life, or the readiness to leave certain parts of nature unexplored and unexploited. This literature is decidedly conservative, and one of its most conspicuous characteristics is the strong language it uses to make its point. Thus, there is no value predicate more frequent in the writings of bioconservatives than the predicate "dehumanising". In its report *Beyond Therapy*, the President's Council on Bioethics more than once asks the rhetorical question whether a possible future practice of taking drugs in order to enhance human functioning is not "dehumanising" in the sense of "compromising the lived humanity of our efforts" (President' Council 2005: 149). Readers of Leon Kass will be reminded of this particular use of "dehumanising" from some of the essays he wrote before he became the Council's president. In 1997, for example, Leon Kass wrote that reproductive cloning is "profoundly dehumanising, no matter how good the product" (Kass 1997: 23). Used in this way, "dehumanising", "abolition" or "posthuman" (as in Francis Fukuyama's title *Our Posthuman Future)* are not meant to refer to any biological transformation involving species change but to a cultural process involving the erosion of certain values held to be both characteristic of human existence and constitutive of its special dignity and worth. In these contexts, the predicate "non-human" is not the opposite of "human" in the biological sense, but the opposite of "truly human" (Lewis 1943: 49) or "fully human" (Kass *ibid*) in a normative sense. What is at stake here is a possible cultural, not a possible biological change.

There are others, however, who envision a radical biological change. Among them is biologist Lee Silver who speculates about changes that a future and technologically more advanced mankind may bring about in the biological analogue of the human essence, the genome. Similarly to certain science fiction plots (see, e.g. Butler 1989) this author develops a scenario in which the members of one layer of society, called "GenRich" succeed in improving the cognitive capacities of their offspring by means of gene technology to such an extent that the GenRich define themselves as members of a species of their own. Later on in this scenario, the GenRich split again so that what used to be one species multiplies into an indefinite number of new species (Silver 1987: 288 f).

Does this speculation show that the genetically "improved" race of GenRich would in fact constitute a new, "posthuman" species? Asking this question means opening a Pandora's box of difficulties and uncertainties. Even within biology, there is no agreed criterion of species membership. In some cases species membership is defined by similarity of phenotype, sometimes by sexual criteria such as the ability to parent common offspring. Thus, wolves, foxes and dogs are customarily classified as members of one common species (because each of the group is able to engender offspring by sexual intercourse with any other), whereas with some plants, minute differences in phenotype, e.g. in the form of leaves, are held to be sufficient for species differentiation.

With humans, the criterion of species membership is even less clear. On the breeding criterion, man does not seem to be a species of its own at all. The genomes of man and chimpanzee have so much common (in fact, 98.5%) that procreation by sexual intercourse between man and chimpanzee does not seem biologically impossible. If we insist, as we certainly want to, that man constitutes a species of his own, we have to rely on some other criterion. But it is not at all clear how this might be specified. There does not seem to be an agreed set of necessary and sufficient conditions. True, there are some necessary conditions. These, however, are neither individually nor cumulatively sufficient to differentiate humans from other animals and from potential intelligent machines. A necessary condition of a being's humanity is that its body contains at least a substantial portion of biotic, organismic tissue. Perfect Robots that functionally mimic humans, or artificially produced "replicants" with human traits and human behaviour but on a non-biotic substrate, will not be serious candidates, whereas "naturally" born humans without the capacity for consciousness or even s. acephalics, children born without any brain, will. This leaves us with the delicate question *how much* biotic tissue a being must possess to be classified as human. A man-machine system which, among others, harbours a complete human brain will presumably be classified as belonging to the human species even if all of its remaining body consists of non-biotic matter. On the other hand, a man-machine system with a brain consisting entirely of silicium chips and other non-biotic components will presumably not be classified as a human being even if the remaining body has normal human organs and limbs. Obviously, a purely quantitative criterion of how much of a compound quasi-organism made of human and inorganic elements should be human will not be adequate. Given that a *substantial* portion of an organism should be human if the whole is to count as human, "substantial" must be interpreted in some qualitative way. Saying this, however, invites further difficulties.

It seems that *homo sapiens* is what has been termed a *cluster concept*, or a concept corresponding to Wittgenstein's model of *family resemblances* rather than a concept definable by a purely conjunctive set of necessary and sufficient conditions (cf. Boyd 1999: 145). In other words, *if* there are sufficient conditions of membership in the human species, it seems doubtful that there is only one set of them and not a number of alternative conditions. This was already adumbrated by Locke in his discussion of real and nominal essences in his *Essay*. On the concept of man he wrote as early as 1690: "We shall not find the nominal essence of any one species of substances in all men the same." (Locke 1961, vol. 2: 55 (III, Chapter VI, 26)).

This diagnosis is confirmed by surveying the three traditional non-disjunctive criteria that have been held to distinguish membership in the human species from membership in others: the essentialist, the genealogical and the genomic criterion. None of these seems satisfactory if applied in isolation.

1. The *essentialist* criterion says that humans share a common metaphysical essence which is present in each of its members and in none of the non-members. An essentialist criterion poses well-known epistemological and logical problems some of which were already pointed out by Locke (cf. Locke 1961, vol. 2: 56f (III, Chapter VI, 27)). Even if we accept the existence of a metaphysical essence of man, this would give us no criterion for identifying this metaphysical essence in doubtful cases. A criterion must have an empirical content in order to be applicable. Moreover, there are logical problems arising from the reality of inter-species hybrids (such as the hybrids from goat and sheep produced by biotechnological means in the 1990s) and the biological possibility of inter-species hybrids between man and ape. Do these hybrids have only one essence, or both? If only one, which of both? Given the inscrutability of essences any answer will be arbitrary.
2. A *genealogical* criterion says that all natural descendants of a being of species S will be of the same species S. This criterion is obviously incomplete because it can only be applied after an initial species has been defined. Moreover, it is unclear whether we would want to include the totality of our biological descendants in the human species no matter what they turn out to be like. To test your intuitions, consult an interesting piece of fiction: In H. G. Wells' novel *The Time Machine* the time traveler comes across rat-like descendants of the human race. They seem to him to have so little in common with today's humans that he does not find it at all adequate to include them in his own species and decides to assign them to a "successor-species" (Wells 1924: 86f).
3. The *genomic* criterion will be the one which comes to mind first and seems the most plausible at first sight. The trouble with a genomic criterion is, however, that it seems impossible to fix a limit of genetic variation. Though 99.9% of the genomes of all humans are identical this is true only in a relative and not in an absolute sense. There seems to be no fixed class of genes that is common to all human genomes (cf. Robert & Baylis 2003: 4). Moreover, it is not at all clear that we know where the human species ends and some other species begins, especially if we think of the many ways in which future generations may attempt to modify the human genome by means of a more developed gene technology. One thing we know for sure is that the addition of one identical chromosome does not make any difference with regard to species membership, since we are familiar with a number of trisomies that remain within the limits of the species. But it is difficult to anticipate what we will say about a being in which one or more chromosomes are replaced by artificial chromosomes with significantly different genetic information. And it is hard to believe that we would assign the resultant being to one species or the other merely on the basis of genetic information and independently of phenotypical criteria. Indeed, one of Locke's

arguments against essentialism seems to hold also for a genomic criterion, namely that "we could not reasonably think that the ranking of things under general names was regulated by those internal real constitutions, or anything else but their obvious appearances" (Locke 1961, vol. 2: 55 (III, Chapter VI, 25)). The idea, which at present may rightly be rejected as utopian, that we will be able at some future time to introduce significant changes into the human genome at will without excessive risks, does not necessarily imply that the beings thus generated will be of a different species.

It follows that if a satisfactory definition of the human species can be given at all, it can only be one that fulfils four general conditions: It has to be empirical instead of metaphysical, it cannot be merely genealogical, it will have to be to be disjunctive rather than conjunctive, and it will have to include phenotypical features alongside purely genomic ones. But even if a definition fulfils these conditions, it is still an open question whether it provides a clear demarcation between what is human and what is not. First, technological progress of the kind adumbrated by transhumanist thinkers might produce "marginal" cases (such as man-machine-hybrids) for which it is controversial whether they are members of the human species. Second, it must be expected that the definition of the species is sufficiently dynamic to reflect and to incorporate the changes introduced by "transhumanist" technologies, so that in a potential future era of posthumanist technologies what is now seen as "posthuman" will be subsumed under the term "human" without further ado. In any case, it is doubtful whether there exists the clear boundary between humanity and what is beyond humanity suggested by the terms "transhumanism" and "posthumanity".

6.3 Human Nature and Its Ambiguities

So much for the first puzzle raised by the expressions "posthumanity" and "transhumanism". The second puzzle goes deeper and touches the very core of the vision of a "posthuman" future. We can express this puzzle by asking in what exact ways "posthumanity", if it is not a step beyond the limits of the human *species*, is at least a step beyond *human nature* as we know it from the history of mankind up to now. The difficulty is that "human nature" is deeply ambiguous (cf. Bayertz 2003: 137). In one of its principal senses, it refers to the purely "natural" aspects of man in contrast to his cultural and social aspects. "Human nature" in this sense is, inevitably, an abstraction, since we do not know of very many human beings that lived in complete isolation from cultural and social factors, such as the few human beings raised by wolves. Nevertheless, this concept of human nature has a limited function. Whenever we speak of "natural needs", "natural urges", "natural gifts" etc. we usually refer to these purely biological aspects no matter how they can be identified in isolation from cultural factors. "Human nature" in this sense, even if based on pure speculation, has always been important as the image of a kind of human existence unspoiled by cultural factors, such as in Rousseau's construct of the "noble savage".

More often, however, the term "human nature" is used in a broader sense not referring specifically to the purely biological aspects of man but to the sum of his typical features including cultural ones. "Nature" is then used in what has been termed the *formal* sense, the sense in which we can also speak of the nature of artificial objects like hammers, or in which Cicero spoke of the nature of the gods in *De natura deorum*. In this sense, "nature" refers to the essential, necessary or constitutive features of a thing. Taken in this sense, the "nature of man", even on a minimalistic understanding, involves a number of non-biological factors such as the ability to make and to use tools, to use language, to build complex social structures and to regulate his behaviour by a system of internalised norms.

To distinguish between the two principal meanings of "human nature" does not mean that a sharp line can be drawn between "nature" and "nurture", or that there are products of their complex interaction that can be assigned to only one of these factors. Even the cultural phenomena seemingly the farthest removed from man's biological substrate are not independent of his biological make-up and biological ancestry. Think, for example, of scientific curiosity, which originates from the "natural" propensity of young children to explore their surroundings, a tendency shared, during childhood at least, by most other intelligent mammals. Ironically, some of the technologies most fiercely rejected by adherents of a principle of naturalness, such as assisted reproduction, satisfy some of the most "natural" needs of mankind, the need to reproduce. Modern reproductive medicine, however artificial in its means, serves the same purposes as nature in its unconscious regulation of mating behaviour, by choosing the most productive and efficient investment of time and energy in terms of number and health of offspring.

It should be observed that changes in "human nature" in the first sense do not necessarily imply changes in "human nature" in the second sense. This is so because human nature in the second, comprehensive sense can be defined in a way that includes, among others, the perpetual self-modification of man's natural make-up by cultural means. Culture has an impact primarily on *ontogenesis*, on how the biological substratum of man is modified, transformed, developed and differentiated in concrete life. But is has an impact also on *phylogenesis*, e.g. by marriage regulations, by rules that restrict the choice of marriage partners, and by encouraging or discouraging births. The genetic make-up of each generation is as much the result of cultural factors as it is the result of biological factors. Changing the natural substratum of man by cultural factors, either genotypically by determining an individual's genetic make-up, or phenotypically by bringing him up in a given social and cultural framework, is part and parcel of human nature in the second, comprehensive sense.

The consequences of this are evident: If it is true that "man is by nature a cultural animal", man's very nature (in a comprehensive sense) consists, among others, in changing his nature (in the restricted sense). Modifying or transforming his own nature more directly and deliberately by means of technology does not constitute a radical change in human nature taken in its comprehensive sense but affirms this nature. Neither technologies that modify the natural processes of reproduction such as gene technology or reproductive cloning nor technologies that open up new ways of making use of man's natural heritage during his lifetime such as brain chips or artificial organs constitute radical changes in human nature.

This leaves open the question how far the use of technologies that "improve" human functioning must go to justify talk of a "change" of human nature in its comprehensive sense. There does not seem an easy answer because there is no consensus on how human nature in this sense should be defined. While the controversy about the definition of what constitutes human nature in its *biological* sense is a *scientific* controversy involving biologists, anthropologists and psychologists, the controversy about the definition of what constitutes human nature in its *comprehensive* sense is a *cultural* controversy involving philosophers, theologians and educators. While the scientific question of what constitutes human nature can in principle be answered by reference to objective fact, the criteria for answering the cultural question are far less clear. On the backdrop of the long history of philosophical constructions of what constitutes the "essence" of man it may be doubted whether a consensus even on the "key constituents" of human nature (Fukuyama 2002: 173) is at all likely. But only if we have a definition of what this "core" is can we hope to have a criterion by which to tell whether the vision of the "transhumanists" is in fact a vision of a mankind *beyond* humanity, i.e. of a mankind that has left behind, in some way or other, the essentials of the human condition.

The question, then, is, whether there is a definition that on the one hand is sufficiently concrete to serve as a criterion for what is within and what is beyond "human nature" and that is at the same time sufficiently open to be acceptable to both parties. Is there such a definition? A brief look into the options open to us will show that any attempt to find such a definition runs into a dilemma: Either the definition is too unspecific to rule out any transformation man might undergo or impose on himself with the help of present and future technologies, or it is too partisan to be acceptable to all parties. Not surprisingly this dilemma is of the same structure as the dilemma confronting the anthropologist in regard to a biological definition of humanity. Either the defining features are too unspecific to give a satisfactory set of sufficient conditions, or they are too specific to account for the great variety of human life forms.

It is clear that human nature cannot be satisfactorily defined either by the *universal* or by the *specific* properties of man as a species. *Universal* properties like embodiment, mortality or vulnerability are too unspecific to single human nature out from the "natures" of other kinds of animals, and they are unlikely to be transcended even by the wildest posthumanist dreams. Even if the life-span of a "posthuman" humanity exceeds that of present humanity by a considerable time or if their health and safety far exceed ours, "posthumans" will still be embodied, mortal and vulnerable. Nor can the "core" of human nature be defined by what is *specific* to man. Though specific abilities like self-consciousness, elaborated language and a complex morality are likely to be contained in any proposed concept of human nature, these abilities will not exhaust the concept. It will also contain features not exclusively characteristic of mankind, such as emotionality and the ability to establish and to maintain personal relationships. But however this may be, a concept of human nature defined by what is specific for humans will in any case be irrelevant to the controversy. It is unlikely that any transhumanist dream will go beyond a human nature defined by what distinguishes man from other species. These features are too trivial to be of interest.

A better candidate for defining human nature in its comprehensive sense is what is *typical* of man as a biological species. Typical properties will have two features: they will be the properties that are exemplified by *most* people most of the time; and they will be properties to which we attach special *importance*. To be typical of mankind, a property must be frequent enough to constitute a standard of normality. In this sense it is normal that humans have five senses, that they depend, in early childhood, on a longish period of care to develop speech, reflection and moral norms, and that they are liable to infectious diseases. But to be typical of mankind, a property must also be in some way important. It must not only concern minute details of man's biochemistry, say, without an impact on his personal or social life. As a rule, typical properties are neither universal nor specific properties. Sentience and emotionality are both typical human properties, but they are neither universal nor specific. There are human beings born without the capacity to have consciousness, and sensation and cognitively simple emotions are to be found in many other animal species. The same holds for other typical human properties such as the property of belonging to one of the two sexes or to live with a family during childhood.

Can we think of the emancipation from human nature implied by the term "posthumanity" as a process of emancipation from what is *typical* of man as a species?

I think that a positive answer would close the question too early. There are at least two difficulties standing in the way of a wholehearted adoption of this position. The *first* difficulty is the inevitable *historical relativity* of judgements about what is typical of a species reaching indefinitely into the future. Any empirical statement about what constitutes human nature is based on the past history of man and on what we have learnt by inspecting the record of man's performance up to the present. Therefore, any statement about human nature, whether in its biological or in its comprehensive sense, will be highly provisional. Statements about human nature in the biological sense are more adequately interpreted as statements about the biological evolution of man *up to the present*. Statements about human nature in its comprehensive sense are more adequately interpreted as statements about the cultural and social evolution of man *up to the present*. What we now call the biological nature of man is the nature of man as it has evolved through millions of years in a hunter-and-gatherer society. In its biological sense, human nature is, at least to a large extent, stone-age human nature. Analogously, what we judge to be *typical* of man as a cultural being covers only a brief period in man's biological and social evolution. It is a "snapshot" of an open process running through thousands of generations (Fukuyama 2002: 152). In both senses, human nature must be expected to change in the future, though at very a different pace. It is as certain that man's biological nature will change in the far future, as it is certain that man's cultural nature will change in the near future. In the long run, it can be expected to adapt to the then existing environment in the same way as it has adapted to the environment of the Stone Age. On the other hand, what is now thought to be "typical" of man need not be typical of man as he evolves in a future characterised by a steadily growing technological and medical potential. From this perspective, any philosophical claim to the effect that we can judge from our limited experience of man's doings and sufferings what is "typical" of man or what his "essence" is, invites the criticism inherent in Mme. de Staël's dictum that "les philosophes veulent enchaîner le futur".

There are not only epistemological, but also moral risks in the attempt to make past history the standard of human nature. This is so because philosophical statements about human nature are easily given a normative function. "Human nature" is often taken to define what should be regarded as "normal", with the consequence that any feature or behaviour that does not correspond to "human nature" stands in danger of being discriminated against. A famous example in this respect is the traditional justification of discriminatory behaviour against women by reference to their inherently dependent and vulnerable "nature". John Stuart Mill, for one, successfully attacked this justification by pointing out the limited evidence: "What is now called the nature of women is an eminently artificial thing - the result of forced repression in some direction, unnatural stimulation in others" (Mill 1969, vol 21: 276).

One consequence of the historical relativity of "human nature" is that "posthumanity" must correspondingly be interpreted in a thoroughly relativistic sense. If to be "posthuman" means to be without some of the features that are held to be *typical* of the human race, this use of "typical" must be taken to refer to the features that *have been* typical of mankind in the recorded past. "Posthumanism" contains an implicit time-index, referring to a continually changing present as its anchoring-point. "Posthumans" are beyond human nature as it is *now*. They are not beyond human nature period.

Another consequence follows from the fact that the attempt to improve his own nature (together with the attempt to improve the nature of his environment) has been at least one of the typical human features up to now. By changing their human nature, potential "posthumans" will not to change *all* properties typical of mankind as we have known it. At least one typical property will be confirmed and strengthened by the process of self-transformation, namely the second order property of self-transcendence and creativity, the property to assume new and possibly unknown properties.

The *second* difficulty in an identification of human nature with what is typical for humans is that there does not seem to be a culture-independent standard of what is important and what is unimportant. Concepts such as "human nature" or "human normality" presuppose a standard defining what is expected from a "full" or "fully developed" human being against which the non-normal, the deviant and retarded can be identified. There is, however, no unique standard by which "normality" can be judged, especially not in pluralist societies with a variety of moral cultures. There is, on the contrary, a certain variety of "Menschenbilder", each carrying with it its own standard of what is important and normal in a human being. A typically Christian standard will, for example, give human weakness and vulnerability a more prominent place in its conception of "normality" than a humanist conception giving more weight to education, self-discipline and perfectibility. Not surprisingly, we find much more skepticism in regard to "transhumanism" in Christian authors than in humanist authors. For many Christians, any attempt at improvement that is not primarily directed at man's living conditions but at man himself threatens to jeopardise man's vulnerability, weakness and dependence which are held, from a Christian perspective, to be central to human nature. From this point of view, "transhumanism" is in fact what it claims to be: an endeavour to transform human nature. From this point of view, this endeavour at the same time poses a deadly threat. It threatens to lose what is believed to be most important in man and in human existence.

For a secular humanist, on the other hand, the prospect of the gradual self-transformation of human nature is far less bleak. The humanist will have no reason to elevate the human condition as it has presented itself to past generations into an eternal principle and to declare the technological advances of the future as somehow incompatible with "human nature". For him, it is nothing else than the completion of a process that has been going on since the Stone Age and is now gaining additional momentum from the acceleration of technological progress. From this perspective, "posthumanism" is not a threat but a hyperbolic name for the effort at self-perfection that has accompanied mankind from its very beginnings. From this point of view, self-improvement, not only by education but also by technology, is not only in perfect conformity with "human nature". For humanists like John Stuart Mill it was also a kind of obligation. In his essay "Nature" he wrote: "The duty of man is the same in respect to his own nature as in respect to the nature of all other things, namely not to follow but to amend it" (Mill 1969, vol 10: 397). Even if one does not want to go as far as Mill and make self-improvement an obligation (to whom? it may be asked), there is nothing, in the humanist framework, to make the transition from humanity to "posthumanity" inherently problematic. Post- and transhumanism are just parts of humanism.

6.4 Conclusion

The controversy surrounding the terms "posthumanity" and "transhumanism" is mainly a controversy about values. For "transhumanists", "posthumanity" is the positive vision of a future in which certain limits inherent in the human condition as we know it are overcome by means of further advances in science, technology, and medicine. For "bioconservatives" this kind of vision is a threat rather than a promise because they think that the substance of humanity, its "core", will be lost, or at least jeopardised, in the process. Instead of dealing with these substantial ethical issues, this chapter has focused on the conceptual issues raised by the terminology in which this controversy is couched. Its argument has been that there are good reasons to take "posthumanity" and "transhumanism" as slogans rather than as well-defined concepts. First, both expressions are inherently paradoxical if taken literally. They suggest that there is a clear demarcation between what is human and what is non-human whereas not even biology is able to provide a clear demarcation between what is specifically human and what is not. In addition, the concept of humanity is dynamic and not static. In a long-term perspective it is probable that the boundaries of the human species will be extended so that they include technical innovations such as man-machine-hybrids that appear "posthuman" only as long as they are not realised. Second, there is a suggestion in both terms that future technologies will bring about changes in human nature. This suggestion is problematic given the fact that human nature is characterised, among other things, by a systematic openness to cultural changes and modifications. What is now thought to be "typical" of man (and thereby constitutive of man's "essence") need not be thought to be typical of man as he evolves in a future characterised by a steadily growing potential of technological and medical self-modification. From this perspective, "posthumanism" is an unduly hyperbolic (and misleading) name for the next stage in a continued effort at self-perfection that has accompanied mankind from its very beginnings.

References

Alexander S (1927) Space, time, and deity. 2nd edition, vol 2, Macmillan, London
Bayertz K (2003) Human nature: How normative might it be? Journal of Medicine and Philosophy 28: 131–150
Bostrom N (2003) Human genetic enhancements: A transhumanist perspective. Journal of Value Inquiry 37: 493–506
Bostrom N (2005) In defense of posthuman dignity. Bioethics 19: 202–214
Boyd R (1999) Homeostasis, species and higher taxa. In: Wilson R A (ed) Species. New Interdisciplinary Essays. MIT Press, Cambridge
Butler O E (1997) Dawn. Warner Books, New York
Fukuyama F (2002) Our posthuman future. Consequences of the biotechnology revolution. Farrar, Strous & Giroux, New York
Huxley J (1957) New bottles for new wine. Chatto & Windus, London
Kass L R (1997) The wisdom of repugnance. The New Republic 2(6): 17–26
Lewis C S (1943) The abolition of man. Collins, Oxford
Locke J (1961) An essay concerning human understanding. In: Yolton J W (ed) Everyman's Library, London, New York
Mill J S (1969) Collected works of John Stuart Mill. University of Toronto Press, Toronto
President's Council on Bioethics (2003) Beyond therapy. Biotechnology and the pursuit of happiness. Dana, New York/Washington DC
Robert J S, Baylis F (2003) Crossing species boundaries. American Journal of Bioethics 3: 1–13
Silver L M (1997) Remaking Eden: How genetic engineering and cloning will transform the American family. Avon Books, New York
Wells H G (1924) The time machine (The Works of H. G. Wells vol 1). Charles Scribner's Sons, New York

Chapter 7
Why I Want to be a Posthuman when I Grow Up

Nick Bostrom

I am apt to think, if we knew what it was to be an angel for one hour, we should return to this world, though it were to sit on the brightest throne in it, with vastly more loathing and reluctance than we would now descend into a loathsome dungeon or sepulchre[1]

Berkley (1685–1753)

7.1 Introduction

Extreme human enhancement could result in "posthuman" modes of being. After offering some definitions and conceptual clarification, I argue for two theses. First, some posthuman modes of being would be very worthwhile. Second, it could be very good for human beings to become posthuman.

7.2 Setting the Stage

The term "posthuman" has been used in very different senses by different authors.[2] I am sympathetic to the view that the word often causes more confusion than clarity, and that we might be better off replacing it with some alternative vocabulary. However, as the purpose of this paper is not to propose terminological reform but to argue for certain substantial normative theses (which one would naturally search for in the literature under the label "posthuman"), I will instead attempt to achieve intelligibility by clarifying the meaning that I shall assign to the word. Such terminological clarification is surely a minimum precondition for having a meaningful discussion about whether it might be good for us to become posthuman.

---

[1] Berkeley et al. 1897: 172.

[2] The definition used here follows in the spirit of Bostrom (2003). A completely different concept of "posthuman" is used in e.g. Hayles 1999.

B. Gordijn, R. Chadwick (eds.) *Medical Enhancement and Posthumanity*,

I shall define *a posthuman* as a being that has at least one posthuman capacity. By *a posthuman capacity*, I mean a general central capacity greatly exceeding the maximum attainable by any current human being without recourse to new technological means. I will use *general central capacity* to refer to the following:

- *Healthspan* – the capacity to remain fully healthy, active, and productive, both mentally and physically
- *Cognition* – general intellectual capacities, such as memory, deductive and analogical reasoning, and attention, as well as special faculties such as the capacity to understand and appreciate music, humor, eroticism, narration, spirituality, mathematics, etc.
- *Emotion* – the capacity to enjoy life and to respond with appropriate affect to life situations and other people

In limiting my list of general central capacities to these three, I do not mean to imply that no other capacity is of fundamental importance to human or posthuman beings. Nor do I claim that the three capacities in the list are sharply distinct or independent. Aspects of emotion and cognition, for instance, clearly overlap. But this short list may give at least a rough idea of what I mean when I speak of posthumans, adequate for present purposes.

In this paper, I will be advancing two main theses. The first is that some possible posthuman modes of being would be very good. I emphasize that the claim is not that *all* possible posthuman modes of being would be good. Just as some possible human modes of being are wretched and horrible, so too are some of the posthuman possibilities. Yet it would be of interest if we can show that there are some posthuman possibilities that would be very good. We might then, for example, specifically aim to realize those possibilities.

The second thesis is that it could be very good *for us* to become posthuman. It is possible to think that it could be good to be posthuman without it being good *for us* to become posthuman. This second thesis thus goes beyond the first. When I say "good for us", I do not mean to insist that for every single current human individual there is some posthuman mode of being such that it would be good for that individual to become posthuman in that way. I confine myself to making a weaker claim that allows for exceptions. The claim is that for *most* current human beings, there are possible posthuman modes of being such that it could be good for these humans to become posthuman in one of those ways.

It might be worth locating the theses and arguments to be presented here within a broader discourse about the desirability of posthumanity. Opponents of posthumanity argue that we should not seek enhancements of a type that could make us, or our descendants, posthuman. We can distinguish at least five different "levels" on which objections against posthumanity could be launched (Table 7.1).

This paper focuses on levels 3 and 4. I am thus setting aside issues of feasibility, costs, risks, side-effects, and social consequences. While those issues are obviously important when considering what we have most reason to do all things considered, they will not be addressed here.

Table 7.1 Levels of objection to posthumanity

Level 0. "It can't be done"
Objections based on empirical claims to the effect that it is, and will remain, impossible or infeasible to create posthumans.
Level 1. "It is too difficult/costly"
Objections based on empirical claims that attempts to transform humans into posthumans, or to create new posthuman beings, would be too risky, or too expensive, or too psychologically distracting. Concerns about medical side-effects fall into this category, as do concerns that resources devoted to the requisite research and treatment would be taken away from more important areas.
Level 2. "It would be too bad for society"
Objections based on empirical claims about social consequences that would follow from the successful creation of posthuman beings, for example concerns about social inequality, discrimination, or conflicts between humans and posthumans.
Level 3. "Posthuman lives would be worse than human lives"
Objections based on normative claims about the value of posthuman lives compared to human lives.
Level 4. "We couldn't benefit"
Objections based on agent-relative reasons against human beings transforming themselves into posthuman beings or against humans bringing new posthuman beings into existence. Although posthuman lives might be as good as or better than human lives, it would be bad for us to become posthuman or to create posthumans.

Some further terminological specifications are in order. By *a mode of being* I mean a set of capacities and other general parameters of life. A posthuman mode of being is one that includes at least one posthuman capacity.

I shall speak of the value of particular modes of being. One might hold that primary value-bearers are some entities other than modes of being; e.g. mental states, subjective experiences, activities, preference-satisfactions, achievements, or particular lives. Such views are consistent with this paper. The position I seek to defend is consistent with a wide variety of formal and substantive theories of value. I shall speak of the value of modes of being for the sake of simplicity and convenience, but in doing so I do not mean to express a commitment to any particular controversial theory of value.

We might interpret "the values" of modes of beings as proxies for values that would be realized by particular lives instantiating the mode of being in question. If we proceed in this way, we create some indeterminacy. It is possible for a mode of being (and even more so for a *class* of modes of being) to be instantiated in a range of different possible lives, and for some of these lives to be good and others to be bad. In such a case, how could one assign a value to the mode of being itself?

Another way of expressing this concern is by saying that the value of instantiating a particular mode of being is context-dependent. In one context, the value might be high; in another, it might be negative. Nevertheless, it is useful to be able to speak of values of items other than those we accord basic intrinsic value. We might for example say that it is valuable to be in good health and to have some money. Yet neither having good health nor having some money is guaranteed to make a positive difference to the value of your life. There are contexts in which the opposite is true. For instance, it could be the case that because you had some money you got robbed and murdered, or that because you were always in rude health you lacked a particular (short, mild) disease experience that would have transformed your mediocre novel into an immortal masterpiece. Even so, we can say that health and money are good things without thereby implying that they are intrinsically valuable or that they add value in all possible contexts. When we say that they are valuable we might merely mean that these things would *normally* make a positive contribution to the value of your life; they would add value in a very wide range of plausible contexts. This mundane meaning is what I have in mind when I speak of modes of being having a value: i.e., in a very wide range of plausible contexts, lives instantiating that mode of being would tend to contain that value.[3]

A life might be good or bad because of its causal consequences for other people, or for the contribution it makes to the overall value of a society or a world. But here I shall focus on the value that a life has for the person whose life it is: how good (or bad) it is for the subject to have this life. The term "well-being" is often used in this sense.[4]

When I speak of the value of a life here, I do not refer to the moral status of the person whose life it is. It is a separate question what the moral status would be of human and posthuman beings. We can assume for present purposes that human and posthuman persons would have the same moral status. The value of a life refers, rather, to how well a life goes for its subject. Different human lives go differently well, and in this sense their lives have different values. The life of a person who dies from a painful illness at age 15 after having lived in extreme poverty and social isolation is typically worse and has less value than that of a person who has an 80-year-long life full of joy, creativity, worthwhile achievements, friendships, and love. Whatever terminology we use to describe the difference, it is plain that the latter kind of life is more worth having. One way to express this platitude is by

[3] Compare this take on "mundane values" with the notion of mid-level principles in applied ethics. The principle of respecting patient autonomy is important in medical ethics. One might accept this if one holds that respect for patient autonomy is an implication of some fundamental ethical principle. But equally, one might accept patient autonomy as an important mid-level principle even if one merely holds that this is a way of expressing a useful rule of thumb, a sound policy rule, or a derived ethical rule that is true in a world like ours because of various empirical facts even though it is not necessarily true in all possible worlds. For the role of mid-level principles in applied ethics, see e.g. Beauchamp and Childress 2001.

[4] I am thus not concerned here with global evaluations into which individuals' well-being might enter as a factor, e.g. evaluations involving values of diversity, equality, or comparative fairness.

saying that the latter life is more valuable than the former.[5] This is consistent with assigning equal moral status to the two different persons whose lives are being compared.

Some pairs of possible lives are so different that it is difficult – arguably impossible – to compare their value. We can leave aside the question of whether, for every pair of possible lives, it is true either than one is better than the other, or that they are equally good; that is, whether all pairs of possible lives have commensurable value. We shall only assume that at least for some pairs of possible lives, one is definitely better than the other.

To supply our minds with a slightly more concrete image of what becoming posthuman might be like, let us consider a vignette of how such a process could unfold.

7.3 Becoming Posthuman

Let us suppose that you were to develop into a being that has posthuman healthspan and posthuman cognitive and emotional capacities. At the early steps of this process, you enjoy your enhanced capacities. You cherish your improved health: you feel stronger, more energetic, and more balanced. Your skin looks younger and is more elastic. A minor ailment in your knee is cured. You also discover a greater clarity of mind. You can concentrate on difficult material more easily and it begins making sense to you. You start seeing connections that eluded you before. You are astounded to realize how many beliefs you had been holding without ever really thinking about them or considering whether the evidence supports them. You can follow lines of thinking and intricate argumentation farther without losing your foothold. Your mind is able to recall facts, names, and concepts just when you need them. You are able to sprinkle your conversation with witty remarks and poignant anecdotes. Your friends remark on how much more fun you are to be around. Your experiences seem more vivid. When you listen to music you perceive layers of structure and a kind of musical logic to which you were previously oblivious; this gives you great joy. You continue to find the gossip magazines you used to read amusing, albeit in a different way than before; but you discover that you can get more out of reading Proust and *Nature*. You begin to treasure almost every moment of life; you go about your business with zest; and you feel a deeper warmth and affection for those you love, but you can still be upset and even angry on occasions where upset or anger is truly justified and constructive.

As you yourself are changing you may also begin to change the way you spend your time. Instead of spending four hours each day watching television, you may

[5] I do not assume that the value of a life, or well-being, supervenes on the mental experiences of a person, nor that it supervenes on a thin time-slice of a person's life. It could represent a wider and more global evaluation of how well a person's life is going.

now prefer to play the saxophone in a jazz band and to have fun working on your first novel. Instead of spending the weekends hanging out in the pub with your old buddies talking about football, you acquire new friends with whom you can discuss things that now seem to you to be of greater significance than sport. Together with some of these new friends, you set up a local chapter of an international non-profit to help draw attention to the plight of political prisoners.

By any reasonable criteria, your life improves as you take these initial steps towards becoming posthuman. But thus far your capacities have improved only within the natural human range. You can still partake in human culture and find company to engage you in meaningful conversation. Consider now a more advanced stage in the transformation process....

You have just celebrated your 170th birthday and you feel stronger than ever. Each day is a joy. You have invented entirely new art forms, which exploit the new kinds of cognitive capacities and sensibilities you have developed. You still listen to music – music that is to Mozart what Mozart is to bad Muzak. You are communicating with your contemporaries using a language that has grown out of English over the past century and that has a vocabulary and expressive power that enables you to share and discuss thoughts and feelings that unaugmented humans could not even think or experience. You play a certain new kind of game which combines VR-mediated artistic expression, dance, humor, interpersonal dynamics, and various novel faculties and the emergent phenomena they make possible, and which is more fun than anything you ever did during the first 100 years of your existence. When you are playing this game with your friends, you feel how every fiber of your body and mind is stretched to its limit in the most creative and imaginative way, and you are creating new realms of abstract and concrete beauty that humans could never (concretely) dream of. You are always ready to feel with those who suffer misfortunes, and to work hard to help them get back on their feet. You are also involved in a large voluntary organization that works to reduce suffering of animals in their natural environment in ways that permit ecologies to continue to function in traditional ways; this involves political efforts combined with advanced science and information processing services. Things are getting better, but already each day is fantastic.

As we seek to peer farther into posthumanity, our ability to concretely imagine what it might be like trails off. If, aside from extended healthspans, the essence of posthumanity is to be able to have thoughts and experiences that we cannot readily think or experience with our current capacities, then it is not surprising that our ability to imagine what posthuman life might be like is very limited. Yet we can at least perceive the outlines of some of the nearer shores of posthumanity, as we did in the imaginary scenario above. Hopefully such thought experiments are already enough to give plausibility to the claim that becoming posthuman could be good for us.

In the next three sections we will look in a little more detail at each of the three general central capacities that I listed in the introduction section. I hope to show that the claim that it could be very good to be posthuman is not as radical as it might appear to some. In fact, we will find that individuals and society already in some ways seem to be implicitly placing a very high value on posthuman capacities – or at least, there are strong and widely accepted tendencies pointing that way.

I therefore do not regard my claim as in any strong sense revisionary. On the contrary, I believe that the denial of my claim would be strongly revisionary in that it would force us to reject many commonly accepted ethical beliefs and approved behaviors. I see my position as a conservative extension of traditional ethics and values to accommodate the possibility of human enhancement through technological means.

7.4 Healthspan

It seems to me fairly obvious why one might have reason to desire to become a posthuman in the sense of having a greatly enhanced capacity to stay alive and stay healthy.[6] I suspect that the majority of humankind already has such a desire implicitly.

People seek to extend their healthspan, i.e. to remain healthy, active, and productive. This is one reason why we install air bags in cars. It may also explain why we go to the doctor when we are sick, why higher salaries need to be paid to get workers to do physically dangerous work, and why governments and charities give money to medical research.[7] Instances of individuals sacrificing their lives for the sake of some other goal, whether suicide bombers, martyrs, or drug addicts, attract our attention precisely because their behavior is unusual. Heroic rescue workers who endanger their lives on a dangerous mission are admired because we assume that they are putting at risk something that most people would be very reluctant to risk, their own survival.

For some three decades, economists have attempted to estimate individuals' preferences over mortality and morbidity risk in labor and product markets. While the tradeoff estimates vary considerably between studies, one recent meta-analysis puts the median value of the value of a statistical life for prime-aged workers to about $7 million in the United States (Viscusi & Aldy 2003). A study by the EU's Environment Directorates-General recommends the use of a value in the interval €0.9–€3.5 million (Johansson 2002). Recent studies by health economists indicate that improvements in the health status of the U.S. population over the 20th century have made as large a contribution to raising the standards of living as all other forms of consumption growth combined (Murphy & Topel 2003; Nordhaus 2003). While the exact numbers are debatable, there is little doubt that most people place a very high value on their continued existence in a healthy state.

---

[6] Having such a capacity is compatible with also having the capacity to die at any desired age. One might thus desire a capacity for greatly extended healthspan even if one doubts that one would wish to live for more than, say, 80 years. A posthuman healthspan capacity would give one the option of much longer and healthier life, but one could at any point decide no longer to exercise the capacity.

[7] Although on the last item, see Hanson (2000) for an alternative view.

Admittedly, a desire to extend one's healthspan is not necessarily a desire to become posthuman. To become posthuman by virtue of healthspan extension, one would need to achieve the capacity for a healthspan that greatly exceeds the maximum attainable by any current human being without recourse to new technological means. Since at least some human beings already manage to remain quite healthy, active, and productive until the age of 70, one would need to desire that one's healthspan were extended greatly beyond this age in order that it would count as having a desire to become posthuman.[8]

Many people will, if asked about how long they would wish their lives to be, name a figure between 85 and 90 years (Cohen & Langer 2005). In many cases, no doubt, this is because they assume that a life significantly longer than that would be marred by deteriorating health – a factor from which we must abstract when considering the desirability of healthspan extension. People's stated willingness to pay to extend their life by a certain amount does in fact depend strongly on the health status and quality of that extra life (Johnson et al. 1998). Since life beyond 85 is very often beset by deteriorating health, it is possible that this figure substantially underestimates how long most people would wish to live if they could be guaranteed perfect health.

It is also possible that a stated preference for a certain lifespan is hypocritical. Estimates based on revealed preferences in actual market choices, such as fatality risk premiums in labor markets or willingness to pay for health care and other forms of fatality risk reduction might be more reliable. It would be interesting to know what fraction of those who claim to have no desire for healthspan extension would change their tune if they were ever actually handed a pill that would reliably achieve this effect. My conjecture would be that when presented with a real-world choice, most would choose the path of prolonged life, health, and youthful vigor over the default route of aging, disease, and death.

One survey asked: "Based on your own expectations of what old age is like, if it were up to you, how long would you personally like to live – to what age?" Only 27% of respondents said they would like to live to 100 or older (Cohen & Langer 2005). A later question in the same survey asked: "Imagine you could live to 100 or older, but you'd have to be very careful about your diet, exercise regularly, not smoke, avoid alcohol, and avoid stress. Would it be worth it, or not?" To this, 64% answered in the affirmative! Why should *more* people want to live beyond 100 when restrictions on activity are imposed? Is it because it frames the question more as if it were a real practical choice rather than as an idle mind game? Perhaps when the question is framed as a mind game, respondents tend to answer in ways which they believe expresses culturally approved attitudes, or which they think signal socially desirable personal traits (such as having "come to terms" with one's own mortality), while this tendency is diminished when the framing suggests a practical choice with real consequences. We do not know for sure, but this kind of anomaly suggests that we should not take people's stated "preferences"

[8] At least one human, Jeanne Calment, lived to 122. But although she remained in relatively fair health until close to her death, she clearly suffered substantial decline in her physical (and presumably mental) vigor compared to when she was in her 20s. She did not retain the capacity to be *fully* healthy, active, and productive for 122 years.

about how long they would wish to live too seriously, and that revealed preferences might be a more reliable index of their guiding values.

It is also worth noting that only a small fraction of us commit suicide, suggesting that our desire to live is almost always stronger than our desire to die.[9] Our desire to live, *conditional on our being able to enjoy full health*, is even stronger. This presumption in favor of life is in fact so strong that if somebody wishes to die soon, even though they are seemingly fully healthy, with a long remaining healthy life expectancy, and if their external circumstances in life are not catastrophically wretched, we would often tend suspect that they might be suffering from depression or other mental pathology. Suicidal ideation is listed as a diagnostic symptom of depression by the American Psychiatric Association.[10]

Even if a stated preference against healthspan extension were sincere, we would need to question how well considered and informed it is. It is of relevance that those who know most about the situation and are most directly affected by the choice, namely the elderly, usually prefer life to death. They usually do so when their health is poor, and overwhelmingly choose life when their health is at least fair. Now one can argue that a mentally intact 90-year-old is in a better position to judge how their life would be affected by living for another year than she was when she was 20, or 40. If most healthy and mentally intact 90-year-olds prefer to live for another year (at least if they could be guaranteed that this extra year would be one of full health and vigor), this would be evidence against the claim that it would be better for these people that their lives end at 90.[11] Similarly, of course, for people of even older age.

One can compare this situation with the different case of somebody becoming paraplegic. Many able-bodied people believe that their lives would not be worth living if they became paraplegic. They claim that they would prefer to die rather than continuing life in a paraplegic state. Most people who have actually become paraplegic, however, find that their lives are worth living.[12] People who are paraplegic are typically better judges of whether paraplegic lives are worth continuing than are people who have never experienced what it is like to be paraplegic. Similarly, people who are 90 years old are in a better position to judge whether their lives are worth continuing than are younger people (including themselves at any earlier point in their lives).[13]

One study assessed the will to live among 414 hospitalized patients aged 80–98 years, presumably representing the frailer end of the distribution of the "old old".

[9] For some, the reluctance to commit suicide might reflect a desire not to kill oneself rather than a desire not to die, or alternatively a fear of death rather than an authentic preference not to die.

[10] DSM-IV (American Psychiatric Association 2000).

[11] This is a kind of Millian best-judge argument. However, if fear of death were irrational, one could argue that people who are closer to death are on average worse judges of the value for them of an extra year of life, because their judgments would tend to be more affected by irrational fear.

[12] This basic result is reflected in many chronic disease conditions (Ubel et al. 2003). The discrepancy of attitudes seems to be due to non-patient's failure to realize the extent to which patients psychologically adapt to their condition (Damschroder et al. 2005).

[13] The analogy with paraplegia is imperfect in at least one respect: when the issue is healthspan extension, we are considering whether it would be worth living an extended life in perfect health and vigor. If anything, this discrepancy strengthens the conclusion, since it is more worth continuing living in perfect health than in poor health, not less worth it.

40.8% of respondents were unwilling to exchange any time in their current state of health for a shorter life in excellent health, and 27.8% were willing to give up at most 1 month of 12 in return for excellent health (Tsevat et al. 1998).[14] (Patients who were still alive one year later were even less inclined to give up life for better health, but with continued large individual variations in preferences.) The study also found that patients were willing to trade significantly less time for a healthy life than their surrogates assumed they would.

Research shows that life-satisfaction remains relatively stable into old age. One survey of 60,000 adults from 40 nations discovered a slight upward trend in life-satisfaction from the 20s to the 80s in age (Diener & Suh 1998). Life satisfaction showed this upward trend even though there was some loss of positive affect. Perhaps life-satisfaction would be even higher if positive affect were improved (a possibility we shall discuss in a later section). Another study, using a cross-sectional sample (age range 70–103 years), found that controlling for functional health constraints reversed the direction of the relationship between age and positive affect and produced a negative association between age and negative affect (Kunzmann et al. 2000). These findings suggest that some dimensions of subjective well-being, such as life-satisfaction, do not decline with age but might actually increase somewhat, and that the decline in another dimension of subjective well-being (positive affect) is not due to aging per se but to health constraints.

Most people reveal through their behavior that they desire continued life and health,[15] and most of those who are in the best position to judge the value of continued healthy life, at any age, judge that it is worth having. This constitutes prima facie support for the claim that extended life is worth having even when it is not fully healthy. The fact that this holds true at all currently realized ages suggests that it is not a strongly revisionary view to hold that it could be good for many people to become posthuman through healthspan extension. Such a view might already be implicitly endorsed by many.

7.5 Cognition

People also seem to be keen on improving cognition. Who wouldn't want to remember names and faces better, to be able more quickly to grasp difficult abstract ideas, and to be able to "see connections" better? Who would seriously object to being able to appreciate music at a deeper level? The value of optimal cognitive functioning is so obvious that to elaborate the point may be unnecessary.[16]

---

[14] See also McShine et al. 2000. For a methodological critique, see Arnesen and Norheim 2003.

[15] This is fully consistent with the fact that many people knowingly engage in risky behaviors such as smoking. This might simply mean that they are unable to quit smoking, or that they desire the pleasure of smoking more than they desire a longer healthier life. It does not imply that they do not desire longer healthier life.

[16] One might even argue that a desire for cognitive improvement is a constitutive element of human rationality, but I will not explore that hypothesis here.

This verdict is reflected in the vast resources that society allocates to education, which often explicitly aims not only to impart specific items of knowledge but also to improve general reasoning abilities, study skills, critical thinking, and problem solving capacity.[17] Many people are also keen to develop various particular talents that they may happen to have, for example musical or mathematical, or to develop other specific faculties such as aesthetic appreciation, narration, humor, eroticism, spirituality etc. We also reveal our desire for improving our cognitive functioning when take a cup of coffee to increase our alertness or when we regret our failure to obtain a full night's sleep because of the detrimental effects on our intellectual performance.

Again, the fact that there is a common desire for cognitive improvement does not imply that there is a common desire for becoming posthuman. To want to become posthuman through cognitive improvement, one would have to want a great deal of cognitive improvement. It is logically possible that each person would only want to become slightly more intelligent (or musical, or humorous) than he or she currently is and would not want any very large gain. I will offer two considerations regarding this possibility.

First, it seems to me (based on anecdotal evidence and personal observations) that people who are already endowed with above-average cognitive capacities are at least as eager, and, from what I can tell, actually *more* eager to obtain further improvements in these capacities than are people who are less talented in these regards. For instance, someone who is musically gifted is likely to spend more time and effort trying to further develop her musical capacities than is somebody who lacks a musical ear; and likewise for other kinds of cognitive gifts.

This phenomenon may in part reflect the external rewards that often accrue to those who excel in some particular domain. An extremely gifted musician might reap greater rewards in terms of money and esteem from a slight further improvement in her musicality than would somebody who is not musically gifted to begin with. That is, the difference in external rewards is sometimes greater for somebody who goes from very high capacity to outstandingly high capacity than it is for somebody who goes from average capacity to moderately high capacity. However, I would speculate that such differences in external rewards are only part of the explanation and that people who have high cognitive capacities are usually also more likely (or at least no less likely) to desire further increases in those capacities than are people of lower cognitive capacities even when only the intrinsic benefits of capacities are considered. Thus, if we imagine a group of people placed in solitary confinement for the remainder of their lives, but with access to books, musical instruments, paints and canvasses, and other prerequisites for the exercise of capacities, I would hypothesize that those with the highest pre-existing capacity in a given domain would be more likely (or at least not less likely) to work hard to further develop their capacities in that domain, for the sake of the intrinsic benefits that the possession and exercise of those capacities bestow, than would those with

[17] U.S. *public* expenditure on education in 2003 was 5.7% of its GDP (World Bank 2003).

lower pre-existing capacities in the same domain.[18] While $100 brings vastly less utility to a millionaire than to a pauper, the marginal utility of improved cognitive capacities does not seem to exhibit a similar decline.

These considerations suggest that there are continuing returns in the "intrinsic" (in the sense of non-instrumental, non-positional) utility of gains in cognitive capacities, at least within the range of capacity that we find instantiated within the current human population.[19] It would be implausible to suppose that the current range of human capacity, in all domains, is such that while increments of capacity within this range are intrinsically rewarding, yet any further increases outside the current human range would lack intrinsic value. Again, we have a prima facie reason for concluding that enhancement of cognitive capacity to the highest current human level, and probably beyond that, perhaps up to and including the posthuman level, would be intrinsically desirable for the enhanced individuals. We get this conclusion if we assume that those who have a certain high capacity are generally better judges of the value of having that capacity or of a further increment of that capacity than are those who do not possess the capacity in question to the same degree.

7.6 Emotion

It is straightforward to determine what would count as an enhancement of healthspan. We have a clear enough idea of what it means to be healthy, active, and productive, and the difference between this state and that of being sick, incapacitated, or dead. An enhancement of healthspan is simply an intervention that prolongs the duration of the former state. It is more difficult to define precisely what would count as a cognitive enhancement because the measure of cognitive functioning is more multifaceted, various cognitive capacities can interact in complex ways, and it is a more normatively complex problem to determine what combinations of particular cognitive competences are of value in different kinds of environments. For instance, it is not obvious what degree of tendency to forget certain kinds of facts and experiences is desirable. The answer might depend on a host of contextual factors. Nevertheless, we do have some general idea of how we might value various increments or decrements in many aspects of our cognitive functioning – a sufficiently clear idea, I suggest, to make it intelligible without much explanation what one might mean by phrases like "enhancing musical ability", "enhancing abstract reasoning ability" etc.

---

[18] Complication: if high capacity were solely a result from having spent a lot of effort in developing that capacity, then the people with high capacity in some domain might be precisely those that started out having an unusually strong desire for having a strong capacity in that domain. It would then not be surprising that those with high capacity would have the strongest desire for further increases in capacity. Their stronger desire for higher capacity might then not be the result of more information and better acquaintance with what is at stake, but might instead simply reflect a prior inclination.

[19] It would be more difficult to determine whether the marginal intrinsic utility of gains in capacity are constant, or diminishing, or increasing at higher levels of capacity, and if so by what amount.

It is considerably more difficult to characterize what would count as emotional enhancement. Some instances are relatively straightforward. Most would readily agree that helping a person who suffers from persistent suicidal depression as the result of a simple neurochemical imbalance so that she once again becomes capable of enjoyment and of taking an interest in life would be to help her improve her emotional capacities. Yet beyond cases involving therapeutic interventions to cure evident psychopathology it is less clear what would count as an enhancement. One's assessment of such cases often depends sensitively on the exact nature of one's normative beliefs about different kinds of possible emotional constitutions and personalities.

It is correspondingly difficult to say what would constitute a "posthuman" level of emotional capacity. Nevertheless, people often do strive to improve their emotional capacities and functioning's. We may seek to reduce feelings of hate, contempt, or aggression when we consciously recognize that these feelings are prejudiced or unconstructive. We may take up meditation or physical exercise to achieve greater calm and composure. We may train ourselves to respond more sensitively and empathetically to those we deem deserving of our trust and affection. We may try to overcome fears and phobias that we recognize as irrational, or we may wrestle with appetites that threaten to distract us from what we value more. Many of us expend life-long effort to educate and ennoble our sentiments, to build our character, and to try to become better people. Through these strivings, we seek to achieve goals involving modifying and improving our emotional capacities.

An appropriate conception of emotional capacity would be one that incorporates or reflects these kinds of goal, while allowing perhaps for there being a wide range of different ways of instantiating "high emotional capacity", that is to say, many different possible "characters" or combinations of propensities for feeling and reacting that could each count as excellent in its own way. If this is admitted, then we could make sense of emotional enhancement in a wide range of contexts, as being that which makes our emotional characters more excellent. A posthuman emotional capacity would be one which is much more excellent than that which any current human could achieve unaided by new technology.

One might perhaps question whether there are possible emotional capacities that would be *much* more excellent than those attainable now. Conceivably, there might be a maximum of possible excellence of emotional capacity, and those people who currently have the best emotional capacities might approach so closely to this ideal that there is not enough potential left for improvement to leave room for a posthuman realm of emotional capacity. I doubt this, because aside from the potential for fine-tuning and balancing the various emotional sensibilities we already have, I think there might also be entirely new psychological states and emotions that our species has not evolved the neurological machinery to experience, and some of these sensibilities might be ones we would recognize as extremely valuable if we became acquainted with them.

It is difficult intuitively to understand what such novel emotions and mental states might be like. This is unsurprising, since by assumption we currently lack the required neurological bases. It might help to consider a parallel case from within the normal range of human experience. The experience of romantic love is something that many of us place a high value on. Yet it is notoriously difficult for a child or a prepubescent teenager to comprehend the meaning of romantic love or why adults should make so much fuss about this experience. Perhaps we are all currently in the situation of children relative to the emotions, passions, and mental states that posthuman beings could experience. We may have no idea of what we are missing out on until we attain posthuman emotional capacities.

One dimension of emotional capacity that we can imagine enhanced is subjective well-being and its various flavors: joy, comfort, sensual pleasures, fun, positive interest and excitement. Hedonists claim that pleasure is the only intrinsic good, but one need not be a hedonist to appreciate pleasure as one important component of the good. The difference between a bleak, cold, horrid painful world and one that is teeming with fun and exciting opportunities, full of delightful quirks and lovely sensations, is often simply a difference in the hedonic tone of the observer. Much depends on that one parameter.

It is an interesting question how much subjective well-being could be enhanced without sacrificing other capacities that we may value. For human beings as we are currently constituted, there is perhaps an upper limit to the degree of subjective well-being that we can experience without succumbing to mania or some other mental unbalance that would prevent us from fully engaging with the world if the state were indefinitely prolonged. But it might be possible for differently constituted minds to have experiences more blissful than those that humans are capable of without thereby impairing their ability to respond adequately to their surroundings. Maybe for such beings, gradients of pleasure could play a role analogous to that which the scale ranging between pleasure and pain has for us (Pearce 2004). When thinking the possibility of *posthumanly happy* beings, and their psychological properties, one must abstract from contingent features of the human psyche. An experience that would consume us might perhaps be merely "spicy" to a posthuman mind.

It is not necessary here to take a firm stand on whether posthuman levels of pleasure are possible, or even on whether posthuman emotional capacities more generally are possible. But we can be confident that, at least, there is vast scope for improvements for most of individuals in these dimensions because even within the range instantiated by currently exiting humans, there are levels of emotional capacities and degrees of subjective well-being that, for most of us, are practically unattainable to the point of exceeding our dreams. The fact that such improvements are eagerly sought by many suggests that if posthuman levels were possible, they too would be viewed as highly attractive.[20]

[20] The quest for subjective well-being, in particular, seems to be a powerful motivator for billions of people even though arguably none of the various means that have been attempted in this quest has yet proved very efficacious in securing the goal (Brickman & Campbell 1971).

7.7 Structure of the Argument, and Further Supporting Reasons

It might be useful to pause briefly to reflect on the structure of the argument presented so far. I began by listing three general central capacities (healthspan, cognition, and emotion), and I defined a posthuman being as one who has at least one of these capacities in a degree unattainable by any current human being unaided by new technology.

I offered some plausibility arguments suggesting that it could be highly desirable to have posthuman levels of these capacities. I did this partly by clarifying what having the capacities would encompass and by explaining how some possible objections would not apply because they rely on a misunderstanding of what is proposed. Furthermore, I tried to show that for each of the three capacities we find that many individuals actually desire to develop the capacities to higher levels and often undertake great effort and expense to achieve these aims. This desire is also reflected in social spending priorities, which devote significant resources to e.g. healthspan-extending medicine and cognition-improving education. Significantly, at least in the cases of healthspan extension and cognitive improvement, the persons best placed to judge the value and desirability of incremental improvements at the high end of the contemporary human capacity distribution seem to be especially likely to affirm the desirability of such additional improvements of capacity. For many cognitive faculties, it appears that the marginal utility of improvements *increases* with capacity levels. This suggests that improvements beyond the current human range would also viewed as desirable when evaluated by beings in a better position to judge than we currently are.

That people desire X does not imply that X is desirable. Nor does the fact that people find X desirable, even when this judgment is shared among those who are in the best position to judge the desirability of X, prove that X is desirable or valuable. Even if one were to assume some version of a dispositional theory of value, it does not follow from these premises that X is valuable. A dispositional theory of value might assert something like the following:

> X is valuable for A if and only if A would value X if A were perfectly rational, perfectly well-informed, and perfectly acquainted with X.[21]

The people currently best placed to judge the desirability for an individual of enhancement of her general central capacities are neither perfectly rational, nor perfectly well-informed, nor perfectly acquainted with the full meaning of such enhancements. If these people were more rational or obtained more information or became better acquainted with the enhancements in question, they would perhaps no longer value the enhancements. Even if everybody judged becoming posthuman as desirable, it is a logical possibility that becoming posthuman is not valuable, even given a theory of value that defines value in terms of valuing-dispositions.

---

[21] See e.g. Lewis 1989.

The argument presented in the preceding sections is not meant to be deductive. Its ambition is more modest: to remind us of the plausibility of the view that (1) enhancements along the three dimensions discussed are possible in principle and of significant potential intrinsic value, and (2) enhancements along these dimensions large enough to produce posthuman beings could have very great intrinsic value. This argument is defensible. One way in which it could be defeated would be by pointing to further information, rational reasoning, or forms of acquaintance, not accounted for by current opinion, and which would change current opinion if it were incorporated. Critics could for example try to point to some reasoning mistake that very old people commit when they judge that it would be good for them to live another year in perfect health. However, I think the considerations I have pointed to provide prima facie evidence for my conclusions.

There are other routes by which one could reach the position that I have advocated, which supports the above arguments. For instance, one might introspect one's own mind to determine whether being able to continue to live in good health longer, being able better to understand the world and other people, or being able more fully to enjoy life and to react with appropriate affect to life events would seem like worthwhile goals for oneself if they were obtainable (see e.g. Bostrom 2005). Alternatively, one might examine whether having these capacities to an enhanced or even posthuman degree could enable one to realize states and life paths that would have great value according to one's favorite theory of value. (To me, both these tests deliver affirmative verdicts on (1) and (2).)

Yet another route to making the foregoing conclusions plausible is by considering our current ignorance and the vastness of the as-yet unexplored terrain. Let S_H be the "space" of possible modes of being that could be instantiated by someone with current human capacities. Let S_P be the space of possible modes of being that could be instantiated by someone with posthuman capacities. In an intuitive sense, S_P is enormously much larger than S_H. There is a larger range of possible life courses that could be lived out during a posthuman lifespan than during a human lifespan. There are more thoughts that could be thought with posthuman cognitive capacities than with human capacities (and more musical structures that could be created and appreciated with posthuman musical capacities etc.). There are more mental states and emotions that could be experienced with posthuman emotional faculties than with human ones. So why, apart from a lack of imagination, should anybody suppose that the S_H already contains all the most valuable and worthwhile modes of being?

An analogy: For as long as anybody remembers, a tribe has lived in a certain deep and narrow valley. They rarely think of what lies outside their village, and on the few occasions when they do, they think of it only as a mythical realm. One day a sage who has been living apart from the rest, on the mountainside, comes down to the village. He explains that he has climbed to the top of the mountain ridge and from there he could see the terrain stretching far away, all the way to the horizon. He saw plains, lakes, forests, winding rivers, mountains, and the sea. Would it not be reasonable, he says, in lieu of further exploration, to suppose that this vast space is likely to be home to natural resources of enormous value? – Similarly, the sheer size and diversity of S_p is in itself a prima facie reason for thinking that it is likely to contain some very great values (Bostrom 2004).

7.8 Personal Identity

Supposing the previous sections have succeeded in making it plausible that being a posthuman could be good, we can now turn to a further question: whether becoming posthuman could be good *for us*. It may be good to be Joseph Haydn. Let us suppose that Joseph Haydn had a better life than Joe Bloggs so that in some sense it is better to be Haydn and living the life that Haydn lived than to be Bloggs and living Bloggs' life. We may further suppose that this is so from Bloggs' evaluative standpoint. Bloggs might recognize that on all the objective criteria which he thinks makes for a better mode of being and a better life, Haydn's mode of being and life are better than his own. Yet it does not follow that it would be good for Bloggs to "become" Haydn (or to become some kind of future equivalent of Haydn) or to live Haydn's life (or a Haydn-like life). There are several possible reasons for this which we need to examine.

First, it might not be possible for Bloggs to become Haydn without ceasing to be Bloggs. While we can imagine a thought experiment in which Bloggs' body and mind are gradually transformed into those of Haydn (or of a Haydn-equivalent), it is not at all clear that personal identity could be preserved through such a transformation. If Bloggs' personal identity is essentially constituted by some core set of psychological features such as his memories and dispositions, then, since Haydn does not have these features, the person Bloggs could not become a Haydn-equivalent. Supposing that Bloggs has a life that is worth living, any transformation that causes the person Bloggs to cease to exist might be bad for Bloggs, including one that transforms him into Haydn.

Could a current human become posthuman while remaining the same person, or is the case like the one of Bloggs becoming Haydn, the person Bloggs necessarily ceasing to exist in the process? The case of becoming posthuman is different in an important respect. Bloggs would have to lose all the psychological characteristics that made him person Bloggs in order to become Haydn. In particular, he would have to lose all his memories, his goals, his unique skills, and his entire personality would be obliterated and replaced by that of Haydn. By contrast, a human being could retain her memories, her goals, her unique skills, and many important aspects of her personality even as she becomes posthuman. This could make it possible for personal identity to be preserved during the transformation into posthuman.[22]

[22] See also DeGrazia 2005. DeGrazia argues that identity-related challenges to human enhancement largely fails, both ones based on considerations of personal identity and ones based on narrative identity (authenticity), although he mainly discusses more moderate enhancements than those I focus on in this paper.

It is obvious that personal identity could be preserved, at least in the short run, if posthuman status is achieved through radical healthspan enhancement. Suppose that I learnt that tonight after I go to bed, a scientist would perform some kind of molecular therapy on my cells while I'm sleeping to permanently disable the aging processes in my body. I might worry that I would not wake up tomorrow because the surgery might go wrong. I would *not* worry that I might not wake up tomorrow because the surgery succeeded. Healthspan enhancement would help *preserve* my personal identity. (If the psychological shock of discovering that my life-expectancy had been extended to a thousand years were so tremendous that it would completely remold my psyche, it is possible that the new me would not be the same person as the old me. But this is not a necessary consequence.[23])

Walter Glannon has argued that a lifespan of 200 years or more would be undesirable because personal identity could not be persevered over such a long life (Glannon 2002). Glannon's argument presupposes that personal identity (understood here as a determinant of our prudential concerns) depends on psychological connectedness. On this view, we now have prudential interests in a future time segment of our organism only if that future time segment is psychologically connected to the organism's present time segment through links of backward-looking memories and forward-looking projects and intentions. If a future time segment of my brain will not remember anything about what things are like for me now, and if I now have no projects or intentions that extend that far into the future, then that future time segment is not part of my person. Glannon asserts that these psychological connections that hold us together as persons could not extend over 200 years or so.

There are several problems with Glannon's argument, even if we accept his metaphysics of personal identity. There is no reason to think it impossible to have intentions and projects that range over more than 200 years. This would seem possible even with our current human capacities. For example, I can easily conceive of exciting intellectual and practical projects that may take me many hundreds of years to complete. It is also dubious to assume that a healthy future self several hundred years older than I am now might would be unable remember things from current life stage. Old people often remember their early adulthood quite well, and it is not clear that these memories always decline significantly over time. And of course, the concern about distant future stages being unable to remember their earlier stages disappears completely if we suppose that enhancements of memory capacity becomes available.[24] Furthermore, if Glannon was right, it would follow that it is "undesirable" for a small child to grow up, since adults do not remember

[23] It is not even a psychologically plausible consequence even within the limitations of current human psychology. Compare the case to that of a man on death row who has a remaining life-expectancy of 1 day. An unexpected pardon suddenly extends this to 40 years – an extension by a factor of 14,610! He might be delighted, stunned, or confused, but he does not cease to exist as a person. If he did, it would presumably be *bad* for him to be pardoned. Even if one believed (erroneously in my view) that mortality or aging were somehow essential features of the persons we are, these features are consistent with vastly extended healthspan.

[24] It is clear that in order for an *extremely* long life to not become either static or self-repeating, it would be necessary that mental growth continues.

what it was like to be a small child and since small children do not have projects or intentions that extend over time spans as long as decades. This implication would be counterintuitive. It is more plausible that it can be desirable for an agent to survive and continue to develop, rather than to die, even if psychological connections eventually become attenuated. In the same way, it could be desirable for us to acquire the capacity to have a posthuman healthy lifespan, even if we could not remain the same person over time scales of several centuries.

The case that personal identify could be preserved is perhaps less clear-cut with regard to radical cognitive or emotional enhancement. Could a person become radically smarter, more musical, or come to possess much greater emotional capacities without ceasing to exist? Here the answer might depend more sensitively on precisely which changes we are envisaging, how those changes would be implemented, and on how the enhanced capacities would be used. The case for thinking that both personal identity and narrative identity would be preserved is arguably strongest if we posit that (a) the changes are in the form of addition of new capacities or enhancement of old ones, without sacrifice of preexisting capacities; and (b) the changes are implemented gradually over an extended period of time; (c) each step of the transformation process is freely and competently chosen by the subject; and (d) the new capacities do not prevent the preexisting capacities from being periodically exercised; (e) the subject retains her old memories and many of her basic desires and dispositions; (f) the subject retains many of her old personal relationships and social connections; and (g) the transformation fits into the life narrative and self-conception of the subject. Posthuman cognitive and emotional capacities could in principle be acquired in such a way that these conditions are satisfied.

Even if not all the conditions (a)–(g) were fully satisfied in some particular transformation process, the normatively relevant elements of a person's (numerical or narrative) identity could still be *sufficiently* preserved to avoid raising any fundamental identity-based objection to the prudentiality of undergoing such a transformation. We should not use a stricter standard for technological self-transformation than for other kinds of human transformation, such as migration, career change, or religious conversion.

Consider again a familiar case of *radical* human transformation: maturation. You currently possess vastly greater cognitive capacities than you did as an infant. You have also lost some capacities, e.g. the ability to learn to speak a new language without an accent. Your emotional capacities have also changed and developed considerably since your babyhood. For each concept of identity which we might think has relevant normative significance – personal (numerical) identity, narrative identity, identity of personal character, or identity of core characteristics – we should ask whether identity in that sense has been preserved in this transformation.

The answer may depend on exactly how we understand these ideas of identity. For each of them, on a sufficiently generous conception of the identity criteria, identity was completely or in large part preserved through your maturation. But then we would expect that identity in that sense would also be preserved in many other transformations, including the ones that are *no more profound* as that of a child growing into an adult; and this would include transformations that would make you posthuman. Alternatively, we might adopt conceptions that impose more stringent criteria for the preservation of identity. On these conceptions, it might be impossible to become posthuman without wholly or in large part disrupting one form of identity or another. However, on such restrictive conceptions, identity would also be disrupted in the transformation of child into adult. Yet we do not think it is bad for a child to grow up. Disruptions of identity in those stringent senses form part of a normal life experience and they do not constitute a disaster, or a misfortune of any kind, for the individual concerned.

Why then should it bad for a person to continue to develop so that she one day matures into a being with posthuman capacities? Surely it is the other way around. If this had been our usual path of development, we would have easily recognized the failure to develop into a posthuman as a misfortune, just as we now see it as a misfortune for a child to fail to develop normal adult capacities.

Many people who hold religious beliefs are already accustomed to the prospect of an extremely radical transformation into a kind of posthuman being, which is expected to take place after the termination of their current physical incarnation. Most of those who hold such a view also hold that the transformation *could* be very good for the person who is transformed.

7.9 Commitments

Apart from the concern about personal identity, there is a second kind of reason why it might be bad for a Bloggs to become a Haydn. Bloggs might be involved in various projects, relationships, and may have undertaken commitments that he could not or would not fulfill if he became Haydn. It would be bad for Bloggs to fail in these undertakings if they are important to him. For example, suppose that Mr. Bloggs is deeply committed to Mrs. Bloggs. His commitment to Mrs. Bloggs is so strong that he would never want to do anything that contravenes any of Mrs. Bloggs' most central preferences, and one of her central preferences is that Mr. Bloggs not become posthuman. In this case, even though becoming posthuman might in some respects be good for Mr. Bloggs (it would enable him to understand more, or to stay healthy longer, etc.) it might nevertheless be bad for him all things considered as it would be incompatible with fulfilling one of the commitments that are most important to him.[25]

This reason for thinking that it might be bad for a person to become posthuman relies on the assumption that it can be very bad for a person to forfeit on

---

[25] We may include under this rubric any "commitments to himself" that Mr. Bloggs might have. For example, if he has a firm and well-considered desire not to become posthuman, or if he has solemnly sworn to himself never to develop any posthuman capacities, then it could perhaps on grounds of these earlier desires or commitments be bad for Mr. Bloggs to become posthuman.

commitments that would be impossible to fulfill as a posthuman.[26] Even if we grant this assumption, it does not follow that becoming a posthuman would necessarily be bad for us. We do not generally have commitments that would be impossible to fulfill as posthumans. It may be impossible for Mr. Bloggs to become posthuman without violating his most important commitment (unless, of course, Mrs. Bloggs should change her mind), but his is a special case.

Some humans do not have any commitments of importance comparable to that of Mr. Bloggs to his wife. For such people the present concern does not apply. But even for many humans who do have such strong commitments, becoming posthuman could still be good for them. Their commitments could still be fulfilled if they became posthuman. This is perhaps clearest in regard to our commitments to projects and tasks: most of these we could complete – indeed we could complete them better and more reliably – if we obtained posthuman capacities. But even with regard to our specific commitments to people, it would often be possible to fulfill these even if we had much longer healthspans or greatly enhanced cognitive or emotional capacities.

7.10 Ways of Life

In addition to concerns about personal identity and specific commitments to people or projects, there is a third kind of reason one might have for doubting that it could be good for us to become posthuman. This third kind of reason has to do with our interpersonal relations more broadly, and with the way that the good for a person can be tied to the general circumstances and conditions in which she lives. One might think that the very concept of a good life for a human being is inextricably wound up in the idea of flourishing within a "way of life" – a matrix of beliefs, relationships, social roles, obligations, habits, projects, and psychological attributes outside of which the idea of a "better" or "worse" life or mode of being does not make sense.

The reasoning may go something like this: It would not be good for a clover to grow into a rhododendron, nor for a fly to start looking and behaving like a raven. Neither would it, on this view, be good for a human to acquire posthuman capacities and start living a posthuman life. The criterion for how well a clover is doing is the extent to which it is succeeding in realizing its own particular nature and achieving the natural "telos" inherent in the clover kind; and the equivalent might be said of the fly. For humans, the case may be more complicated as there is a greater degree

[26] One may also hold that a person in Mr. Bloggs' situation has additional reasons for not becoming posthuman that don't rely on it being worse for him to become posthuman. For instance, he might have moral reasons not to become posthuman even if it would be good for him to become one. Here I am concerned with the question whether it would necessarily be bad *for* Bloggs to become posthuman, so any moral reasons he might have for declining the transition would only be relevant insofar as they would make the outcome worse *for Mr. Bloggs*.

of relevant individual variation among humans than among other species. Different humans are pursuing different "ways of life", so that what counts as flourishing for one human being might differ substantially from what counts as such for another. Nevertheless, as we are all currently pursuing human ways of life, and since what is good for us is defined by reference to our way of life, it is not the case for any human that it would be good for her to become posthuman. It might be good for posthumans to be posthumans, but it would not be good for humans to become posthuman.

This third concern seems to be a conglomerate of the two concerns we have already discussed. Why could it not be good for a human to become posthuman? One possible reason is if her personal identity could not be preserved through such a transformation. The comparison with the clover appears to hint at this concern. If a clover turned into a rhododendron, then the clover would presumably cease to exist in the process. If a fly started looking and behaving like a raven, would it still be a fly? So part of what is going on here seems to be that the assertion that the relevant form of identity could not be preserved in the transformations in question. But we have already addressed this concern insofar as it pertains to humans becoming posthuman.

There might be more at stake with this third concern than identity. The problem with a clover becoming a rhododendron is not just that the clover might cease to exist in the process, but that it seems a mistake to think that being a rhododendron is in any sense better than being a clover. There might be external criteria of evaluation (such as economic or aesthetic value to the human owner) according to which a rhododendron is better or more valuable than a clover. But aside from such extrinsic considerations, the two plants seem to be on a par: a thriving clover thrives just as much as a thriving rhododendron, so if the good for a plant is to thrive then neither kind is inherently better off or has a greater potential for realizing a good life than the other. Our challenger could claim that the same holds vis-à-vis a human and a posthuman.

I think the analogy is misleading. People are not plants, and the concept of a valuable mode of being for a person is fundamentally different from that of the state of flourishing for a plant. In a metaphorical sense we can ascribe interests to plants and other non-sentient objects: this clover "could use" some water; that clock "needs" winding up; the squeaky wheel "would benefit" from a few drops of oil. Defining interests relative to a functionalist basis might be the only way we can make sense of these attributions. The function of the clock is to indicate the time, and without being wound up the clock would fail to execute this function; thus it "needs" to be wound up. Yet sentient beings may have interests not only in a metaphorical sense, based on their function, but in a quite literal sense as well, based on what would be normatively good for them. A human being, for example, might have interests that are defined (partially) in terms of what she is actually interested in, or would be interested in given certain conditions.[27] So from the fact that we

---

[27] Compare the dispositional theories of value, discussed above.

could not make sense of the claim that it would be good for a clover to become a rhododendron, it does not follow that we would similarly be unable to make sense of the claim that it would be good for a human to become a posthuman. Even if the successful execution of "the function" of a human were not facilitated by becoming posthuman, there would be other grounds on which one could sensibly attribute to a human an interest in becoming posthuman.

It is at any rate highly problematic that something as complex and autonomous as a human being has any kind of well-defined "function". The problem remains even if we relativize the function to particular ways of life or particular individuals. We might say that the function of the farmer is to farm, and that of the singer is to sing, etc. But any particular farmer is a host of other things as well: e.g. a singer, a mother, a sister, a homeowner, a driver, a television watcher, and so forth *ad infinitum*. Once she might have been a hairdresser; in the future she might become a shopkeeper, a golfer, a person with a disability, a transsexual, or a posthuman. It is difficult to see how any strong normative conclusions could be drawn from the fact that she currently occupies a certain set of roles and serves a certain set of functions. At most we could conclude that when and insofar as she acts as a farmer, she ought to tend to her crops or livestock; but from the fact that she is a farmer, nothing follows about whether she ought to be or remain a farmer. Likewise, the most we could conclude from the fact that she is currently a human person is that she ought to do things that are good for humans – brush her teeth, sleep, eat, etc. – but only so long as she remains human. If she became a posthuman who did not need to sleep, she would no longer have any reason so sleep. And the fact that she currently has a reason to sleep is not a reason for her not to become a sleepless posthuman.

At this point, an objector could attempt an alternative line of argumentation. Maybe there are some crucial interests that we have that are not conditional on us occupying particular social roles or having particular personal characteristics or serving particular functions. These interests would be unlike our interest in sleep, which does not provide us with a reason not to change in such a way that we no longer need to sleep. Rather these unconditional ("categorical") interests would be such as to give us reason not to change in ways that would make us no longer have those interests.

I have already admitted that individuals can have such interests, and in some cases this might make it the case for some possible individuals that it would not be good for them to become posthuman. I discussed this above as the "second concern". This is not a problem for my position since it is compatible with it being true for other individuals (and perhaps for the overwhelming majority or even all actual human persons) that it could be good for them to become posthuman. But our hypothetical objector might argue that there are certain categorical interests we all have *qua* humans. These interests would somehow derive from human nature and from the natural ends and ideals of flourishing inherent in this essential nature. Might not the existence of such universally shared categorical human interests invalidate the thesis that it could be good for us to become posthuman?

7.11 Human Nature

Let us consider two different candidate ideas of what a human "telos" might be. If we seek a telos for human individuals within a naturalistic outlook, one salient candidate would be the maximization of that individual's inclusive fitness. Arguably, the most natural way to apply a functional characterization of a human individual from an evolutionary perspective is as an inclusive fitness maximizer (tuned for life in our ancestral environment). From this perspective, our legs, our lungs, our sense of humor, our parental instincts, our sex drive and romantic propensities subserve the ultimate function of promoting the inclusive fitness of an individual. Now if we define the telos of a human individual in this way, as vehicle for the effective promulgation of her genes, then many of the seemingly most attractive posthuman possibilities would be inconsistent with our successfully realizing this alleged telos, in particular those possibilities that involve radical alteration of the human genome. (Replacing our genes with other genes does not seem to be an effective way to promulgate the genes we have.)

As a conception of the human good, however, the telos of maximizing inclusive fitness is singularly lacking in plausibility. I do not know of any moral philosopher who advocates such a view. It is too obvious that what is good for a person can, and usually does, diverge from what would maximize that person's inclusive fitness.[28] Those who attempt to derive a theory of the human good from the telos inherent in a conception of human functioning will need to start from some conception of human functioning other than the evolutionary one.

One starting point that has had more appeal is the doctrine that a human being is essentially a rational animal and that the human telos is the development and exercise of our rational faculties. Views of this sort have a distinguished pedigree that can be traced back at least to Aristotle. Whatever the merits of this view, however, it is plainly not a promising objection to the claims I advance in this paper, since it would be perfectly possible for a posthuman to realize a telos of rationality as well as a human being could. In fact, if what is good for us is to develop and exercise our rational nature, this implies that it would be good for us to become posthumans with appropriately enhanced cognitive capacities (and preferably with extended healthspan too, so that we may have more time to develop and enjoy these rational faculties).

One sometimes hears it said that it is human nature to attempt to overcome every limit and to explore, invent, experiment, and use tools to improve the human condition.[29] I don't know that this is true. The opposite tendency seems to be at least as

---

[28] For example, for a contemporary man the life plan that would maximize inclusive fitness might be to simply donate as much sperm to fertility clinics as possible.

[29] The quest for posthuman capacities is as old as recorded history. In the earliest preserved epic, the Sumerian *Epic of Gilgamesh* (approx. 1700 B.C.), a king sets out on a quest for immortality. In later times, explorers sought the Fountain of Youth, alchemists labored to concoct the Elixir of Life, and various schools of esoteric Taoism in China strove for physical immortality by way of control over or harmony with the forces of nature. This is in addition to the many and diverse religious traditions in which the hope for a supernatural posthuman existence is of paramount importance.

strong. Many a great invention was widely resisted at the time of its introduction, and inventors have often been viciously persecuted. If one wished to be provocative, one might even say that humanity has advanced technologically *in spite of anti-technological tendencies in human nature*, and that technological advancement historically has been due more to the intrinsic utility of technological inventions and the competitive advantages they sometimes bestow on their users than to any native preference among the majority of mankind for pushing boundaries and welcoming innovation.[30] Be that as it may; for even if it were "part of human nature" to push ever onward, forward, and upward, I do not see how anything follows from this regarding the desirability of becoming posthuman. There is too much that is thoroughly unrespectable in human nature (along with much that is admirable), for the mere fact that X is a part of human nature to constitute any reason, even a prima facie reason, for supposing that X is good.

7.12 Brief Sketches of Some Objections and Replies

Objection: One might think that it would be bad for a person to be the only posthuman being since a solitary posthuman would not have any equals to interact with.

Reply: It is not necessary that there be only one posthuman.

I have acknowledged that capacities may not have basic intrinsic value and that the contribution to well-being that having a capacity makes depends on the context. I suggested that it nevertheless makes sense to talk of the value of a capacity in a sense similar to that in which we commonly talk of the value of e.g. money or health. We can take such value ascriptions as assertions that the object or property *normally* makes a positive contribution to whatever has basic value. When evaluating posthuman attributes, the question arises what we should take to be the range of circumstances against which we assess whether something "normally" makes a positive contribution. As we do not have a concrete example in front of us of a posthuman civilization, there is a certain indeterminacy in any assertion about which things or attributes would "normally" make a positive contribution in a posthuman context. At this point, it may therefore be appropriate to specify some aspects of the posthuman context that I assume in my value-assertions. Let me here postulate that the intended context is one that includes a society of posthuman beings.

What dialectical constraints are there on what I am allowed to stipulate about the posthuman context? The main cost to making such stipulations is that if I end up defining a gerrymandered "posthuman context", which is also extremely unlikely

[30] As J.B.S. Haldane wrote: "The chemical or physical inventor is always a Prometheus. There is no great invention, from fire to flying, which has not been hailed as an insult to some god. But if every physical and chemical invention is a blasphemy, every biological invention is a perversion. There is hardly one which, on first being brought to the notice of an observer from any nation which has not previously heard of their existence, would not appear to him as indecent and unnatural" (Haldane 1924).

ever to materialize, then the significance of any claims about what would normally be valuable in that context would tend to wane. It is simply not very interesting to know what would "normally" be valuable in some utterly bizarre context defined by a large number of arbitrary stipulations. I do not think that by postulating a society of posthumans I am significantly hollowing out my conclusions. I do, in fact, assume throughout this paper more generally that the postulated posthuman reference society is one that is adapted to its posthuman inhabitants in manners similar to the way current human society is adapted to its human inhabitants.[31] I also assume that this reference society would offer many affordances and opportunities to its posthuman inhabitants broadly analogous to those which contemporary society offers humans. I do not intend by this postulation to express any prediction that this is the kind of posthuman society that is most likely to form, nor do I mean to imply that being a posthuman could not be valuable even outside of the context of such a kind of society. The postulation is merely a way of delimiting the claims I am trying to defend in this paper.

Objection: The accumulated cultural treasures of humanity might lose their appeal to somebody whose capacities greatly exceeded those of the humans who produced them. More generally, challenges that seemed interesting to the person while she was still human might become trivial and therefore uninteresting to her when she acquires posthuman capacities. This could deprive posthumans of the good of meaningful achievements.

Reply: It is not clear why the ability to appreciate what is more complex or subtle should make it impossible to appreciate simpler things. Somebody who has learnt to appreciate Schoenberg may still delight in simple folk songs, even bird songs. A fan of Cézanne may still enjoy watching a sunrise.

Even if it were impossible for posthuman beings to appreciate some simple things, they could compensate by creating new cultural riches. I am assuming that the reference society would offer opportunities for doing this – see above.

If some challenges become too easy for posthumans, they could take on more difficult challenges. One might argue that an additional reason for developing posthuman cognitive capacities is that it would increase the range of interesting intellectual challenges open to us. At least within the human range of cognitive capacity, it seems that the greater one's capacity, the more numerous and meaningful the intellectual projects that one can embark on. When one's mind grows, not only does one get better at solving intellectual problems – entirely new possibilities of meaning and creative endeavor come into view.

Objection: A sense of vulnerability, dependence, and limitedness can sometimes add to the value of a life or help a human being grow as a person, especially along moral or spiritual dimensions.

Reply: A posthuman could be vulnerable, dependent, and limited. A posthuman could also be able to grow as a person in moral and spiritual dimensions without those extrinsic spurs that are sometimes necessary to affect such growth in humans.

---

[31] But I do not assume that the reference society would only contain posthuman beings.

The ability to spontaneously develop in these dimensions could be seen as an aspect of emotional capacity.

Objection: The very desire to overcome one's limits by the use of technological means rather than through one's own efforts and hard work could be seen as expressive of a failure to open oneself to the unbidden, gifted nature of life, or as a failure to accept oneself as one is, or as self-hate.[32]

Reply: This paper makes no claims about the expressive significance of a desire to become posthuman, or about whether having such a desire marks one as a worse person, whether necessarily or statistically. The concern here rather is about whether being posthuman could be good, and whether it could be good for us to become posthuman.

Objection: A capacity obtained through a technological shortcut would not have the same value as one obtained through self-discipline and sacrifice.

Reply: I have argued that the possession of posthuman capacities could be extremely valuable even were the capacities are effortlessly obtained. It is consistent with what I have said that achieving a capacity through a great expenditure of blood, sweat, and tears would further increase its value. I have not addressed what would be the *best* way of becoming posthuman. We may note, however, that is unlikely that we *could* in practice become posthuman other than via recourse to advanced technology.

Objection: The value of achieving a goal like winning a gold medal in the Olympics is reduced and perhaps annulled if the goal is achieved through inappropriate means (e.g. cheating). The value of possessing a capacity likewise depends on how the capacity was acquired. Even though having posthuman capacities might be extremely valuable if the capacities had been obtained by appropriate means, there are no humanly possible means that are appropriate. Any means by which humans could obtain posthuman capacities would negate the value of having such capacities.

Reply: The analogy with winning an Olympic medal is misleading. It is in the nature of sports competitions that the value of achievement is intimately connected with the process by which it was achieved. We may say that what is at stake in the analogy is not really the value of a medal, nor even the value of winning a medal, but rather (something like) winning the medal by certain specified means in a fair competition, in a non-fluke-like way, etc. Many other goods are not like this. When we visit the doctor in the hope of getting well, we do not usually think that the value of getting well is strongly dependent on the process by which health is achieved; health and the enjoyment of health are valuable in their own right, independently of how these states come about. Of course, we are concerned with the value of the means to getting well – the means themselves can have negative value (involving perhaps pain and inconvenience), and in evaluating the value of the consequences of an action, we take the value of the means into account as well as the value of the goal that they achieve. But usually, the fact that some means have negative value does not reduce the value of obtaining the goal state.

---

[32] Compare Sandel 2004, although it is not clear that Sandel has an expressivist concern in mind.

One possible exception to this is if the means are in a certain sense *immoral*. We might think that a goal becomes "tainted", and its value reduced, if it was achieved through deeply immoral means. For example, some might hold that the value of medical findings obtained by Nazi doctors in concentration camps have reduced or no value because of the way the findings were produced. Yet this radical kind of "taint" is a rather special case.[33] Having to use bad means might be good reason not to pursue a goal, but *typically* this is not because the use of bad means would reduce the value of the attainment of the goal, but rather it is either because the means themselves have more negative value than the goal has positive value, or (on a non-consequentialist view) because it is morally impermissible to use certain means independently of the total value of the consequences.[34]

The values that I have alleged could be derived from posthuman capacities are not like the value of an Olympic gold medal, but rather like the value of health. I am aware of no logical, metaphysical, or "in principle" reason why humans could not obtain posthuman capacities in ways that would avoid recourse to immoral means of the sort that would "taint" the outcome (much less that would taint the outcome to such a degree as to annul its extremely high surplus value). It is a further question to what extent it is *practically feasible* to work towards realizing posthuman capacities in ways that avoid such taint. This question lies outside the scope of the present paper. My conclusion may therefore be understood to implicitly contain the proviso that the posthuman capacities of which I speak have been obtained in ways that are non-Faustian.

Objection: Posthuman talent sets the stage for posthuman failure. Having great potential might make for a great life if the potential is realized and put to some worthwhile use, but it could equally make for a tragic life if the potential is wasted. It is better to live well with modest capacities than to life poorly with outstanding capacities.

Reply: We do not lament that a human is born talented on grounds that it is possible that she will waste her talent. It is not clear why posthuman capacity would be any more likely to be wasted than human capacity. I have stipulated that the

[33] Even in the Nazi doctor example, it is plausibly the *achievement* of the doctors (and of Germany etc.) that is tainted, and the *achievement's* value that is reduced. The value of the *results* is arguably unaffected, although it might always be appropriate to feel uncomfortable when employing them, appropriate to painfully remember their source, regret the way we got them, and so forth.

[34] It might help to reflect that we do not deny the value of our current human capacities on grounds of their evolutionary origin, even though this origin is (a) largely not a product of human achievement, and (b) fairly drenched in violence, deceit, and undeserved suffering. People who are alive today also owe their existence to several thousands of years of warfare, plunder, and rape; yet this does not entail that our capacities or our mode of existence is worthless. Another possibility is that the result has positive value X, the way you get it has negative value Y, but the "organic whole" comprising both the result and the way it was obtained has an independent value of its own, Z, which also might be negative. On a Moorean view, the value of this situation "on the whole" would be $X + Y + Z$, and this might be negative even if X is larger than $(-Y)$ (Moore 1903). Alternatively, Z might be incommensurable with $X + (-Y)$. In either case, we have a different situation than the one described above in the text, since here X could invariant under different possible ways in which the result was obtained. However, I do not know of any reason to think that this evaluative situation, even if axiologically possible, would necessarily obtain in the sort of case we are discussing. (I'm indebted to Guy Kahane for this point.)

posthuman reference society would offer affordances and opportunities to its posthuman inhabitants broadly analogous to those that contemporary society offers humans. If posthumans are more prone to waste their potential, it must therefore be for internal, psychological reasons. But posthumans need not be any worse than humans in regard to their readiness to make the most of their lives.[35]

7.13 Conclusion

I have argued, first, that some posthuman modes of being would be extremely worthwhile; and, second, that it could be good for most human beings to become posthuman.

I have discussed three general central capacities – healthspan, cognition, and emotion – separately for most of this paper. However, some of my arguments are strengthened if one considers the possibility of combining these enhancements. A longer healthspan is more valuable when one has the cognitive capacity to find virtually inexhaustible sources meaning in creative endeavors and intellectual growth. Both healthspan and cognition are more valuable when one has the emotional capacity to relish being alive and to take pleasure in mental activity.

It follows trivially from the definition of "posthuman" given in this paper that we are not posthuman at the time of writing. It does not follow, at least not in any obvious way, that a posthuman could not also remain a human being. Whether or not this is so depends on what meaning we assign to the word "human". One might well take an expansive view of what it means to be human, in which case "posthuman" is to be understood as denoting a certain possible type of human mode of being – if I am right, an exceedingly worthwhile type.[36]

References

American Psychiatric Association (2000) Diagnostic Criteria from DSM-IV-TR. American Psychiatric Association, Washington, DC

Arnesen T M, Norheim O F (2003) Quantifying quality of life for economic analysis: time out for time trade off. Medical Humanities 29(2): 81–86

Beauchamp T L, Childress J F (2001) Principles of Biomedical Ethics. Oxford University Press, New York

[35] If they have enhanced emotional capacity, they may be *more* motivated and more capable than most humans of realizing their potential in beautiful ways.

[36] I am grateful to Ross Beaton, Bert Gordijn, Guy Kahane, Toby Ord, David Pearce, David Rodin, Anders Sandberg, Julian Savulescu, Harrosh Shlomit, and Elena Patigo Solana for helpful comments. Earlier versions of this paper were presented at the James Martin Advanced Research Seminar (Oxford, 30 January 2006), and at the Institute for Science, Innovation and Society (Nijmegen, 21 February 2006).

Berkeley G, Sampson G et al. (1897) The Works of George Berkeley DD, Bishop of Cloyne. G Bell, London
Bostrom N (2003) The transhumanist FAQ: v 2.1. World Transhumanist Association. Available from http://transhumanism.org/index.php/WTA/faq
Bostrom N (2004) Transhumanist Values. In: Adams F (ed) Ethical Issues for the 21st Century. Philosophical Documentation Center Press, Charlottesville, VA
Bostrom N (2005) The Fable of the Dragon-Tyrant. Journal of Medical Ethics 31(5): 273–277
Brickman P, Campbell D T (1971) Hedonic Relativism and Planning the Good Society. In: Apley M H (ed) Adaptation Level Theory: A Symposium. Academic, New York: 287–302
Cohen J, Langer G (2005) Most Wish for a Longer Life - Despite Broad Aging Concerns. ABC News/USA Today Poll. Available from http://abcnews.go.com/images/Politics/995a1Longevity.pdf
Damschroder L J, Zikmund-Fisher B J et al. (2005) The impact of considering adaptation in health state valuation. Social Science & Medicine 61(2): 267–277
DeGrazia D (2005) Enhancement technologies and human identity. Journal of Medicine and Philosophy 30: 261–283
Diener E, Suh E M (1998) Subjective well-being and age: an international analysis. Annual Review of Gerontology and Geriatrics 17: 304–324
Glannon W (2002) Identity, prudential concern, and extended lives. Bioethics 16(3): 266–83
Haldane J B S (1924) Daedalus; or, Science and the Future. K Paul, Trench, Trubner, London
Hanson R (2000) Showing that You Care: The Evolution of Health Altruism. Available from http://hanson.gmu.edu/showcare.pdf
Hayles N K (1999) How we became posthuman: virtual bodies in cybernetics, literature, and informatics. University of Chicago Press, Chicago, IL
Johansson P O (2002) On the definition and age-dependency of the value of a statistical life. Journal of Risk and Uncertainty 25(3): 251–263
Johnson F R, Desvousges W H et al. (1998) Eliciting stated health preferences: an application to willingness to pay for longevity. Medical Decision Making 18(2): 57–67
Kunzmann U, Little T et al. (2000) Is age-related stability of subjective well-being a paradox? Cross-sectional and longitudinal evidence from the Berlin Aging Study. Psychology and Aging 15(3): 511–426
Lewis D (1989) Dispositional Theories of Value. Proceedings of the Aristotelian Society, supp63: 113–137
McShine R, Lesser G T et al. (2000) Older Americans hold on to life dearly. British Medical Journal 320(7243): 1206–1207
Moore G E (1903) Principia Ethica. Cambridge University Press, Cambridge
Murphy K, Topel R (2003) The Economic Value of Medical Research. Measuring the Gains from Medical Research: An Economic Approach. University of Chicago Press, Chicago, IL
Nordhaus W (2003) The Health of Nations: The Contribution of Improved Health to Living Standards. Measuring the Gains from Medical Research: An Economic Approach. University of Chicago Press, Chicago, IL
Pearce D (2004) The Hedonistic Imperative. Available from http://www.hedweb.com/hedab.htm
Sandel M (2004) The case against perfection. The Atlantic Monthly: 293(3)
Tsevat J, Dawson N V et al. (1998) Health values of hospitalized patients 80 years or older. Jama-Journal of the American Medical Association 279(5): 371–375
Ubel P A, Loewenstein G et al. (2003) Whose quality of life? A commentary exploring discrepancies between health state evaluations of patients and the general public. Quality of Life Research 12(6): 599–607
Viscusi W K, Aldy J E (2003) The value of a statistical life: a critical review of market estimates throughout the world. Journal of Risk and Uncertainty 27(1): 5–76
World Bank (2003) EdStats - The World Bank's Comprehensive Database of Education Statistics. 2006. Available from http://www1.worldbank.org/education/edstats/index.html

Chapter 8
What is the Good of Transhumanism?[1]

Charles T. Rubin

8.1 Introduction

Broadly speaking, transhumanism is a movement seeking to advance the cause of post-humanity. It advocates using science and technology for a reconstruction of the human condition sufficiently radical to call into question the appropriateness of calling it "human" anymore. While there is not universal agreement among transhumanists as to the best path to this goal, the general outline is clear enough. Advances in genetic engineering, artificial intelligence, robotics and nanotechnology will make possible the achievement of the Baconian vision of "the relief of man's estate," as they allow us to conquer disease, eliminate unhappiness, end scarcity and postpone, perhaps indefinitely, death itself. But fulfilling such long-standing dreams is only the beginning of what our new powers will make possible. Left to itself, the present trajectory of technological development necessarily aims at a future incomprehensible to beings such as we are – at no distant date an evolutionary leap in the way intelligence is embodied, and what it can accomplish. Transhumanism seeks to make sure no atavistic scruple obstructs this momentum, and to maximize its benefits and minimize its admitted risks.

While there is no lack of illuminating print works advocating transhumanism, that its public face should be on the World Wide Web is as much a matter of course as once would have been the use by similar movements of the printed broadside or the public lecture. On the websites of the World Transhumanist Association (www.transhumanism.org) and the Extropy Institute (www.extropy. org) – premier among transhumanism's many organizations – one finds authoritative statements explaining and justifying the transhumanist project. If transhumanism were primarily an academic school or a professional association, it would not be entirely fair to turn to these admittedly popular presentations for a critical look at the transhumanist vision. But as these are the documents by which transhumanism presents itself to the public as a movement, and through which it hopes to gain adherents, it is legitimate to make

[1] The author wishes to thank the Scaife Foundation for its support of this research, along with Leslie Rubin, Steve Balch, Tom Short, Bert Gordijn and Ruth Chadwick for their intellectual and/or editorial assistance.

B. Gordijn, R. Chadwick (eds.) *Medical Enhancement and Posthumanity*,

them the primary, though not exclusive, focus of this analysis of transhumanism's vision of the way things ought to be.

This chapter will argue that however rhetorically effective it might be for transhumanism to present its opponents as obscurantists, the real debate between transhumanism and its thoughtful critics is not about further developments in science and technology *per se* but about the substantive goals for which science and technology will be employed. While at first glance transhumanism appears to aim at increasing health and wealth and extending life, a deeper look shows that the promise to reconstruct humanity necessarily will change the meaning behind these familiar aims in ways we cannot necessarily now comprehend. That ignorance is covered over by transhumanism's belief in diversity, a belief that proves to be perfectly consistent with human extinction. But the willingness to support diverse modes of not being human over being human ultimately illustrates a nihilistic aspect of transhumanist norms.

8.2 Progress, Competition and Restraint

Transhumanism advocates progress in scientific research and technological development, and reason as a foundation for both. Max More's "Principles of Extropy (3.11)" explains, "Extropy entails strongly affirming the value of science and technology" (More 2003: Section 4). The second of the substantive six parts of Nick Bostrom's "The Transhumanist FAQ: A General Introduction (2.1)" is about "Technologies and Projections," the ways in which cryonics, nanotechnology, genetic engineering, artificial intelligence and virtual reality will advance transhumanist goals (Bostrom 2003b: 7–19). The human condition can be improved through "applied reason" (Bostrom 2003b: 4). Thus, following Francis Bacon's early lead, the knowledge achieved through the use of reason is valued as a means to further ends. We want to know what these up and coming technologies are "good for" (Bostrom 2003b: 7).

The instrumental good of reason has important consequences with respect to the other side of the coin – the critical stance transhumanism takes against those it often calls "Bioluddites," people who make efforts to restrict developments in certain areas of science and technology because of fears about how they will be used (Hughes 2004: *passim*). While the indignation deployed against such efforts might make one think that transhumanists were standing up on behalf of reason and knowledge for its own sake, and therefore under all circumstances, that is not simply true. Transhumanists acknowledge that scientific and technological reason could produce frightening outcomes; "the gravest existential risks facing us in the coming decades," the FAQ say, "will be of our own making" (Bostrom 2003b: 22). But transhumanism makes what amounts to a prudential judgement that the best way of dealing with such risks is by anticipating them and creating the proper conditions for their avoidance or minimization. Generally that means that the very technologies that will pose the risks are the ones we will also have to rely on to reduce them. Thus, for example, we can anticipate that genetic engineering might create the possibility of weaponised disease outbreaks. But we will need to rely on genetic engineering to produce cures or prophylactic measures. If "we" (however defined) choose to restrain relevant research, that will only leave us vulnerable to those who choose not to restrain themselves. Indeed, "we" had best be sure that we are well ahead of "them" in our abilities. Similarly, if nanotechnology can be imagined to have attractive commercial possibilities, "we" will lose market share to "them," or encourage a black market, if "we" operate under restrictions that "they" don't (Naam 2005: 39).

This arms race logic is central to transhumanism's effort to invest so far only imagined technologies and their consequences with an aura of inevitability. It is a powerful argument, and in the real world cannot be ignored. Yet while it certainly suggests the difficulty of control and restraint of technological development, it does not prove its impossibility or undesirability. It abstracts from difficult but necessary questions about restricting access to information and techniques even in a world where, on balance, we want research and development to be reasonably free. As a result, if it proves anything it proves too much, as Ray Kurzweil – a major intellectual ally of transhumanism – must have realized when he was moved to write a joint editorial with Bill Joy – a major critic – against the decision to publish the genome of the virus that caused the 1918 flu pandemic (Kurzweil & Joy: 2005).

Freedom of research and development does not always have to mean the widest dissemination of all results; that something has a market does not always mean it should be freely marketed. Restraint of development is more plausible the larger the "we" among whom there is a consensus grows and the more there is effective enforcement, social and/or legal, of that norm. This point is acknowledged when the FAQ speak on behalf of "expanding the rule of law to the international plane" (Bostrom 2003b: 33). Bostrom adds, "Global security is the most fundamental and nonnegotiable requirement of the transhumanist project" (Bostrom 2003a: Section 4). While such statements are quite vague (if the transhumanist project must wait on global security it could wait a very long time indeed), they suggest that at least all transhumanists are not advocating the anarchy under which the arms race logic is most compelling.

While some will use enforcement costs and lack of complete success at enforcing restraint as an argument for removing it altogether, that is an argument that can be judged on its particular merits – even when the risks of enforcement failures are extremely great. The fact that nuclear non-proliferation efforts have not been entirely successful has not yet created a powerful constituency for putting plans for nuclear weapons on the Web, and allowing free sale of the necessary materials. In the event, transhumanists, like "Bioluddites," want to make distinctions between legitimate and illegitimate uses of "applied reason," even if as we will see they want to minimize the number of such distinctions because, as we will note later, they see diversity as a good. Of course, those who want to restrict some technological developments likewise look to some notion of the good. This disagreement about goods is the important one, untouched by "Bioluddite" name-calling. The mom-and-apple-pie defense of reason, science and technology one finds in transhumanism is rhetorically useful, within the framework of modern societies which have already bought into this way of looking at the world, to lend a sense of familiarity and necessity to arguments that are designed eventually to lead in very unfamiliar directions. But it is secondary to ideas of what these enterprises are good for, to which we now turn, and ultimately to questions about the foundation on which transhumanist ideas of the good are built.

8.3 Health, Happiness and Longevity

Transhumanism sees the good of scientific research and technological development in their proven ability to facilitate wealthier, healthier, longer and happier lives. "Principles of Extropy" says, "Science and technology are essential to eradicate constraints on lifespan, intelligence, personal vitality, and freedom" (More 2003: Section 1). As stated in the FAQ, transhumanism is "The intellectual and cultural movement that affirms the possibility and desirability of fundamentally improving the human condition through applied reason, especially by developing and making widely available technologies to eliminate aging and to greatly enhance human intellectual, physical, and psychological capacities" (Bostrom 2003b: 4). As "Principles of Extropy" puts it, "Pursuing extropy means seeking continual improvement in ourselves, our cultures, and our environments. Perpetual progress involves improving ourselves physically, intellectually, and psychologically" (More 2003: Section 1). It means, "Living vigorously, effectively, and joyfully" (More 2003: Section 3).

On the surface, we are again seeing little more than a restatement and elaboration of the fundamental Baconian project of "the relief of man's estate" that has been so definitive for the creation of the modern world. And so too there is something familiar about the transhumanist diagnosis of the roadblocks in the way of achieving such goals: nature, tradition and religion. The FAQ note how "Changing nature for the better is a noble and glorious thing for humans to do." They acknowledge that "the qualification 'for the better' " is crucial (Bostrom 2003b: 35) – but it seems that for transhumanism that is not a hard standard to reach. Hitting on all three of the roadblocks, the FAQ describe how, "the pre-industrial age was anything but idyllic. It was a life of poverty, misery, disease, heavy manual toil from dawn to dusk, superstitious fears, and cultural parochialism" (Bostrom 2003b: 29). "Principles of Extropy" likewise argues that "Perpetual progress calls for us to question traditional assertions that we should leave human nature fundamentally unchanged in order to conform to 'God's will' or to what is considered 'natural' ". Or again, "Valuing perpetual progress is incompatible with acquiescing in the undesirable aspects of the human condition. Continuing improvements means challenging natural and traditional limitations on human possibilities" (More 2003: Section 1).

Despite this rejection of so many traditional sources for grounding or deriving values, the FAQ suggest that "it is perfectly possible to be a transhuman – or, for that matter, a transhumanist – and still embrace most traditional values and principles of personal conduct" (Bostrom 2003b: 7). Since people hold in their heads all kinds of contradictory beliefs at the same time, doubtless there is that much truth to this careful formulation. But David Pearce, a cofounder of the World Transhumanist Association presents in his "hedonistic imperative" a more consistent picture of the relationship between transhumanism and traditional values and principles. He draws conclusions that, while doubtless not universally accepted among transhumanists, open the door to seeing some problems within the broader argument about the meaning of "for the better."

"Nature is barbarous and futile beyond belief," Pearce believes.

> Warfare, rape, famine, pestilence, infanticide and child-abuse have existed since time immemorial. They are quite 'natural,' whether from a historical, cross-cultural or sociobiological perspective. The implicit, and usually highly selective, equation of the 'natural' with the morally good is dangerously facile and simplistic. The popular inclination to ascribe some kind of benign wisdom to an anthropomorphized Mother Nature serves, in practice, only to legitimate all manner of unspeakable cruelties (Pearce 1998: 4.6).

So Nature has dealt human beings a pretty bad hand. But Pearce believes that advances in understanding and manipulating the brain chemically and genetically will eventually make it possible for people to be happy all the time. Indeed, people will be so unimaginably (to us) happy that previous human psychology, based as it was on the naturally given, will be seen in this hedonic future as tragic, perhaps incomprehensible, mental illness. On the basis of a particular variant of utilitarianism, Pearce concludes that we have a moral obligation to seek out this euphoria for ourselves, and indeed to reconstruct the natural order entirely so that any other beings capable of suffering will likewise be happy. "It is not, needless to say, the fault of cats that they are prone to torturing mice; but then, given the equations of physics, it isn't the fault of Nazis they try to persecute Jews. This is no reason to let them continue to do so" (Pearce 1998: 1.10). But more: "For ethically it is imperative that the sort of unspeakable suffering characteristic of the last few hundred million years on earth should never recur elsewhere. If such horror might exist anywhere else in the cosmos, presumably in the absence of practical intelligence sufficiently evolved to eliminate its distal roots, then this suffering too must be systematically sought out. It needs to be extirpated just as hell-states will have been on earth" (Pearce 1998: 4.13).

Imagine this rescue fleet arriving on *our* doorstep; it seems likely that its promise of the complete reconstruction of human psychology and terrestrial ecology would be greeted with alarm. For Pearce that atavistic reaction is merely an indicator of the raw deal we have from Darwinian evolution, which has not selected for the prevalence of brain states that we call happiness. It is also built on an unwillingness to confront the fact, as he presents it, that happiness as we experience it is entirely a matter of brain chemistry. If I am happy because I'm in love with a biological person or with a virtual person whose computer program is stimulating the appropriate nerve centers in my brain, or born with a sunny disposition, or properly medicated or genetically enhanced, it is essentially the same thing as far as what goes on in the brain is concerned. Conditions in our brain such as that which we label happiness are products of the laws of physics, and as such open to deliberate and self-conscious manipulation.

Three observations need to be made about this effort to revise our understandings of the human good. First, Pearce promises us freedom from the *particulars* of the naturally given (the way our brains happen to have evolved) while at the same time completely subsuming the human into the naturally given *in general* (the chemistry and physics of the brain that make us what we are). That would seem to accord with the view of the FAQ: "There is no fundamental dichotomy between humanity and the rest of the world. One could say that nature has, in humanity, become conscious and self-reflective" (Bostrom 2003b: 38). So the Blind Watchmaker has by chance created not just a watch but a Sighted Watchmaker; intelligence and intentionality replace chance. Yet even the Sighted Watchmaker remains bound by the fundamental constraints through which the Blind Watchmaker makes watches. Transhumanism generally is committed to the same proposition, essentially accepting the Baconian dictum that "nature to be commanded must be obeyed." This position suggests that our sense of freedom may always have been an illusion of consciousness, or based on ignorance. What we think of as our choice to conquer nature is dictated to us by nature.

Hence (in the second place), the theme of overcoming nature requires more attention. Pearce may be at an extreme in his willingness to present such a thoroughgoing moral condemnation of the naturally given. The FAQ seem to stand in contrast, sometimes speaking with a more conventional voice of environmental concern. ("Not only are transhumanist technologies ecologically sound, they may be the only environmentally viable option for the long term" (Bostrom 2003b: 38)). But ecological soundness and environmental viability do not have to be taken as phrases that could only characterize present or historically given ecosystems or environments. "Nature" in this respect could be modified along with human beings. There is no reason to think the FAQ suggest any more serious scruples about the macrocosm than it does about the microcosm, however much lip service must be paid to the environmental awareness necessary for coalition building.

Still, it is certainly true that nature often falls short of human moral aspirations, just as it is true that human beings can exhibit a depravity that is hard to see in the rest of nature. How to understand the human relationship to nature, which arises as a question out of the fact that we are the only beings we know to have arisen out of the naturally given with the ability to significantly alter that given, is a question too important to be allowed to run to the extremes such as Pearce's thoroughgoing condemnation, or more conventional environmentalist veneration.[2]

Yet third, despite his ability to speak the language of happiness – and after all, who does not want to be happy? – Pearce knows he has an uphill battle to get his readers on board with statements like, a "symbiotic union of biologically programmed euphoria and mature virtual reality software engineering, however, is an awesomely good prospect" (Pearce 1998: 3.5). "Accounts like this," he admits, "inevitably sound cold, technocratic and Brave New Worldish. It should be recalled

[2] Rejection of/reliance on nature is not unique to transhumanism and is of a piece with understanding nature within the limits of the framework set by modern assumptions – a particularly illuminating instance of which is Mill 1969: 373–402.

that the developments they describe should avert suffering on a scale which a single mind cannot possibly comprehend; and make a lot of people blissfully well" (Pearce 1998: 3.3). "Blissfully well" here means not achieving the mean or being saintly, for example; reasoning teaches Pearce that it means rather possessed of a brain genetically engineered to produce certain chemical states beyond what the unengineered brain produces while being electronically stimulated by a computer in such a way as to be experiencing sensations that do not correspond to the actual location or activity of the body. Indeed, so "awesomely good" is this prospect that Pearce uses it to suggest why in fact the alien happiness rescue fleet has not done its moral duty and arrived on our doorstep from a far more advanced civilization that has already taken the step he contemplates. As the "motivational incentives to choose the inconvenient kinds of experience involved in (non-virtual) space-exploration etc. are somewhat diminished…the very possibility of vulgar physical star hopping may just never arise" (Pearce 1998: 3.5). Forget "Star Trek" or "Firefly," with their conflicted and often unhappy people; while Pearce thinks he has arguments that suggest why constant happiness might lead to ever greater human achievement, his premises are always drawing him back to a "wirehead" future.

Pearce's transhumanism suggests in a particularly dramatic way how the transhumanist promise of wealth, health, happiness and longevity has specific content which will not necessarily correspond to people's pre-existing understandings of what makes for a good life. Of course longer, healthier and more productive lives, are going to command wide endorsement as good things. Yet our existing understandings of these goods do not comprehend how we can use the laws of nature to free ourselves from norms drawn from natural, traditional or religious constraints that up to the present have defined this goodness. At the same time, they tend not to be built on the strong determinism about the source and meaning of our choices such as is found in Pearce's doubtless intentionally shocking statement (even given Art Spiegelman's *Maus*) equating cats and Nazis, instead presupposing some degree of moral freedom.

Again, not all transhumanists would draw Pearce's particular consequences so sharply. But despite the fact that the FAQ and "Principles of Extropy" do not enter into discussions of their underlying principles so deeply as Pearce, it is hard to see how some form of the same premises one finds in Pearce could fail to inform transhumanism's picture of happiness more generally. Outside of the FAQ, Bostrom acknowledges that transhumanism "has its roots in secular humanist thinking" (Bostrom 2003a: Section 1). The manner in which science, technology and reason are described and endorsed would certainly lead one to think that transhumanism is committed to the modern, scientific materialism that sees nature, including human nature, as malleable; happiness will be defined by the manipulation of stuff whether inside or outside the brain. Otherwise, the whole discussion of overcoming limits via technology would hardly make sense. But as a consequence, a good many traditional views must fall by the wayside – any that depend on the existence of a soul, for example, or divine revelation or on a given human nature, or even on existent social constellations. Among "traditional" norms, then, which could *consistently* be combined with transhumanist aspirations as readily as some sort of pragmatic utilitarianism of the sort Pearce adduces?

For a "loosely defined movement" seeking to expand its base of adherents, it would not necessarily serve to press such consistency too hard. When it comes to presenting its vision of the good, one often finds in transhumanism a rhetoric of compassion to supplement its rhetoric of development and discovery. One finds an initial emphasis on the techniques that will allow healing of those suffering from specific disability and disease, apparently accepting the existence of something like a norm of health (Naam 2005: *passim*). But this acceptance is only provisional, because the same techniques that will cure disease and disability will also prove useful to enhance and reconstruct. We may create direct brain/machine interfaces in order to help restore the ability to move and manipulate to paralyzed people; the more we know the more such linkages will become commonplace for all. Eventually, to fail to have such a hookup may be regarded as a disability.

Broadly speaking, then, what is promised is not the same as what is delivered. Transhumanism stands foursquare behind the now traditional modern project for improvement of the human condition. The FAQ, for example, pose the question "Shouldn't we concentrate on current problems such as improving the situation of the poor, rather than putting our efforts into planning for the 'far' future?" The answer, of course, is "We should do both" (Bostrom 2003b: 27). But the paths it chooses to such goals are determined by its vision of the technologically imaginable, rather than by some determinate idea of a good life, because it advocates overcoming the existing limitations that define the human condition, and a world that is in some way unimaginable to the merely human.

To put it another way, what "healthier," "wealthier," "happier," and even "longer" lives look like, what the very terms themselves mean, becomes a new problem once we start to move from transhumans to posthumans, as the bars of achievement and ability rise to unprecedented heights. Of course, there have always been disagreements about what makes a good life. Transhumanism is not the first, even secular, movement to put the force of necessity behind projections of an end to human ills, nor to imagine beyond that some unimaginable future destiny. It is even not unique in rejecting nature, religion, tradition or history as relevant standards by which a good life may be defined. But such extreme open-endedness creates a problem. This principled uncertainty about the meaning of the posthuman is relevant to the judgement of cases today; it influences essential elements of the transhumanist case for what we should be doing now. For already to some extent today and all the more so even in the near term, all kinds of things are or will be possible that, from the non-transhumanist point of view, don't look like good ideas. Objections to cloning or electrically induced happiness can't only be answered by claims that we *must* develop these technologies; technological might makes right no more than any other variety. Yet justification in terms of achieving some ineffable posthuman condition is not exactly a reasoned defense, and the very incomprehensibility of the posthuman makes it look like allegiance to it is an article of faith. In light of that problem, transhumanism makes a virtue of a necessity, and celebrates a future built up from the maximization of choice, a future of diversity and inclusion. It aspires to the higher selfishness, a world in which "it looks good to me" commands moral respect and is a key principle of social organization.

8.4 Diversity, Choice and Inclusion

"Self-direction" is one of the seven keys "Principles of Extropy"; technology creates new possibilities of choice that must be appreciated without the burden of ideas inapplicable to these new circumstances.

> Self-direction calls on us to rise above the surrender of independent judgement that we see – especially in religion, politics, morals, and relationships. Directing our lives asks us to determine for ourselves our values, purposes, and actions. New technologies offer more choices not only over what we do but also over who we are physically, intellectually, and psychologically. By taking charge of ourselves we can use these new means to advance ourselves according to our personal values (More 2003: Section 6).

Hence "Each individual should be free and responsible for deciding for themselves in what ways to change or to stay the same... Pursuing extropy means vigorously resisting coercion from those who try to impose their judgements of safety and effectiveness of various means of self-experimentation" (More 2003: Section 6).

By using the phrase "safety and effectiveness," More likely aims this last shot at the United States Food and Drug Administration, for it is tasked by statute precisely with making those judgements. In any case, for More doubtless any regulatory regime so tasked is inappropriate when it comes to transhuman enhancements. This position is disputed by less libertarian transhumanist advocates, who see an ongoing role for government regulation in such matters. Indeed, there is some tension within the "Principles of Extropy" themselves, evident in the assertion that "Coercion of mature, sound minds outside of the realm of self-protection, whether for the purported 'good of the whole' or for the paternalistic protection of the individual, is unacceptable" (More 2003: Section 6). For when is coercion for self-protection not paternalistic? But the basic preference for maximization of free choice and individual responsibility for such choice is clear enough – choice, however, whose maturity is presumably indicated by the extent to which it is "rational," "reflective" and "informed."

"Since self-direction applies to everyone, this principle requires that we respect the self-direction of others ... Appreciating that other persons have their own lives, purposes, and values implies seeking win-win cooperative solutions rather than trying to force our interests at the expense of others" (More 2003: Section 6). So there is no illusion here about the diversity of choices likely to be made and the potential for conflict contained therein, but a hope that such situations can be met with a "benevolent disposition" which "embodies more emotional stability, resilience, and vitality than cynicism, hostility or meanness," approaching others in a spirit of "friendship cooperation and pleasure" (More 2003: Section 6).

The end result is an "open society," another of the main points of the "Principles of Extropy." The concept of

> Open societies avoids utopian plans for 'the perfect society,' instead appreciating the diversity in values, lifestyle preferences, and approaches to solving problems. In place of the static perfection of a utopia, we might imagine a dynamic 'extropia' — an open, evolving

> framework allowing individuals and voluntary groupings to form the institutions and social forms they prefer. Even where we find some of those choices mistaken or foolish, open societies affirm the value of a system that allows all ideas to be tried with the consent of those involved (More 2003: Section 5).

Of course, libertarians have espoused ideals such as this since long before transhumanism came on the scene. But to those who have, in light of their reading of human nature or history, hitherto greeted them with slack-jawed amazement, Extropy has the reply that now we can talk about such arrangements in light of a complete human redesign. Benevolent dispositions can be manufactured. Still, there is some tension lurking between allowing all ideas to be tried as a mechanism to achieve posthumanity, and requiring posthumanity to allow all ideas to be tried, a tension that again speaks to the confusing freedom that transhumanism promises. If I am born benevolent by someone's clever redesign, then a whole realm of moral choice is denied to me. If, as is imagined by James Hughes, executive director of the World Transhumanist Association, I can turn benevolence on and off as one among a variety of programmable dispositions, we are back to square one, wondering where the disposition to flick that switch as opposed to others Hughes imagines ("Kohlberg's Stage Six, Islamic Sharia, or Ayn Randian selfishness" (Hughes 2004: 255)) is coming from – since of course even without such enhancements one is able to choose to be benevolent. Or not, if Pearce is correct, in which case this freedom promised by transhumanism is as illusory as any other.

The FAQ, while somewhat less libertarian in emphasis, further complicate the picture of what diversity will mean as a practical matter, suggesting that it will have to accommodate challenges from two directions. "Transhumanists reject speciesism, the (human racist) view that moral status is strongly tied to membership in a particular biological species, in our case homo sapiens" (Bostrom 2003b: 31). That means that on the one hand, animals that may not be sufficiently in our moral circle will have to be included, since "all beings that can experience pain have some moral status" (Bostrom 2003b: 31). On the other hand, "posthuman" creations will likewise need to be included; indeed, there are already serious discussions even of the rights and legal status of sentient computers. (A further complication: if Pearce is correct, will the euphoric beings of the future feel pain at all, or as we do – since there will no longer be any reason for it to produce unhappiness?)

How will societies deal with this expanded range of moral inclusion? From the side of the posthuman it is difficult to say because "we must bear in mind that we are likely to base our expectations on the experiences, desires, and psychological characteristics of humans. Many of these expectations may not hold true of posthuman persons. When human nature changes, new ways of organizing a society may become feasible" (Bostrom 2003b: 32). It may be that transhumanists recognize the echoes of 20th century totalitarianism in this promise of what becomes possible if only we can change human nature. Perhaps as a way of avoiding the same terrible results, the FAQ suggest that:

> The ideal social organization may be one that includes the possibility for those who so wish to form independent societies voluntarily secluded from the rest of the world, in order to pursue traditional ways of life or to experiment with new forms of communal living.

> Achieving an acceptable balance between the rights of such communities for autonomy, on the one hand, and the security concerns of outside entities and the just demands for protection of vulnerable and oppressed individuals inside these communities on the other hand, is a delicate task and a familiar challenge in political philosophy (Bostrom 2003b: 32).

The state of the world today may suggest that this challenge can be "familiar" without having been definitively met, despite the efforts of political philosophy hitherto. One might speculate that it is a problem that worsens as human power increases. Yet the modes of political and social organization that in practice seem to work relatively well in a highly diverse nation such as the United States work within the framework of "human racist" assumptions about the meaning of equality such as are suggested in the Declaration of Independence. Furthermore, contrary to the hopes of Extropy, these modes of organization do not by and large depend decisively on benevolence and niceness but rather assume, with James Madison, that men are not angels. Indeed, the somewhat glib protestations about new social forms more than anything else call attention to the possibility that posthumans will be as little concerned for those mere humans choosing "traditional ways of life" as those humans have been about other animals.

That this possibility is real is acknowledged by transhumanists. Speaking of the possibility of super-intelligent, sentient computers, the FAQ note that:

> The would-be creator of a new life form with such surpassing capabilities would have an obligation to ensure that the proposed being is free from psychopathic tendencies and, more generally, that it has humane inclinations. For example, a superintelligence should be built with a clear goal structure that has friendliness to humans as its top goal. Before running such a program, the builders of a superintelligence should be required to make a strong case that launching it would be safer than alternative courses of action (Bostrom 2003b: 34).

FAQ Version 1 was more open on the topic than FAQ 2, for in FAQ 1 we find explicit admission that "if the posthumans are not bound by human-friendly laws and they don't have a moral code that says it would be wrong, they might then decide to take actions that would entail the extinction of the human species" (Hughes 2004: 247). FAQ 2, on the other hand, professes to find the concern about such conflict overblown.

> It is a common theme in fiction because of the opportunities for dramatic conflict, but that is not the same as social, political, and economic plausibility in the real world. It seems more likely that there would be a continuum of differently modified or enhanced individuals, which would overlap with the continuum of as-yet unenhanced humans. The scenario in which 'the enhanced' form a pact and then attack 'the naturals' makes for exciting science fiction but is not necessarily the most plausible outcome. Even today, the segment containing the tallest 90 percent of the population could, in principle, get together and kill or enslave the shorter decile. That this does not happen suggests that a well-organized society can hold together even if it contains many possible coalitions of people sharing some attribute such that, if they unified under one banner, would make them capable of exterminating the rest (Bostrom 2003b: 33).

Here again we have the familiar Madisonian notion that societies with a great degree of social and economic diversity can limit the formation of dangerous factions. Yet that idea works best on the basis of an ideal of human equality which was itself rather hard won in the face of a range of actual inequalities that pale in comparison with those which will be introduced by trans- and posthumanity. So it is extremely curious that in the context of a criticism of fiction for being unrealistic, FAQ 2 pass over the known history of relations between human beings and animals, between human beings at vastly different levels of technological development, indeed between human groups that are in any manner "strange" to one another and instead has us celebrate the social accomplishment that today taller people have not killed or enslaved shorter people.[3]

While it is strictly speaking true, given our complete ignorance of the constraints that will operate on posthuman beings, that efforts on their part to bring about human extinction is "not necessarily the most plausible outcome" one could with equal or greater truth say it is "not necessarily the most implausible outcome."

Such concern is justified because all the characteristics by which we understand and admire diversity in the world we now know are, as the transhumanists are fully aware, human characteristics, based on a human given that limits our potential for good or ill. Since it is just that given which transhumanism proposes to eliminate, all bets about the resulting moral universe are off. The FAQ want to avoid this consequence by distinguishing between being human and being humane:

> If there is value in being human, it does not comes from being 'normal' or 'natural,' but from having within us the raw material for being humane: compassion, a sense of humor, curiosity, the wish to be a better person. Trying to preserve 'humanness,' rather than cultivating humaneness, would idolize the bad along with the good. One might say that if 'human' is what we are, then 'humane' is what we, as humans, wish we were. Human nature is not a bad place to start that journey, but we can't fulfill that potential if we reject any progress past the starting point (Bostrom 2003b: 36).

Here humane attributes are being treated as abstractions only accidentally connected to our humanity. But the positive characteristics mentioned are positive precisely because we are the kind of being that we are. Compassion and empathy, for example, are positive because we do not have a hive mind, and are separated by our bodies, and can suffer. Or again, we admire "the wish to be a better person" because it is hard to be better; we can't just buy upgrades and we have to fight against passions and interests that do not make us better.

So Hughes is quite right to wonder whether it "is possible to imagine a 'liberty-respecting' policy that discourages misanthropy among posthumans" (Hughes 2004: 248). Will the mature, rational and informed choices of humans look the same way to transhumans or posthumans, if as expected their capacities in all these areas are superior to ours? And if not, what respect will they grant them? The

---

[3] Using the persistence of a short minority as an example of social tolerance is odd given that height is well documented to convey advantage even in "well-organized societies"; the shortest are allowed to survive, but at a significant disadvantage. Indeed, the point becomes downright bizarre upon recollection that one of the main areas today in which enhancement of children is already being practiced is providing them with human growth hormone. While by definition there will always be a shortest decile, in fact there are societies already open to making it as tall as possible, "eliminating" the category as defined by today's measurements.

respect that parents give to the choices of children? That humans give to the choices of their pets? That humans give to the choices of nuisance animals?

8.5 Enhancement, Identity and Extinction

While the transhumanists use the traditional language of libertarian inclined progressivism to discuss the good of transhumanism, there is really no way to dispute that they are leading us into completely uncharted moral waters. In that context, it is not foolish to be concerned about the fate of humanity, and not only out of the conventional worry that highly advanced beings might find their precursors an embarrassing nuisance, or that we may fall prey to their incomprehensible projects or conflicts, or that we might be useful to them in some degrading way, or that great power might easily coexist with great malevolence, or that we will simply be outcompeted in an evolutionary struggle. An underappreciated source for human extinction might be found in a corollary to Arthur Clarke's law "any sufficiently advanced technology is indistinguishable from magic": any sufficiently advanced act of benevolence is indistinguishable from malevolence (Rubin 1996: 168). Of course I am doing the right thing by not giving the pan-handler money to buy drugs with – but perhaps he does not see it quite the same way. One need only recall the aforementioned arrival of the fleet of alien ships intent on making all sentient life happy all the time to see the problem here. Indeed, Clarke himself wrote the definitive book on the subject, *Childhood's End*, in which a benevolent race comes to shepherd humanity to the next evolutionary level, literally destroying the world and all remaining human beings as the *successful* result of their mission.

Yet even if, as the FAQ would have us believe, such inter-specific problems can be solved or are overblown, it remains the case that transhumanism is in effect promising the end of humanity. For if they are correct about the appeal of the possibilities inherent in transhumanity and posthumanity, what mature, rational decision could be made to remain human? As transhumanists tend to portray those who oppose them as in thrall to the irrational, as bio-Luddites, as racists, as death-lovers they are in effect saying that they can imagine no good reasons why people would not enhance themselves to the maximum extent possible. But of course if anyone *wants* to decay and die, transhumanism would not, as is supposed of its opponents, impose its views and prevent it.

Or would it? An illuminating point comes up when the FAQ attempt to stand forthrightly against eugenics and for reproductive freedom. Yet:

> Beyond this, one can argue that parents have a moral responsibility to make use of these methods, assuming they are safe and effective. Just as it would be wrong for parents to fail in their duty to procure the best available medical care for their sick child, it would be wrong not to take reasonable precautions to ensure that a child-to-be will be as healthy as possible. This, however, is a moral judgment that is best left to individual conscience rather than imposed by law. Only in extreme and unusual cases might state infringement of procreative liberty be justified. If, for example, a would-be parent wished to undertake a genetic modification that would be clearly harmful to the child or would drastically curtail

> its options in life, then this prospective parent should be prevented by law from doing so. This case is analogous to the state taking custody of a child in situations of gross parental neglect or child abuse (Bostrom 2003b: 21).

Since already today failure to provide necessary blood transfusions can count as "gross parental neglect," is it so difficult to imagine a day when a parental choice *not* to make a generally accepted genetic modification in their child would trigger "state infringement"? In a world where technological enhancement is expected to widen greatly "options in life," will not a parental decision to accept the current norm more and more look like the choice of tragic yet preventable disability?

Nor does the existence posited in the FAQ of a "continuum of differently modified or enhanced individuals" (Bostrom 2003b: 33) between the human and the posthuman really act as intended to change the anti-human dynamic of the argument. First of all, is this continuum really consistent with the supposed necessity on which transhumanism depends that drives scientific and technological development in the first place? Will not these competitive forces move people to seek maximum available enhancement, not to speak of the supposed advantages of so doing in living healthier, happier, wealthier and longer lives? People will surely not always make the same choices of particular enhancements, but if the transhumanist program prevails, they will surely tend to maximize enhancement to the limit of the constantly changing desires and capabilities, about which more below. An analogy: at present, relatively few people in the US have a big plasma TV and the widest cable selection of channels, but nearly everyone has some sort TV, and of those who don't only a tiny fraction are holding out in principle. What from one point of view is a continuum of TV possibilities is from another an isolated minority of non-TV watchers.

Furthermore, the TV continuum is created in part by price discrimination. Transhumanists acknowledge this effect as a short-term issue; early adopters of new possibilities will pay a high price for them. But they also point to the powerful tendency for technology prices to go down over time, and/or call for public support for the provision of otherwise too costly technological benefits (Naam 2005: 63–66). This effort to deal with wealth based inequalities that historically tend to leave the have-nots at the mercy of the haves would be more convincing if it were not for the "perpetual progress" element of transhumanism, which would seem to imply that there will always be an exploitable, expensive advantage to be found at the cutting edge. Of course, here again it is doubtless an error to apply human-based thinking to the transformed beings advocated by transhumanism. Maybe they will find a way to make us free in the face of competitive necessity, and equal in our radical inequality.

The more one appreciates the gap that transhumanism would have us believe will exist between the human and the posthuman, the more it appears that the "ideal," continuum of possibilities or not, will indeed be the opportunity for those wishing to maintain their "traditional" humanity to be voluntarily "secluded" from the rest of the world. The survival of the voluntary element in this seclusion will surely be tested the moment mere humans begin to look like a danger to themselves or to posthumans if left in a mixed milieu.

The foregoing thoughts cannot prove that successful transhumanism will result in human extinction or even a bad deal for the merely human. But they can remind that the advocacy of free choice and the protection of diversity which substitute for a substantive picture of the human good in transhumanism are themselves instrumental to creating a posthuman world which, on assumption, we cannot know to have any room for human values like choice or diversity. In any case, transhumanists appropriately seem clearer that the story of intelligence will pass out of human hands. "The arrival of superintelligence will clearly deal a heavy blow to anthropocentric worldviews. Much more important than its philosophical implications, however, would be its practical effects. Creating superintelligence may be the last invention that humans will ever need to make, since super intelligences could themselves take care of further scientific and technological development. They would do so more effectively than humans. Biological humanity would no longer be the smartest life form on the block" (Bostrom 2003b: 13).

What transhumanism does, then, is to dangle before us the glorious possibilities of human inventiveness, with the ultimate expectation that human inventiveness will be superceded. If what defines our humanity is self-transcendence as a species (Kurzweil 2005: 9), will those who remain human yet uninventive be in effect less than human? Here in about the most artless form imaginable we are being offered a Faustian bargain. "Fulfill your deepest material hopes and dreams – but by the way, the price is human obsolescence." One could call this bargain devilish were it not made with such illuminating, if occasional, candor, as if by some imp under compulsion periodically to blurt out the truth (Todorov 2002: 3). Yet the promise compels nevertheless by the very familiarity of the good things it promises, by the imagination of ring of Gyges-like powers of wish fulfillment to come, by intimation of presently unimaginable pleasures, by the ultimate hope of staving off our mortality.

But to whom exactly is the bargain being offered? One might think from the transhumanist emphasis on individual choice and social diversity, from their effort to claim the moral high-grounds of compassion, benevolence and cooperation, that the choice is being offered to a free moral being. But we have already seen how that is hardly the case. In asserting that Nazi and cat alike act faultlessly out of the "equations of physics," Pearce is simply making explicit the consequences of the scientific materialism on which transhumanism seems committed to building its understanding of human things. From this point of view, we are not free, and what we call our subjectivity is a manipulable object.[4] To think that a perduring "I" is freely accepting or declining enhancement and modification is to fall prey to the error of thinking there is a "ghost in the machine" when in fact such a decision is the in-principle calculable result of determinate bodily biology/chemistry/physics. "The reality is we are constantly changing" (Naam 2005: 59).

[4] The issue of what kind of human freedom, if any, is consistent with scientific materialism is of course not unique to transhumanism – but that does not mean it ought to be elided. There are efforts to try to reconcile scientific materialism with genuine human freedom. See, for example, Wolfram 2002: 750–53 or Hameroff and Penrose 1996.

But there is a tension in transhumanist thinking in this connection. The FAQ talk about "uploads," the prospect of creating posthuman beings by transferring the contents of brains into a computer. The resulting being could be embodied in robot form, or it could inhabit virtual realities. In any case, "it matters little whether you are implemented on a silicon chip inside a computer or in that gray, cheesy lump inside your skull, assuming both implementations are conscious" (Bostrom 2003b: 18). But of course it matters a great deal; the FAQ also admit that downloads raise "philosophical, legal and ethical challenges" galore: "if we imagine that several similar copies are made of your uploaded mind. Which one of them are you? Are they all you, or are none of them you?" (Bostrom 2003b: 18) Such questions do not arise with human beings; they are indicative of a profound change in the meaning of the self, and hence of the moral universe the self inhabits.

It may be that scientific materialism already undermines notions of a unified self, but transhumanism absolutely seeks to explode them (Todorov 2002: 4–5). Not only does the I that chooses become thereby a different I, but in effect it does not choose, the outcome being determined by the temporary physical state of the I prior to the change to a new state. So it is not quite right to suggest that "In a world where we can sculpt our own emotions and personalities, people will no longer be able to say 'I can't help it, that's just the way I am'" (Naam 2005: 60). For there is just as little an I free to sculpt itself in the new world as there is an I free to resolve to change in present world.

8.6 Uncertainty, Faith and Nihilism

Starting from transhumanism's materialism, then, it is the purest conjecture, pure faith, that would make one think that qualities of humaneness derived from the human would have any meaning in a world bent on overcoming the human. Nick Bostrom attempts to defend against this conclusion that transhumanism commits unknowable selves to unknowable values. On the one hand, he notes that not all enhancements need be so radical as to create discontinuity of personal identity, that some posthuman values may be things we already value now, but only with an incomplete understanding of them, and that an "incremental exploration of the posthuman realm may be indispensable for understanding posthuman values" (Bostrom 2003a: Section 3). But what is noteworthy is the relentless pressure that the logic of transhumanism places on such moderate (relatively speaking) formulations. For on the other hand, (a) "Preservation of personal identity, especially if this notion is given a narrow construal, is not everything" (b) "we may favor future people being posthuman rather than human, if the posthumans would lead lives more worthwhile than the alternative humans would" (c) "Transhumanism promotes the quest to develop further so that we can explore *hitherto inaccessible realms of value*" [emphasis added]. So "worthwhile" may well mean "worthwhile in terms of some now inaccessible realm of value". Finally, (d) "if the mode of being of a posthuman being is radically different from that of a human being, then we may doubt whether a posthuman being could be the same person as a human being, even if the posthuman being originated from a human being" (Bostrom 2003a: Section 3).

In connection with this last point, Bostrom makes what he doubtless feels is a telling *tu quoque* argument. "Depending on what our views are about what constitutes personal identity, it could be that certain modes of being, while possible, are not possible for us, because any being of such a kind would be so different from us that they could not be us. Concerns of this kind are familiar from theological discussions of the afterlife." In "Christian theology," souls only enter heaven after a period of purification. "Skeptics may doubt that the resulting minds would be sufficiently similar to our current minds for it to be possible for them to be the same person" (Bostrom 2003a: Section 3).

Leave aside the equivocation about the corrosive effect of scientific materialism on concepts of personal identity, the confusion between mind and soul, and the theological argument that the soul becomes more essentially itself as it is purified. Note instead that Bostrom tacitly admits a generic likeness between transhumanism, which we thought was a product of reasoning, and arguments based on faith. This insight is important. When the goal of transhumanism becomes the incomprehensible posthuman, discussion of it, as of the afterlife, becomes a matter of faith.

Not simply faith, of course. If the transhumanists are correct, their faith will be incrementally justified by works – scientific and technological achievements – until such time that intelligence ascends to levels inaccessible to those who are left behind. Those works will doubtless fall out along a continuum, from those which are said to be good from the point of view of the mundane human, to others (technically speaking, no longer on a continuum) which will appear good only to those whose faith allows them to see from *sub specie* the posthuman apotheosis. Since the very notions of transhumanity and posthumanity point so firmly to this extreme, we may once again wonder what it means to define a good in terms of the unknowable.

Biblical theologies that point to an equally unknowable end will not help illuminate this question, because in them the route to that end is through defined, humanly comprehensible acts of self-discipline called forth by a providential order in which human power is vanishingly small. Transhumanism seeks to liberate the diverse wills of the choosing individuals to remake their worlds, even as it turns those free choices into outcomes determined by laws of nature – but also only limited by laws of nature. So where Biblical theologies face the unknowable in an attitude of submission, transhumanism uses it to liberate what Thomas Hobbes long ago called a "restless desire of power after power that ceaseth only in death" (Hobbes 1968: 161), assuming death cannot be indefinitely delayed. How do we judge the extent of our power? By our ability to negate what is given by nature or tradition, to be sure, but also power to negate *whatever* is for the moment given in the name of possibilities foreseen or unforeseen. That is the deeper meaning behind the bland pragmatism in the "Principles of Extropy" discussion of "perpetual progress" ("conserving what works for as long as it works and altering that which can be improved"): "no mysteries are sacrosanct, no limits unquestionable" (More 2003: Section 1).

Negation can be good. To negate suffering and disease is well worth attempting; the effort to negate death is at least understandable. But finally, transhumanism does not seek to negate suffering and disease in the name of human happiness and health, but rather in the name of the willful achievement of any imaginable and unimaginable alternative. Pious caveats about safety and humaneness and equality of access will ultimately have no traction in the face of this assumption. Promoting discussion of the future and "an interdisciplinary approach to understanding and evaluating the opportunities for enhancing the human condition and the human organism" (Bostrom 2003a: Section 1) seem a weak reed with which to hold off the will to power (Garreau 2005: 241).

So without firm ground to stand on, there is more than a hint of nihilism in transhumanist negation. The rationality which it values so highly is itself moored to nothing but the will of the individual reasoner. According to the "Principles of Extropy" reason helps us "understand the Universe" and "advance our knowledge," but its essentially critical function cannot allow even such claims to stand unqualified: we have to "remain wary of the human propensity to settle for and defend any comfortable explanation" (More 2003: Section 7). We have gone far beyond Socratic doubt, here. "Rational thinkers accept no final intellectual authorities. No individual, no institution, no book, and no single principle can serve as the source or standard of truth. All beliefs are fallible and must be open to testing and challenging. Rational thinkers do not accept revelation, authority, or emotion as reliable sources of knowledge. Rational thinkers place little weight on claims that cannot be checked. In thinking rationally, we rely on the judgement of our own minds while continually re-examining our own intellectual standards and skills" (More 2003: Section 7). In making everything perpetually provisional, the reason of transhumanism means we can do anything we want so long as we maintain a critical distance from the doing of it – a utopia of irony.

Transhumanists are doubtless decent folk, struggling to do right in the world as they see the right. So the conclusion that the good of transhumanism is finally "everything is permitted" will probably be objectionable to many, who would never dream of themselves offending against the "values, standards and principles" of their milieus. But how could it be otherwise when the very goal of the movement is overcoming the constraints of the human, constraints which define the character of our moral world, a goal which constantly pushes it to extremes? When nature is shorn of goals or purposes that would imbue it with moral significance? When tradition, religion, and custom all are to be tried at the bar of the willful individual reasoner? When it must have faith in the desirability of a future that it admits we cannot understand?

8.7 Conclusion

The transhumanist program to rebuild humanity leaves it morally adrift. Despite the fact that it begins from the familiar goals of healthier, happier, wealthier and longer lives, removing those goals from their human context makes their meaning and, to the extent some of them are instrumental, their purposes, uncertain. The libertarian effort to substitute the goal of diversity for this uncertainty means transhumanism can only have faith that the future it advocates, a future that may well have no room for human beings, will be desirable. To the extent that transhuman and posthuman diversity is achieved by negation of whatever is given, it appears in fact to represent a variety of nihilism.

The problems inherent in transhumanism should make us look again at what it means to help people lead better human lives, and question whether this project has in fact become obsolete in the face of our latest scientific and technical achievements. The supposed necessity, in light of our powers, that we take the path to posthumanity is really a result of a failure to make moral distinctions based on a substantive picture of the human good, and to think that such distinctions can matter. In his brilliant science fiction novel *The Diamond Age*, Neal Stephenson imagines a world where nano- and information technology open the door to all kinds of transhuman possibilities – some of which are indeed exploited. He departs from the transhumanists, however, in a key premise of the book: as "nearly anything" becomes possible because of the new technology in his fictional world, the "cultural role in deciding what *should* be done with it had become far more important than imagining what *could* be done" (Stephenson 1995: 31). The most successful societies in this world cultivate rather than reject restraint. Transhumanism is too entranced by the "could" to pay serious attention to the "should" beyond assertions that because this transformation is going to happen we better talk about ways to deal with it. But because culture is all about making distinctions between what should and should not be done, Stephenson's science *fiction* is more realistic than the transhumanist *science* fiction about a posthuman world. Transhumanists may be correct that we are on a slippery slope to a new world, but a choice can still be made about joining them in pouring on more oil.

References

Bostrom N (2003a) Transhumanist Values. http://www.transhumanism.org/index.php/WTA/more/transhumanist-values Last accessed 5/23/06

Bostrom N (2003b) The Transhumanist FAQ: A General Introduction (Version 2.1). http://www.transhumanism.org/resources/FAQv21.pdf. Last accessed 12/1/05

Garreau J (2005) Radical Evolution: The Promise and Peril of Enhancing Our Minds, Our Bodies–And What It Means to Be Human Doubleday, New York

Hameroff S, Penrose R (1996) Orchestrated Objective Reduction of Quantum Coherence in Brain Microtubules: The 'Orch OR' Model for Consciousness. www.quantumconsciousness.org/penrose-hameroff/orchOR.html Last accessed 12/12/05

Hobbes T (1968) Leviathan.Penguin Books, Baltimore, MD

Hughes J (2004) Citizen Cyborg: Why Democratic Societies Must Respond to the Redesigned Human Future. Westview, Cambridge

Kurzweil R (2005) The Singularity Is Near. Viking, New York

Kurzweil R, Joy B (2005) Recipe for Destruction. The New York Times, October 17: A23

Mill J S (1969) Nature. In: Essays on Ethics, Religion and Society. University of Toronto Press, Toronto

More M (2003) Principles of Extropy Version 3.11. http://www.extropy.org/principles.htm Last accessed 5/23/06

Naam R (2005) More Than Human: Embracing the Promise of Biological Enhancement. Broadway Books, New York

Pearce D (1998) The Hedonic Imperative. http://www.hedweb.com/hedethic/hedonist.htm Last accessed 5/23/06

Rubin C T (1996) First contact: Copernican moment or nine day's wonder? In: Kingsley S A, Lemarchand G A (eds) The Search for Extraterrestrial Intelligence (SETI) in the Optical Spectrum II. The International Society for Optical Engineering, Bellingham, WA

Stephenson N (1995) The Diamond Age or, A Young Lady's Illustrated Primer. Bantam Books, New York

Todorov T (2002) Imperfect Garden: The Legacy of Humanism. Princeton University Press, Princeton, NJ

Wolfram S (2002) A New Kind of Science. Wolfram Media Champaign, Champaign, Ilinois

Part III
Current Developments

Chapter 9
Cosmetic Surgery

Mary Devereaux

9.1 Introduction

The rapid expansion of medical knowledge and biotechnology in recent decades has fostered utopian hopes for medicine. No longer are our hopes limited to the wish that chronic diseases such as diabetes and high blood pressure will soon go the way of polio and smallpox. Advances in areas such as genetics, neuroscience, psychopharmacology, and stem cell science foster the dream that in the not too distant future medicine will put us in command of our biological processes, psychological states, even our physical appearance.

For the immediate present, medicine's ability to deliver on this promise remains largely unrealized. But that is changing. With each passing decade, medicine has more and more to offer in the way of physiological improvements, techniques and procedures such as organ transplants that extend the previous limits of human health and function. Medicine's stable of aesthetic enhancements such as Botox injections and liposuction continues to grow and with it the power to reshape the appearance of the human face and body and forestall physical signs of aging. The pressure for medicine to deliver such enhancements – to move beyond treating sickness and disease to a control of entire biological processes, including, perhaps, mortality itself – will only expand as techniques improve.

It appears then that medicine faces a significant transformation. The basic assumption of traditional medicine is that the limits of the human are biologically fixed. New technologies, including nanotechnology and machine/human interfaces, may put us in the position to change these limits. The effects of this 'radical evolution'[1] will, we can expect, transform our understanding not only of the human body, but also our conception of the self and the trajectory of human life. Yet much of the discussion of these effects remains abstract and highly speculative. Both those who advocate, and those who decry, the anticipated optimization of human biology tend to draw conclusions on the basis of hypothetical projections about what the future is likely to bring. In at least one area, however, we have decades of established clinical practice in biomedical enhancement and hundreds of thousands of completed procedures to draw

[1] I take the term 'radical evolution' from Joel Garreau's book of the same title (Garreau 2005).

B. Gordijn, R. Chadwick (eds.) *Medical Enhancement and Posthumanity*,

upon. That area is cosmetic surgery. Cosmetic surgery thus provides a natural starting point for an investigation of the likely future of medical enhancement (cf. Goering 2001) and its effects on our conception of the human.

In what follows, I take cosmetic surgery as a case study. The aim is to examine features of cosmetic surgery that illuminate some of what we may expect as medicine turns to other forms of human enhancement. I begin with a short discussion of the history and terminology of cosmetic surgery, pointing to how the field developed medical procedures designed to treat the facial wounds incurred in the trenches of World War I and noses ravaged by syphilis, procedures later employed to alter ethnic noses and eradicate signs of aging (Gilman 1999). The aim here is to see in cosmetic surgery a pattern typical of medical technology: techniques developed for medical ends adapted to "making the body beautiful," more socially acceptable, more in line with subjective preferences. Against this background, I devote the bulk of the essay to a critical analysis of the claim that cosmetic surgery qualifies as a form of health care, and hence, a legitimate branch of medicine. The final section raises four specific areas of ethical concern, each of which will likely reappear as medicine adapts to increasing demands for new forms of human enhancement.

9.2 Cosmetic Surgery

The history of cosmetic surgery dates back to the last decades of the 19th century. One feature of that history makes it especially relevant. That is the widely noted tendency of medical procedures developed in one context to get adapted and employed in another context, e.g., off-label drug prescribing. More to the point, procedures developed to treat disease or disability almost inevitably get put to use as enhancements for the healthy or typical, making the normal "even better." So, for example, as Sander Gilman chronicles, surgical techniques developed to repair the facial wounds of war victims or the ravages of diseases such as syphilis were soon adapted for purposes of assimilation, e.g., eradicating the Jewish nose or the 'telltale foreskin' (Gilman 1999: 124–144). It is this pattern that medical observers also see playing out in areas like genetics. Thus, prenatal testing, developed to screen embryos for incurable medical conditions such as Huntington's, now gets employed to screen for medically insignificant conditions or to meet social preferences for a child of a certain gender (Rothschild 2005: 124–126).

The study of the history of cosmetic surgery has been dominated by the tendency to focus primarily on patient-related social and cultural issues. So, for example, Susan Bordo explores the way cosmetic surgery "normalizes," disciplines, and corrects women's bodies and their sense of themselves (Bordo 1993: 31–32). Kathy Davis examines the stories of suffering and transformation women tell about their cosmetic surgeries (Davis 1995: 96ff.). Historians such as Elizabeth Haiken trace the process by which surgical alteration becomes an accepted part of American culture, providing treatment for a newly defined 'inferiority complex' (Haiken 1997: 91–130). Gilman traces how cosmetic surgery reflects 19th and 20th century ideas of race, allowing individuals "to pass" by surgically fashioning a new identity (Gilman 1998, 1999). In short, scholars largely view cosmetic surgery through a cultural lens.

What receives comparatively little attention is the specific impact of cosmetic surgery on the culture of *medicine*. How, for example, does growing patient demand for appearance-enhancing services bear on the definition and professional norms of medicine? Ought we to take for granted that face peels and other beauty procedures belong within the scope of medicine at all? Or might some demands for cosmetic surgery be better met by non-medical interventions such as a change in diet or other forms of medical care such as psychotherapy? How are physicians to navigate the conflicts of interest inherent in obtaining informed consent for risky, but, for them, highly lucrative, operations? Lastly, what effect does the prevalence of cosmetic surgery and other aesthetic enhancements have on prevailing notions of health and disease, aging and death – and how do these changes affect medical training and practice?

It is with these normative issues that medicine faces that I am concerned. What we learn from examining the ethical and professional issues raised by cosmetic surgery may help us see what lies ahead as medicine faces pressures to inaugurate and implement other forms of enhancement.

9.3 Definitions

Some clarification. First, terminology. In common parlance, the term 'plastic' or 'cosmetic' surgery can refer indifferently to procedures aimed at restoration, e.g., repairing bodies torn by war, accident, or disease and/or those aimed at aesthetic improvements such as reducing a subjectively displeasing nose or altering socially stigmatizing features. My concern lies exclusively with the latter enterprise: elective interventions aimed at bettering appearance. To avoid ambiguity, I will use the term 'cosmetic surgery' only to refer to this latter practice.[2] I adopt the standard use of 'reconstructive surgery' for interventions undertaken to reconstruct the body's normal appearance or repair functional deficits.[3]

What distinguishes cosmetic from reconstructive surgery is not its tools (or procedures), but its aim: the absence of a specifically health-related rationale. Breast implant surgery following the loss of a breast to cancer is reconstructive. Its use to make normal, healthy breasts fashionably large belongs to the category of cosmetic

[2] Note that not all of what falls within the common understanding of cosmetic surgery is surgical. Botox injections involve no cutting. A number of newer techniques for face lifts avoid the knife by using lasers or radio frequencies. While my discussion centers primarily on surgical forms of bodily modification, many of these less invasive procedures carry their own medical risks and raise many of the same ethical and social issues.

[3] As Sander Gilman argues, the distinction between reconstructive and "plastic" or cosmetic surgery is as old as the profession itself. The attempt to justify using medicine for the ends of beauty and other non-health-related goals has a fascinating history (Gilman 1998: 4).

surgery. It is difficult to draw a clear dividing line between cosmetic and reconstructive surgery because the line between health-related and non-health-related procedures is not sharp.[4] But for our purposes, a rough distinction will suffice.

9.4 Relation to Healthcare

The very nature of cosmetic surgery gives rise to questions about its legitimacy. Cosmetic surgery employs painful, invasive, potentially risky medical procedures in the absence of disease or impairment and it expends scarce medical expertise and resources in the pursuit of aims that have little or nothing to do with healthcare. Unlike biopsies, heart surgery, or appendectomies, beauty surgery lacks an obvious medical rationale. The "patient" is not sick. The aim is not the treatment or prevention of disease or disability. The improvement of appearance falls outside the usual definition of medicine as fixed by the Hippocratic tradition. While now professionalized and a recognized specialty, cosmetic surgery has not always enjoyed that status.[5] Nor have questions of legitimacy and standing entirely disappeared.[6] I want to consider four attempts to provide a rationale for cosmetic surgery as a legitimate branch of medicine.

9.4.1 It's Just Medicine

The first argument is that cosmetic surgery is just ordinary medicine. In operating on the body, e.g., tightening facial muscles, cosmetic surgeons perform surgery. The surgery they perform differs in no important respect from cardiac surgery or the removal of gall bladder stones. Both kinds of operation require the acquisition and exercise of skills specific to medicine, e.g., knowledge of physiology, surgical technique, the use of anesthetic, and the ability to control infection. Because cosmetic surgery is just another branch of medicine, it needs no special justification.

This line of argument cannot survive scrutiny. Unlike procedures aimed at correcting functional impairment, e.g., a hip replacement, or providing relief from disfigurement, cosmetic interventions expose patients to medical risk for no therapeutic

[4] As a number of medical historians and others have noted, our notion of what constitutes good health (or basic healthcare) alters as biological science and biotechnology advance. A healthy pregnancy now includes prenatal care; measles and chicken pox are no longer an expected part of childhood. Nor are the toothless grins of the aged any longer regarded as normal parts of aging, at least not in those areas of the world able to afford what is now regarded as the standard of care in developed nations. These are complicated issues, about which I will have more to say later.

[5] On the organization of plastic surgery as a profession, see Haiken 1997: 44–90 and Gilman 1999: 4.

[6] Regarding its legitimacy as healthcare, cosmetic surgery is still regarded as 'elective,' hence not covered by medical insurance. While widely popular, hair transplants, buttock implants, and face lifts for younger and younger women – and the advertisements for such in popular magazines – give cosmetic surgery the air of quackery.

benefit. Even successful cosmetic surgery does not improve the health of the patient, except incidentally. Surgery aimed at aesthetic improvement or socially more acceptable features is different from medicine.

This is not to deny that cosmetic procedures can have therapeutic side effects. The American Headache Society reports that several clinical trials have substantiated anecdotal reports that patients receiving Botox injections experience fewer headaches (Nisbel 2003). But Botox is no rival to Bayer. It is not marketed or purchased to alleviate or prevent headaches. It is sold as a way to erase signs of aging and stress. Thus, while some cosmetic procedures may be said to belong within "the core of medical practice," because they confer health benefits, this fact, as Miller, Brody and Chung rightly argue, "has no bearing … on the vast majority of purely cosmetic surgery procedures performed on normal bodies …" (Miller et al. 2000: 358).

Proponents of "it's just medicine" point out that surgical procedures, including those clearly aimed at treating illness and disease, are not risk free. So the element of risk cannot itself make cosmetic surgery problematic. The difference is that in the former case health risks are undergone for the sake of health benefits. As a number of ethicists have rightly insisted, subjecting *healthy* people to medical risks is a morally different proposition from subjecting people who are ill or disabled to the same risks. A medical practice which exposes sound bodies to unnecessary risk stands in considerable tension with the physician's promise to "do no harm." What then justifies cosmetic surgery that does not produce incidental therapeutic benefits?

9.4.2 Meeting Consumer Demand

A second line of argument is that cosmetic surgery satisfies consumer needs. Breast implants, like cell phones and the latest iPods, are consumer goods. They mark status, improve social position, and reflect personal taste. From this perspective, cosmetic surgery is justified because cosmetic surgeons provide a service people want.[7] Cosmetic surgery remains a part of medicine because the techniques it uses, e.g., suturing and other surgical procedures, how to control infection, are taught in medical schools.[8]

One may of course wonder whether physicians should be in the beauty business. Defenders of commercial medicine will answer that the business of physicians is

---

[7] Surgical procedures have come into favor as gifts. So, husbands purchase gift certificates for their wives to have breast implants, daughters arrange face lifts for their mothers, parents provide Rhinoplasty for their children. Extreme instances of patient-driven medicine include the highly controversial Scottish doctor, Robert Smith, who agreed to amputate healthy limbs in response to patient demands. These patients were not physically sick nor were they incompetent according to psychiatrists. For a fascinating discussion of the reasoning behind Smith's actions, see Elliott 2000: 72–84.

[8] Cosmetology, massage and mortuary professionals also require training in areas such as dermatology, physiology and the use of certain medical tools, devices, or products. Medical training and equipment do not by themselves make a doctor.

business. If physicians can meet consumer demand for beautification, why shouldn't they? Like other businesses, medicine follows the market (Sullivan 2001: 79–80). So long as doctors employ safe and effective procedures, and patients know the risks, cosmetic surgery is justified.

The problem with this justification is that it abandons the traditional idea of medicine *as a profession*. What makes a profession a profession is that in contrast to business (a purely commercial enterprise), it has an internal end or telos. An internal end is not only the goal one wants to achieve, but what defines the enterprise itself. In the case of medicine that telos is health. The goal of furthering health is distinct from meeting consumer demand. Medicine also has internal, health-related norms which include standards of expertise (exemplified in Board certification) and standards of care. These technical and ethical standards are part of what makes medicine a profession and part of what makes it the specific profession it is. The normative force of these standards is not contingent upon market forces or consumer demand. Were there a market niche for medical service made cheaper by the elimination of routine hand washing, a doctor would still have to wash her hands.

This is not to say that physicians are required to forego profit. Medicine is a profession not a charity. But there's more to being a doctor than having a set of marketable skills. That this is so is witnessed by the fact that the use of medical skills to administer death by lethal injection conflicts with the requirements of being a doctor. If medicine were just a business, there would be nothing wrong with using physicians to execute prisoners on death row. Ditto the deployment of medical knowledge to facilitate the torture of "enemy combatants." The point is that the conception of medicine as a profession precludes the idea that medicine is just business or that it is just a skill.

The proper aim of medicine is to meet the medical needs of one's patients. The sphere of medical needs is much smaller than the sphere of human wants. Even if medicine satisfies legitimate desires, desire satisfaction as such isn't medicine. So, while my middle-aged patients may beseech me to inject "more and more" Botox or to siphon off yet another quart of accumulated fat, it doesn't follow that I should comply with their requests any more than I ought to provide growth hormones to my short, but healthy, nephew simply to improve his chances at a basketball scholarship. Recommendations for medical treatment ought to be based on medical judgment about medical need. One cannot simply trade satisfying expressed client preferences for professional medical judgment.[9]

To insist that clinical judgment must trump client demand is not to deny that health care, as an institution has become more of a business with the rise of managed care in the US over the past 25 years. The majority of doctors no longer work alone or in small group practices; nor do they necessarily have long-standing relationships with a fixed, familiar patient base. In the contemporary United States, the

[9] On the importance of the shift from "social trustee professionalism" to "expert professionalism," see Thompson 2005: 267ff.

goals of medicine are more often set by the insurance provider or medical organization than the Hippocratic Oath. Doctors make their lives by practicing medicine and so are driven by market forces and the need to meet economic pressures.[10] But it is possible to acknowledge these realities without abandoning the idea of medicine as a profession.

The next two conceptions of cosmetic surgery can be thought of as responses to the recognition of the failure of the two previous approaches. They recognize the ways in which cosmetic surgery is anomalous and attempt to find ways of understanding it that make the practice consistent with traditional understandings of medicine.

9.4.3 Using the Blade to Cure the Soul: Cosmetic Surgery as Psychological Medicine

This third conception represents cosmetic surgery as a form of *psychological* healing. Elective procedures such as Rhinoplasty and breast implants serve psychological ends, e.g., the relief of emotional distress caused by unlucky genes, undesired features or signs of aging. On this view, cosmetic surgery is warranted because it "heals" self-consciousness or low self-esteem. The claim is that 'using the knife' results in "measurable and meaningful improvement in psychosocial functioning and psychological well being in the long term" (Honigman et al. 2001: 1229). Cosmetic surgery, understood in these terms, is in effect a form of psychotherapy. The beauty doctor "creates beauty to cure the soul" (Gilman 1999).

This historically prominent line of argument re-frames cosmetic surgery as a natural extension of the medical arts. After all, modern medicine takes care not only of the body, but also the mind, treating disorders such as agoraphobia, depression, and bipolar disorder. By removing or refashioning what gives distress (the abnormally large nose, rolls of unwanted fat, a sagging jowl), the cosmetic surgeon provides a psychological benefit that justifies the risks of surgery.

There are two problems with this rationale. The first is that not everything that makes people happy or augments their subjective well-being qualifies as a health benefit. Cigarette smoking may improve self-esteem by giving one an air of nonchalance or the image of being cool – or help control weight gain. Money too works wonders in increasing confidence and bolstering self-regard. But a physician who handed his patients fistfuls of money or packs of cigarettes wouldn't be practicing medicine. The point is not that doctors are or should be indifferent to the happiness of their patients, but that subjective well-being – what makes the patient happy – is distinct from healthcare and must take a back seat to the latter. In short, the proper goal of medicine is health, not happiness. The claim that cosmetic surgery makes people happy, even if true, fails as medical justification.

---

[10] Many of those who opt out of the managed care system, often by engaging in fee-for-service specialties such as cosmetic surgery, see themselves as "experts," trained at great personal expense, and expecting a return on investment.

A second concern is that problems of self-esteem or depression born of social or work-related rejection may be better met by therapies that directly address the problems that caused them. Breast implants or Rhinoplasties may buttress the rigid, often demeaning, beauty standards responsible for generating the desire for cosmetic surgery. Cosmetic surgery may foster the very conditions it pretends to alleviate. If, as critics charge, prevailing beauty norms often rest upon insidious gender, racial and ethnic representations, then the price of the psychological well-being cosmetic surgery provides may be the cultivation of a false sense of self.

9.4.4 Optimization

The last line of justification strives to validate cosmetic surgery by going back to the body. Its claim is that cosmetic surgery is a form of optimization, of "making the best of." The unattractive face can be made ordinary or 'average,' the average, beautiful. This conception depends upon an expanded notion of health – one that goes far beyond the idea of health as the attaining or maintaining some average or agreed upon capacities, e.g., a specified resting heart rate, hemoglobin level, blood pressure, or restoring "species-typical functioning." It may define health as the attainment of maximal species-typical functioning or as the transcendence of species-typical limitations altogether.[11] One goal of optimization is to give all of us the capability to run at Olympic speeds and enjoy the skills now possessed by only the very gifted. Another is to transcend even the far range of normal function, allowing human beings to re-grow injured body parts, stay awake for seven days, and enjoy an unwavering feeling of contentment (Garreau 2005).[12] If this seems over the top, it is. Yet these are claims that pro-optimizers actually make.

To the objection that such achievements lie beyond the original brief of medicine, its defenders reply, so what? Why must we restrict ourselves to a traditional conception of medicine? The same benevolent regard that motivates restoration of function also motivates its optimization. Prior to the 20th century, medicine did not include prevention, research into the causes of disease, public health campaigns or education to eradicate the chronic conditions that plagued modern societies (Porter 2002: 157–159). Much of what belongs quite comfortably to contemporary medicine – vaccination programs, epidemiology, psychotherapy, anesthesiology, even regular hand-washing – required an expansion of medicine's reach. Why then not go further? Why stop at restoring health and normal function when the technical know-how exists to do more? Extending memory, lengthening average life span, and while we're at it, removing unsightly bumps and bulges will benefit all of us.

[11] For the notion of "species-typical functioning," see Daniels 1986: 33. For a critique of the idea of using 'typicality' as a medical standard, see Anita Silvers, "A Fatal Attraction to Normalizing: Treating Disabilities as Deviations from 'Species Typical' Functioning" in Parens 1998: 93–123.

[12] Garreau maintains that the acceleration of advances in computing and biology will bring dramatic changes in our lifetimes and almost certainly in the lifetimes of our children.

This is certainly a tempting vision. It promises to make us all faster, smarter, and yes, more fetching.

Philosopher Julian Savulescu goes so far as to contend that enhancing biological and psychological characteristics may be ethically required (Savulescu 2003). Particularly with respect to children, Savulescu insists, choosing not to enhance their functioning is harmful. Just as it would be medically wrong to withhold a good diet or vaccinations for early childhood diseases, so too, he claims, physicians ought not to forestall the benefits of genetic, pharmacological or other medical enhancements as these become available.

Savulescu's reasoning may convince some of the justifiability of a wider use of Ritalin, growth hormones, and other prescription drugs. Others will balk at administering drugs with side effects and unforeseen long-term consequences, especially to the young. Far more controversial are interventions designed to "optimize" appearance rather than function. Children may need the ability to sit still and pay attention in order to learn. They can study perfectly well, however, without a nice nose or surgically pinned ears.

One can easily predict Savulescu's response to this last objection. Although protruding ears may not directly interfere with education or professional success, such features can negatively impact self-confidence and social interaction. In so doing, they "disable" individuals in ways that diminish quality of life and that surgery can fix. So characterized, the smaller (or less ethnic) nose and flatter ears offered by the cosmetic surgeon are motivated by the impulse to do good. The idea is that a change in features will increase self-confidence and the likelihood of success.[13]

Despite its appeal, the optimization rationale faces a number of philosophical and ethical hurdles. First, while some efforts to extend human capabilities may strike us as morally unproblematic (e.g., the possibility of faster runners), others, such as an expanded memory or military endurance gained through the "erasure" of traumatic memories, will give at least some of us pause (Wolpe 2003; Kolber 2006). What the enhancement controversy reveals is the need for a principled means of establishing the boundaries of professional obligation, the limits of private and public healthcare insurance and the proper sphere of biomedical research (Juengst 1998: 29). Traditional medicine has tended to fix these boundaries by appealing to notions of health and disease, or notions such as the aforementioned concept of 'species-typical function.' While problematic, such notions assumed that at some level the limits of the human (and hence of medicine) are biologically fixed. New biotechnologies have opened up the possibility that we may soon be in a position to change many of the biological

[13] At this point, the optimization defense comes very close to the idea that cosmetic surgery is justified because it gives us the means to make us subjectively happy. On the psychological model, a finer appearance makes us feel better about ourselves. The optimization model introduces an intermediary step. Improved appearance leads to personal or professional success, which in turn is presumed to enhance personal satisfaction or "happiness." While this point cannot be pursued here, the biomedical discussion of enhancement would profit from a more philosophical reflection on what constitutes human flourishing and some attention to the history of this discussion.

limits assumed by traditional medicine. But this possibility raises questions about the permissibility and desirability of making such changes. The friends of optimization push hard for these developments. They assume answers to questions they don't pause long enough to ask.

Even if optimization is an acceptable goal for medicine, the employment of scarce medical resources for this purpose raises moral and political questions that Savulescu's commitment to the individual obscures. The basic fact is that the financial and human resources available for healthcare are limited. The use of these resources to meet the demand for optimization means that fewer resources are available for the care of health. With the US population growing and the number of physicians remaining largely constant since 1980 (an artifact of limiting medical school enrollment), one has to consider the repercussions. American medical schools, for example, have a history of limiting enrollment. With the number of graduates remaining largely constant since 1980 and US population increasing, the diversion of large numbers of MDs into cosmetic surgery and boutique specialties has obvious costs to basic healthcare (Wall 2005). Does this distribution of resources reflect good medical judgment? Does it reflect medical judgment at all? Is it just?

The optimization argument is subject to a further – foundational – difficulty: that it trades on a basic error. That error is the idea that cosmetic surgery and other appearance-based modifications actually expand human functionality. This is rarely the case. Breast implants don't increase cancer-resistance or boost lactation. Smaller noses don't improve breathing. Whitening does not strengthen the teeth. What cosmetic surgery delivers is something other than functional improvement. Nor is such improvement the aim. The goal, as both patients and doctors know, is aesthetic (and social) enhancement. The effect of the procedures responsible for these enhancements is often reduced functionality, e.g., decreased breast sensation, paralyzed and expressionless facial muscles. In many standard cosmetic procedures, health is compromised or put at risk in exchange for non-health-related ends.

9.5 Questions and Concerns

We have been focusing on the kind of cosmetic surgery that goes by the name of medical enhancement. The term 'medical enhancement' suggests a practice that *adds* something to health and healthcare. But this assumption merits scrutiny. Presenting cosmetic surgery as something extra, a supplement to basic healthcare provides a misleading and misguided picture. It leads us to make two seriously erroneous assumptions: the first concerning the concept of enhancement, the second concerning its costs.

First, much of the debate over the benefits and risks of medical enhancement centers on the question "How far beyond good health should we go?" Casting the question this way assumes that good health and good healthcare remain fixed while we pursue the dream of improving "human form or functioning beyond what is necessary to sustain or restore good health" (Juengst 1998: 29). What we have seen, however, is that the growth of the practice of medical enhancement may actually lead to a worsening of health. Patients undergo the injury of surgery itself and its short and long term risks. Some forms of cosmetic surgery, e.g., liposuction, raise especially serious questions about whether the benefits are worth the risk. Survey results obtained from board-certified plastic surgeons indicate a 1 in 5,000 mortality rate from liposuction, often from pulmonary thromboembolism (Grazer & de Jong 2000). Other forms of cosmetic surgery, while unlikely to cause death, can result in long term crippling effects, e.g., toe shortening – cutting the foot to fit the shoe rather than the reverse – a procedure that cannot but strike an impartial observer as perverse. Talk of *medical* enhancement thus obscures the fact that the dimension along which things are enhanced is not medical. As these and other cases illustrate, much of what gets called enhancement "enhances" neither health nor function.

One therefore has to ask to what extent medical enhancement can properly be classified as *health*care. The tendency to redefine each new cosmetic procedure as a cure for some freshly minted disease or disorder, e.g., cellulite, dermatochalasis (the presence of excess upper or lower eyelid skin), asymmetrical breasts, gynecomastia (enlargement of the male breast), is evidence of the profession's awareness of the need to provide a medical warrant for the imposition of health risks in the service of refashioning "unfashionable" and "unaesthetic" bodies.

The second error in characterizing cosmetic surgery as 'enhancement' lies in the assumption that its effects on the *healthcare system* are minimal. Putting medical energy and resources into making people pretty and keeping them 'young' when a significant percentage of the national population lacks even basic healthcare has real implications for patients, their caregivers, and society at large. Patient demand for Botox injections and a host of new cosmetic procedures has, as report after report indicates, risen exponentially in the US, UK and other developed countries. The call for so-called designer drugs such as Prozac and Viagra is also mushrooming. If leading scientists are correct that ever more powerful biotechnology, including brain/machine interfaces and cosmetic neurology, will be widely available within 10–15 years (Garreau 2005: 35–38), competitive demand for such services will only increase, putting growing pressure on medical resources already stretched thin.

Changes in patient demands aren't the only explanation of shifts in medical resources. Physicians too find these new and lucrative specialties attractive. In the face of managed care, providing traditional medical services has become a headache. Diminished control and lowered income not surprisingly lead more and more physicians to service specialties such as cosmetic dermatology, areas of medicine that offer regular hours, a better educated clientele, and more remuneration. One result is the increasing competition for residencies in cosmetic specialties. The shift in medical personnel from basic healthcare to "service-oriented," fee-for-service specialties may come to be a public health problem.

I am not claiming that the desire for a surgically altered appearance is always false. Nor am I claiming that cosmetic surgery is always unethical. Still less do I mean to suggest that all plastic surgeons are irresponsible or evil. What I have tried to do is to call attention to the aspects of cosmetic surgery as practiced in the US today that raise ethical concerns and in so doing point to ways in which new forms of enhancement may be ethically problematic.

I want to close by pointing to four specific areas of ethical concern that may be expected to reappear in new guises with the rise of novel non-cosmetic medical enhancers. All of them illustrate the tension between "consumer oriented entrepreneurial practice" and traditional medical ethics as defined by a tradition reaching back to Hippocrates (Miller et al. 2000: 353).

The first issue concerns advertising. Print ads in magazines and newspapers, the internet, Oprah Winfrey, and word of mouth all tout the benefits of anti-aging procedures to younger and younger patient populations, men as well as women.[14] Television lends itself to hype: infomercials for "face lifts in a bottle" or the latest in non-surgical lower eyelid lifts. The exploitation of the fears and social insecurities of the vulnerable is ethically dubious on general grounds. Playing on such insecurities also raises questions grounded in the norms of a profession dedicated to healing, saving lives and public health. This is not to say that the wish for cosmetic surgery is always an artifact of advertising. Many patients describe suffering estrangement from their bodies and report post-surgical relief at achieving an acceptable face or body (Davis 1995: 99–103). But, as critics of the deregulation of medical advertising and the free market promotion of cosmetic surgery caution, such practices erode trust in the doctor/patient relationship and "undermine public confidence in the medical profession" (Ring 2002: 599). Much of what passes for medical information in this context is inaccurate or misleading. Ads for cosmetic surgery, unlike ads for new medications, rarely mention complications, negative outcomes, or the likelihood of post-operative pain and suffering. If patients are to give genuine informed consent, they must be aware of the risks and assume them voluntarily, based on a vivid and visceral sense of the possible outcomes.[15] Breast implants can rupture (Brown et al. 2001) and thromboembolism and death from procedures such as liposuction, while rare, do occur (Clayman & Caffee 2006: 78–81). They must understand that they are risking health for beauty.

A second problem is the conflict of interest inherent in the practice of cosmetic surgery. In helping patients realize their dreams of "a better self" (diagnosing and excising their "defects"), physicians stand to make significant sums of money. Advising a teenage patient that breast enlargements may not make her happier or a middle-aged woman that another face-lift will not nullify the fact that she is growing older generates no income. Although most surgeons no doubt put patient well-being first, the economic structure of cosmetic surgery pulls in the other direction.

[14] Feminists have argued for decades that the marketing strategy for cosmetic surgery rests on the assumption that aging is ugly and ugliness a disease for which cosmetic surgery is the most effective cure (Wolf 1990; Ring 2002: 597).

[15] The 'before' and 'after' pictures ubiquitous in the marketing of cosmetic surgery never include images of what can go wrong. Yet in obtaining genuinely informed consent, physicians should insure that patients know the real risks, something perhaps best conveyed by photographs.

Cosmetic surgeons can reply that they do take the welfare of their potential patients seriously. They act in accordance with the "express preferences" of clients, without presuming paternalistically to have a better understanding of what those preferences are than the patients themselves do. But all too often anti-paternalism provides an excuse for the non-exercise of professional judgment, e.g., the unlicensed but growing practice of hymenoplasty or "revirgination," the surgical reconstruction of the hymen offered by a handful of private surgeons to women who want to "surprise" their husbands with "a special gift" (Walters 2006: 1–2).

This brings us to the related issue of appropriate psychological screening. In an area where patient preferences play such a determining role – in both diagnosis of "the problem" and in measuring "success of outcome "—much depends on the judgment of the client-patient. Should cosmetic surgeons agree to operate on individuals who refuse to undergo psychiatric evaluation to identify clinical depression, body dysmorphic disorder, anorexia nervosa or other psychiatric conditions? These and other "body image" issues may predict a poor outcome and make cosmetic surgery ill advised. Body dysmorphia, the excessive preoccupation with minor or imaginary physical defects that causes clinically significant impairment "in social, occupational or other important areas of functioning," can, for example, sometimes be effectively treated with SSRIs and cognitive behavioral therapy, but only if it is correctly diagnosed. Yet plastic surgeons are neither required to administer psychological tests nor are they trained to do so (Rohrich 2000: 1605–1607). Psychological evaluation is left to the untrained judgment of physicians who have a structural incentive to overlook disqualifying psychological factors. A system that took psychological assessment out of the hands of the treating physician could circumvent this conflict of interest.

The fourth and last issue involves questions about medical credentialing, safety and outcome measures. It's worth noting that not all cosmetic surgeons are board certified in cosmetic plastic surgery. As observed recently by the President of the American Society for Aesthetic Plastic Surgery (ASAPS), "Anyone with an 'MD' can call themselves a cosmetic surgeon and, in fact, some dentists now want to perform cosmetic surgery." (ASAPS 2005). Although properly trained cosmetic surgeons have a guild interest in restricting the franchise, in point of fact, there are few if any restrictions on the title 'cosmetic surgeon.' Critics worry that the explosive growth in demand for such procedures leads physicians with little or no training in the specific techniques to offer such procedures (Singer 2006b: E3). Not only dentists, but also dermatologists, podiatrists, and a variety of other medical specialists want in on the increasingly popular and lucrative cosmetic industry. For their part, patients are left to sort out the issue of proper credentials for themselves. But "buyer beware" is no guarantee of safety.

A related issue is that not all cosmetic surgeries are carried out in accredited facilities. The push is for less invasive cosmetic procedures to move out of the medical office and into the spa or beauty salon, with nurse practitioners providing services such as Botox injections, often without direct physician supervision. Responsible cosmetic surgeons themselves express reservations about the cavalier promotion of surgical treatments provided by non-physicians in settings far from accredited medical facilities (Singer 2006a: E3). Elective surgery is, after all, still surgery and can have unexpected and serious consequences. Even a simple collagen injection (e.g., a needle loaded with bacteria) can cause infection or other complications. Despite such risks, "demedicalization" of at least some cosmetic procedures is driven by commercial interests interested in "getting their share" of what is now a $12 billion a year business.

Aside from issues of safety is the equally important question of whether cosmetic surgery delivers what it promises. Does surgical modification of the body result in demonstrable long-term psychological benefits? A 2004 review of the literature measuring psychosocial outcomes for patients electing cosmetic surgery found generally good results, but noted several methodological limitations in this research (Honigman et al. 2004: 1229–1237). Honigman et al. distinguished, for example, between patient satisfaction with their change in appearance following surgery (being happier about their looks) and "measurable and meaningful improvement in psychosocial functioning and psychological well-being in the long term" (being happier). As they report, studies attempting to measure outcomes reach conflicting conclusions, with some interview-based studies reporting good outcomes, while others note no change or negative consequences (Honigman et al. 2004: 1232). The absence of randomized clinical trials comparing surgical intervention with "no treatment" (or alternatives such as psychotherapy, exercise or expanded social interaction) presents another limitation. Such a study would of course be difficult to enroll or carry out. But even researchers who conclude in favor of the psychological effectiveness of cosmetic surgery acknowledge that without a comparison class it is difficult to know whether the reported improvements resulted from the surgery, other aspects of the intervention, or unrelated changes in circumstance. Nor can the possibility of a "placebo effect" be ruled out (Rankin et al. 1998: 2139–2145).

In short, existing outcome measures fall short of establishing reliability or causality. With the popularity of "makeover" television shows downplaying the risk of body altering cosmetic procedures and touting "extreme" life-altering effects, we may anticipate that unrealistic expectations will lead to increased patient dissatisfaction.

These and other ethical issues raised by cosmetic surgery illustrate what lies ahead. Psychopharmacology and neurobiology already offer to transform the deepest features of the human psyche. Genetic screening and gene therapy stand poised to give us far greater control over our biological inheritance and regenerative medicine may eventually forestall even aging itself. With these and other biomedical advances, concerns about media hype overcoming accurate assessment of medical risks and benefits, physician conflicts of interest, appropriate patient screening, safety and reliability, and the just allocation of scarce healthcare resources will reemerge. The question is whether and how medicine can maintain its own integrity as a profession in the face of pressures from patient-consumers, advancing biotechnology, and its own entrepreneurial impulses. The challenge for physicians is to pause and reflect on what medicine as medicine is – and what it may, at its best and worst, become.[16] This may require resisting the Siren song that promises medicine unimaginable powers in favor of a return to healing the sick.

References

American Society for Aesthetic Plastic Surgery, ASAPS (2005) ASAPS Panel Reviews "State of the Art" in Patient Safety. April 29. www.surgery.org/press/news-release.php?iid=407 Accessed Oct. 24, 2006

Bordo S (1993) Unbearable Weight: Feminism, Western Culture, and the Body. University of California Press, Berkeley, CA/Los Angeles, CA/London

Brown S L, Pennello G, Berg W A, Soo M S, Middleton M S (2001) Journal of Rheumatology May; 28(5):996–1003

Clayman M A, Caffee H H (2006) Office Surgery Safety and the Florida Moratoria. Annals of Plastic Surgery 56 (1), January: 78–81

Daniels N (1986) Just Health Care. Cambridge University Press, New York

Davis K (1995) Reshaping the Female Body: The Dilemma of Cosmetic Surgery. Routledge, New York

Elliott C (2000) A New Way to Be Mad. Atlantic Monthly 286 (6): 72–84

Elliott C (2003) Better than Well: American Medicine Meets the American Dream. W. W. Norton, New York

Garreau J (2005) Radical Evolution: The Promise and Peril of Enhancing Our Minds, Our Bodies and What It Means to Be Human. Doubleday, New York

Gilman S L (1998) Creating Beauty to Cure the Soul: Race and Psychology in the Shaping of Aesthetic Surgery. Duke University Press, Durham, NC/London

Gilman S L (1999) Making the Body Beautiful: A Cultural History of Aesthetic Surgery. Princeton University Press, Princeton, NJ

Goering S (2001) The Ethics of Making the Body Beautiful: What Cosmetic Genetics Can Learn from Cosmetic Surgery. Philosophy & Public Policy Quarterly 21 (1): 21–27

Grazer F M, de Jong R M (2000) Fatal Outcomes from Liposuction: Census Survey of Cosmetic Surgeons. Plastic Reconstructive Surgery 105 (1), January: 436–446

Haiken E (1997) Venus Envy: A History of Cosmetic Surgery. Johns Hopkins University Press, Baltimore, MD/London

Honigman R J, Phillips K A, Castle D J (2004) A Review of Psychosocial Outcomes for Patients Seeking Cosmetic Surgery. Plastic and Reconstructive Surgery, April 1: 1229–1237

Juengst E T (1998) What Does "Enhancement" Mean? In: Parens E (ed) Enhancing Human Traits: Ethical and Social Implications. Georgetown University Press, Washington, DC

Kolber, A J (2006) Therapeutic Forgetting: The Legal and Ethical Implications of Memory Dampening. Vanderbilt Law Review, 59: 1561–1628

Miller F G, Brody H, Chung K C (2000) Cosmetic Surgery and Internal Morality of Medicine. Cambridge Quarterly of Healthcare Ethics 9: 353–364

[16] Some claim that questions about the consequences of medicine moving in these directions comes too late. As Carl Elliott has argued, cosmetic surgery is deeply entrenched in the American psyche. It provides Americans unhappy in their own skins – on Elliott's analysis, most of us – the option to remake themselves, to fit in, to pursue a peculiar kind of American happiness (Elliott 2003: 304). This may be right. But as cosmetic surgery and related procedures become more common, it is even more crucial that they be carried out with appropriate safeguards, fully informed consent and careful thought to short and long term consequences.

Nisbel B (2003) A New Wrinkle for Botox: Headache Relief. University of Michigan Healthsystem Newspage. www.med.umich.edu/opm/newspage/2003/botox.htm
Parens E (1998) (ed) Enhancing Human Traits: Ethical and Social Implications. Georgetown University Press, Washington, DC
Porter R (2002) Blood & Guts: A Short History of Medicine. W. W. Norton, New York
Rankin M, Borah G L, Perry A W, Wey P D (1998) Quality-Of-Life Outcomes After Cosmetic Surgery. Plastic & Reconstructive Surgery 102(6), November: 2139–2145
Ring A L (2002) Using "Anti-Ageing" [sic] to Market Cosmetic Surgery: Just Good Business, or Another Wrinkle on the Face of Medical Practice. MJA 176, June 17
Rohrich R J (2000) The Who, What, When, and Why of Cosmetic Surgery: Do Our Patients Need a Preoperative Psychiatric Evaluation? Plastic and Reconstructive Surgery, December: 1605–1607
Rothschild J (2005) The Dream of the Perfect Child. Indiana University Press, Bloomington, IN
Savulescu J (2003) The Ethics of Enhancement of Human Beings. Unpublished lecture. Delivered at The University of Tokyo, June 30 http://www.practicalethics.ox.ac.uk/introduction/Enhancement%20JAPAN%202.pdf
Singer N (2006a) The Oprah Treatment. New York Times, Thursday, May 11: E1, E3
Singer N (2006b) Love the New Lips! From the Mall? New York Times, Thursday, October 26: E3
Sullivan D A (2001) Cosmetic Surgery: The Cutting Edge of Commercial Medicine in America. Rudgers University Press, New Brunswick, NJ/New York
Thompson D F (2005) Restoring Responsibility: Ethics in Government, Business, and Healthcare. Cambridge University Press, Cambridge
Wall N M (2005) Stealing from the Poor to Care for the Rich. Copyright New York Times http://www.saynotocaps.org/newsarticles/stealingfrompoor.htm
Walters J (2006) Like a Virgin. The Times, February 27. http://women.timesonline.co.uk/article/0,,17909-2057781_1,00.html
Wolf N (1990) The Beauty Myth. Chatto & Windus, London
Wolpe P R (2003) Treatment, Enhancement, and the Ethics of Neurotherapeutics. Brain and Cognition 50: 387–395

Chapter 10
Decelerating and Arresting Human Aging

Walter Glannon

10.1 Introduction

Aging is the bane of our human existence. It is responsible for degenerative diseases of the body and mind and is the cause of much pain, suffering, and diminished quality of life. It is a constant reminder of our mortality. Assuming that mortality is not a disease, and that aging is an intrinsic property of mortality, aging itself is not a disease. But the degenerative features of many diseases are the by-product of aging. Thus it would seem intuitively desirable to intervene in and decelerate or arrest this process. If this intervention were successful, then it could slow the development of and perhaps even prevent diseases and thereby extend the human lifespan. Decelerated and arrested aging could greatly improve the quality of life and increase the well-being of many people.

Biogerontology is the study of the biological mechanisms that control human aging, or senescence. This is the process through which cells stop dividing and all biological functions gradually cease. Two possible interventions that might retard or alter these mechanisms are the generation of new tissues from stem cells and manipulation of the genetic factors regulating aging. In the first type of intervention, new tissues developed from embryonic or other types of stem cells could replace tissues and organs damaged by degenerative diseases. Insulin-producing islet cells for diabetes, cartilage and bone for osteoarthritis and osteoporosis, and neural stem cells for Parkinson's and Alzheimer's disease are just a few examples. These forms of regenerative medicine could control these and other diseases by slowing their progression. They could result in a moderate extension of a person's lifespan beyond the present norm of roughly 80 years. In the second type of intervention, genes regulating the molecular mechanisms of aging could be altered at an early age. By decelerating or arresting aging, this could prevent or at least delay the development of late-onset degenerative diseases such as Parkinson's and Alzheimer's. It might also result in a substantial increase in the human lifespan.

In this chapter, I explore medical, social, and psychological dimensions of these two types of intervention aimed at altering aging. Regenerative medicine may be a mixed blessing. In many cases, it could result in a modest increase in the lifespan. But it could also entail a trade-off between increased quantity and quality of life in

B. Gordijn, R. Chadwick (eds.) *Medical Enhancement and Posthumanity*,

terms of physical function and decreased quality of life in terms of cognitive function. This could cancel out any early benefits of the intervention. A similar trade-off could occur to a greater degree if genetic manipulation of aging mechanisms substantially extended the lifespan. Whether this would benefit us would depend on whether we could retain equal physical and cognitive functioning through the extended period of our lives. In addition, tinkering with genes to decelerate or arrest aging might unleash growth factors normally suppressed by these same genes and result in diseases such as cancer. Even a modest increase in the lifespan for the elderly could be unfair to the young by burdening them in different ways. At a deeper level, such an increase could alter the natural contour of a human life and its component stages. Much of the discussion in this chapter is speculative, especially with respect to the second type of intervention I have described. Nevertheless, given our understanding of the biology of aging and the theoretical possibility of extending the human lifespan, speculation can be the catalyst for consideration of issues raised by intervention in the aging process.

10.2 Medical Factors

It will be helpful to frame the discussion in terms of a fourfold distinction drawn by Eric Juengst et al. in their discussion of biogerontology (Juengst et al. 2003). They describe four possible outcomes of anti-aging medicine: prolonged senescence; compressed morbidity; decelerated aging; and arrested aging. Prolonged senescence would merely extend the lives of the old without mitigating the degenerative effects of aging. Compressed morbidity would shorten the length of time between the onset of aging-related diseases and death. It would allow us to have relatively long lives free of chronic disease and disability and to die quickly from an acute condition such as pneumonia as we reached the limits of the life span. Compressed morbidity may involve accelerated aging, but only for a brief period before death to preclude or at least minimize any disease, pain, or suffering. Decelerated aging would retard but not significantly alter senescence. It would postpone the onset of degenerative diseases, control their progression, and result in a moderate extension of the human lifespan. Arrested aging would involve complete control over the aging process and could prevent many of its deleterious effects. It would negate the effects of senescence by continuously repairing damage to tissues and organs that is the by-product of cell metabolism. Arrested aging could result in a substantial extension of the lifespan.

Prolonged senescence would be the least desirable outcome because it would involve a long period of physical and cognitive decline before death. Arrested aging would be the most desirable outcome. Theoretically, it could enable biologists to not only retard but also reverse the degenerative effects of aging and prevent or cure many diseases. Compressed morbidity arguably would be the second most desirable outcome because it would reduce the likelihood of experiencing the pain and suffering associated with degenerative diseases.[1] This may be even more challenging than arrested aging, since it would require genetically reprogramming a short interval between disease onset and death. This would be extremely difficult, if not impossible, to achieve since ordinarily the length of time between disease onset and death is a function of multiple environmental and biological factors and thus not predictable. Also, these factors are part of an extended process that ordinarily constitutes a substantial interval of time. Decelerated aging would be the most likely and plausible outcome because a moderate life extension through tissue replacement would be the least difficult to achieve.

It may be possible to decelerate aging through a caloric restriction diet involving roughly a 30% reduction in calories. Experiments have shown that such action can extend life in a variety of animal species. In humans, this might slow metabolism and the release of free radicals, the highly reactive oxygen-containing molecules that can expedite senescence. But a dietary change from higher to lower caloric intake does not involve the same intervention in the aging process as tissue regeneration or genetic manipulation, and therefore it does not raise the same biological and ethical concerns. Let's consider the four anti-aging scenarios with respect to the two types of intervention at issue.

Regenerative medicine could decelerate aging by controlling the progression and symptoms of some diseases. Embryonic stem cells may enable researchers to develop tissues to replace those damaged by disease. Ideally, these tissues would derive from one's own somatic cells, which would make them less likely to trigger an adverse immune response in the recipient. Ethical questions about creating and destroying embryos once stem cells had been extracted from them have been discussed at length elsewhere, and accordingly I will leave them aside here.[2] Regenerating islet cells or organs such as pancreases, kidneys, and hearts using stem cells would be difficult enough. Regenerating neurons and neural tissue would be much more difficult because the brain is more plastic and complex than any other organ in the human body. Perhaps the best example of this has been the general failure of neural stem cell transplantation to control and relieve the symptoms of Parkinson's disease. Researchers have not been able to regulate how transplanted neural tissue affects growth factors in the brain. People with regenerated tissues and organs in their bodies may live longer as a result of these interventions. But an equivalent regeneration of brain tissue and restoration or retention of cognitive function would be less likely to occur. A longer life might include many years of dementia, which would offset any gains in restoring or retaining physical function. Decelerated aging could thus result in prolonged senescence. Could altering the genetic mechanisms of senescence avoid this?

Leonard Guarente and other researchers have discovered that increased expression of the SIR2 gene lengthens the lifespan in some species by acting on biological

---

[1] James Fries introduced and analyzed this concept in Fries 1980.

[2] Among others, these discussions include Mahowald 2003, Sandel 2004 and McHugh 2004.

processes that promote survival under conditions of scarcity.[3] This finding is based on research involving the worm *C. elegans*. By tinkering with this and other genes that regulate senescence in humans, it is possible that researchers could not only decelerate but also arrest senescence. Manipulating SIR2 or similar genes might enable researchers to alter the function of telomeres by altering the enzyme telomerase that regulates them. Telomeres are regions of DNA at the ends of chromosomes that control the number of cell divisions and become increasingly shorter the more times cells divide. They are associated with what is known as the "Hayflick Limit," named after biologist Leonard Hayflick, who demonstrated that somatic cells can replicate only a limited number of times (Hayflick & Moorhead 1961; Hayflick 1965, 1977). Manipulation of telomerase in the critical genes might enable researchers to reprogram the genetic mechanisms of senescence and break the Hayflick Limit. Cells might replicate indefinitely and result in an indefinitely extended lifespan.

There is considerable skepticism among biologists and biodemographers of aging as to whether extending the lives of cells beyond the Hayflick Limit is scientifically possible.[4] Many insist that, although the human lifespan has increased significantly over the last two centuries, any additional increase would be modest at best. For the sake of argument, let's suppose that the human lifespan could be substantially increased through genetic means. We need to consider some of the risks.

Any thought of trying to alter the genetic controls on aging for the purpose of greater longevity would have to take into account the theory of antagonistic pleiotropy.[5] Pleiotropy refers to the multiple effects of an organism's phenotype due to a single gene or allele. The same gene can influence the phenotype of more than one part or system of the body. One implication of this theory is that genes protecting us from diseases early in life could make us more vulnerable to diseases later in life. Natural selection favors this trade-off by limiting the number of genetic mutations that can accumulate in cells through reproductive years. This period may be extended to include additional years necessary to nurture offspring so that they can reach reproductive age. But natural selection imposes no such limit beyond these years. By that time, there is no longer any evolutionary reason to limit mutations causing life-threatening diseases because it is beyond the time for transmitting genes to the next generation. There are many examples of genetically controlled physiological processes that illustrate this point. High levels of estrogen in women and of testosterone in men may be favorable for fertility early in life but increase

[3] See Guarente and Kenyon 2000 and Hekimi and Guarente 2003. Also, Kirkland 2002. This process should be contrasted with progeria, the extreme acceleration of aging caused by mutations in a gene on chromosome 1. Progeria is appropriately described as a genetic disease.

[4] Hayflick 2001, 2001–2002. S. Jay Olshansky and Bruce A. Carnes present a similar skeptical view in Olshansky and Carnes 2001. Tom Kirkwood offers a more positive perspective in Kirkwood 2001, 2008.

[5] George Williams first presented and defended this theory in Williams 1957. Another significant paper on this issue is Lithgow and Kirkwood 1996: 80. See also Nesse and Williams 1994 and Greaves 2007.

the risk of breast, ovarian, and prostate cancer later in life. Inflammatory responses may protect us from potentially life-threatening pathogens earlier in life. Yet the cumulative effects of inflammation in the body may result in atherosclerosis and other cardiovascular and neurological diseases later in life.

If antagonistic pleiotropy is a biological fact in humans, then adverse health consequences early in life may be the trade-off for a few additional genetically engineered years later in life. Manipulation of the relevant genes could remove our protection against infectious diseases in youth, adolescence, and early adulthood over a number of generations. One might question these claims, since it is not yet known whether the genes selected to manipulate the mechanisms of aging would have such deleterious side effects. Yet it seems unlikely that none of these genes would be pleiotropic. It is more likely that at least some of them would involve phenotypic traits that would not all be beneficial or benign. It is unclear whether researchers of aging could know in advance which genes would or would not be pleiotropic.

Altering the molecular mechanisms of senescence could affect apoptosis, the programmed cell death ensuring that cells do not replicate out of control. The alteration could disable mechanisms in cells that repair damage to their DNA. In addition, it could unleash growth factors and allow cells and tissues to proliferate, which would have deleterious effects in the body. It could also disarm tumor suppressor genes and cause various cancers. This would not just thwart the desire for a substantial extension of the lifespan. The cancers would prevent people from having even a normal lifespan. Paradoxically, an intervention designed to extend our lives could end up shortening them.

Even if genetic manipulation of aging had only salutary effects on the body, it would leave us with one disturbing possibility. The likely inability to regenerate neural tissue or to genetically prevent neuron death would mean that our cognitive functions would not keep pace with our physical functions. Some centenarians retain a fairly good level of both physical and cognitive functions until just before death. Through genetic good fortune, they enjoy a natural form of compressed morbidity. But these individuals constitute a very small percentage of the human population. For most people, a substantially extended lifespan from genetic manipulation could be much worse than a moderately extended lifespan from regenerative medicine. People might retain physical vigor but also undergo cognitive decline and dementia over many years. It would be the worst possible case of prolonged senescence. Because cognitive and other mental capacities are at least as valuable to us as physical capacities, this scenario would involve an undesirable trade-off between quantity and quality of life.

Francis Fukuyama describes this as a "national nursing home scenario, in which people routinely live to be 150 but spend the last fifty years in a state of childlike dependence on caretakers" (Fukuyama 2002: 69). Alluding to the more moderate life extension that regenerative medicine might afford, Fukuyama further says that "stem cell research might yield new ways to grow body parts … But without a parallel cure for Alzheimer's disease, this wonderful new technology would do no more than allow more people to persist in vegetative states for years longer than is currently possible" (Fukuyama 2002: 69). The difference between what regenerative medicine and genetic manipulation of the molecular mechanisms of aging might do for the body but not for the brain suggests that the prospect of life extension might not be so appealing after all.

Should these two distinct types of intervention be described as therapy or enhancement? How one responds to this question depends on the goal of each intervention. Because new tissues and organs derived from stem cells would replace body parts damaged by degenerative diseases, they would appropriately be described as therapy. These therapies may result in a longer lifespan for people with these diseases. Still, the goal of the intervention would not be to control aging as such but to control the symptoms and progression of diseases. Consequently, people's quality of life might improve. The intervention would restore them to the normal level of quality experienced by other people of the same age or generation who do not have the same diseases. In this regard, improving their quality of life would not be the same as enhancing it, since their diseases would put them below the baseline of acceptable quality of life. It would not raise them above but would restore them to this baseline.

In contrast, the goal of decelerating or arresting aging solely for the purpose of extending the human lifespan beyond the normal 80 years should be described as enhancement. Aging itself is not a disease, and not living for 150 or even 100 years is no disease in any plausible sense of the term. There would be nothing therapeutic about the intervention. Albert Jonsen, Mark Siegler, and William Winslade state that the goals of medicine include the promotion of health and prevention and cure of disease, relief of symptoms, pain, and suffering associated with disease, and prevention of untimely death (Jonsen et al. 2002: 15). The goal of arrested aging would not obviously be consistent with any of these goals. Some might argue that life is intrinsically good and that limiting life to a finite lifespan is intrinsically bad. So extending the lifespan would be intrinsically good as well. Yet there would be nothing therapeutic about a substantial extension of the lifespan for its own sake. Indeed, if a substantial extension of life included a prolonged period of mental decline, then we might be forced to use various therapies to treat the maladies associated with this decline. Our desire for enhancement would be superseded by the need for therapy. From the claim that living for a certain number of years is good, it does not follow that living many more years would be better. Beyond a certain point, a longer life could be worse than a shorter one.

10.3 Social Factors

Extending the lifespan could result in a unique set of intergenerational problems. Fukuyama's "national nursing home" scenario suggests that life extension would entail at least some degree of morbidity, which would gradually worsen with a longer lifespan. Replacing damaged organs and tissues could do much to control the progression and symptoms of some degenerative diseases. But simply living longer would entail a greater risk of developing other diseases. Islet-cell replacement might regulate insulin and the overall effects of diabetes. But it would not prevent other possible endocrine, metabolic, and hematological disorders. As noted, cognitive morbidity would be worse in a longer life, given the lower probability of effective therapies for neurodegenerative diseases.

An elderly population with prolonged morbidity would further strain limited health resources. Prolonged dependence on health care systems for cognitive and physical needs would mean considerable costs for long-term care. These would be avoidable costs if genetically engineered life extension satisfied only a desire, not a legitimate health need arising in the context of a normal lifespan. This normative statement reflects a conceptual difference between life extension as a by-product of regenerative medicine, and life extension for its own sake. The first would meet a medical need, while the second would meet a non-medical desire. This second claim assumes that life extension as such is not one of the goals of medicine.

A disproportionate share of resources would be used to meet the medical needs of the elderly during the long last stage of their lives. If there is public consensus that priority in the allocation of limited medical resources should be given to the health needs of the old, then some health needs of the young could go unmet. Giving priority to very long-term care for the elderly, for example, could limit the ability of a health care system to provide vaccinations, antibiotics, and other medicines necessary to prevent infectious diseases in children and enable them to have a normal lifespan. It could also limit a health care system's ability to pay for preventive screening programs for cancer and other diseases that afflict many people in the prime of life. The medical needs of the old are very different from those of the young, which makes it difficult to compare the two groups and determine whose needs are greater. Insofar as both groups have legitimate medical needs, one could not straightforwardly say that giving priority in allocating health resources to one would be unfair to the other. However, if the medical needs of the old were the result of extending the lifespan through genetic manipulation, then these needs would arise from an intervention that was not medically indicated and served no therapeutic purpose. It would be unfair to the young to deny them medical resources for the sake of older people whose medical needs were the result of a desire to extend life.

Regenerative medicine is more difficult to assess regarding the question of intergenerational fairness. This type of intervention would be medically indicated and therefore therapeutic. The aim would be to control disease progression and symptoms and raise people's quality of life to a decent baseline. Daniel Callahan has argued that health care beyond a normal lifespan of 80 years should aim not to prolong life but to promote quality of life (Callahan 1987, 1990, 1993). It should not involve aggressive and expensive life-sustaining technology that offers little, if any, benefit to people. Insofar as regenerative medicine's primary goals would be to control disease and improve quality of life, in principle it would be consistent with the aims defined by Callahan. Tissue and organ regeneration may result in a moderate extension of life; but this would be a consequence and not the primary purpose of the intervention. Even moderate life extension could limit the amount of medical resources available to meet the health needs of the young. Yet provided that the aim of regenerative medicine is not just to extend life, allocating resources to meet the medical needs of older people with new tissues or organs for their diseases would be justified. This would not involve giving absolute priority to the old. Rather, it would involve weighing different needs between the two age groups and a conditional priority for the old with at least some trade-offs in allocation (Brock 2002; McKerlie 2001).

Children of parents who opted for life extension may have to care for their parents for a considerable period of time. To cite Fukuyama again, this would be a "novel situation in which individuals approaching retirement age today find their own choices constrained by the fact that they still have an elderly parent alive and dependent on them for care" (Fukuyama 2002: 68). A substantial or even a moderate extension of the lifespan of one generation would be unfair to the next in yet another respect. The birth rate in developed countries has been steadily declining for some time. Coupled with an increased lifespan, this will mean a widening ratio of retirees to workers. The solvency of entitlement programs such as social security and health insurance for retirees depends on productivity, inflation, birth rates, and how long beneficiaries will live. A scenario where the number of retirees far exceeded the number of workers would threaten the fiscal viability of these programs. Younger workers would be burdened with substantial payroll taxes to keep entitlement programs solvent. These programs operate on a "pay as you go" basis. Retired beneficiaries of social security paid their fair share into these programs during their working years. In the past, however, most people did not live far beyond retirement age. Interventions associated with regenerative medicine have enabled many to live well beyond that, and many of these same people are spending a greater portion of their lives as beneficiaries of entitlements. Because they did not have to pay the same amount in payroll taxes that younger workers would have to pay to sustain entitlement programs, this situation would also be unfair to the younger generation.

If genetically engineered life-extension was not publicly funded but individuals were allowed to pay for it, then they should not be eligible for public entitlement programs during the extended period of their lives. With a higher percentage of younger workers' incomes taken to sustain these programs, they might not have the financial ability to choose the same life-extending technology that their elders already had chosen. Assuming that the technology was safe and effective, this would be another respect in which the young would have their choices constrained. If genetically engineered life extension were a public program, and non-working people who availed themselves of it received benefits for many years, then entitlement programs could be bankrupt by the time younger workers reached retirement age. For all of the reasons I have cited, life extension for the older generation would be unfair to the younger generation.

One proposed solution to this problem would be to require people to continue working past the current retirement age of 65 in developed countries. Many of these countries are now moving in this direction. There would be at least two issues with the proposal that would make it difficult to gain universal acceptance. First, many people are not happy with but dread their jobs and look forward to the day when they can retire. In many cases, this time cannot come soon enough. To be sure, some find their work meaningful and would want to continue working indefinitely. But this is probably the exception rather than the rule. They would prefer to spend the remainder of their lives free from the restrictions and demands of formal employment. If they were required to continue working, then living longer might only extend the period of constrained choices and decrease their quality of life. Second, most people would not be able to do sustained productive and meaningful work beyond a certain age if cognitive decline could not be reversed or controlled. Increasing the retirement age by five years could in principle ameliorate some of the fiscal problems with entitlements. But a society in which many people lived considerably longer than 65 years would probably generate intractable intergenerational problems.

Although access to interventions that extended the lifespan would be unfair in *inter*generational terms, it is not clear that such access would be unfair in *intra*-generational terms. Assuming that the technology would not be publicly funded, one might object to allowing some to have private access to the technology because it would be based on ability to pay. Some people are financially worse off than others through no fault of their own, and allowing those with a financial advantage to benefit from life-extending technology would seem unfair. It would seem unfair on the assumption that life extension can be both intrinsically and extrinsically good for people by giving them more years of life and increasing their level of well-being.

But attempting life extension through genetic means is not yet feasible and the potential benefits and risks are not known. If the effects of life extension for the first generation to attempt it are not known, then it is not clear that those with access to the technology would be any better off than those without it. Unlike the intergenerational scenario I described, people of the same generation without access to the technology would not be burdened by any harmful consequences of life extension. Without this knowledge, allowing people to pay for genetically manipulated life extension would not be unfair to those who could not pay for it because the latter would not obviously be made any worse off. Indeed, if one accepts antagonistic pleiotropy, then those who availed themselves of the technology could be putting themselves at some risk of developing disease that could thwart their desire and intention to extend their lives.

10.4 Psychological Factors

Leon Kass and others have discussed the value of a lifespan with symbolically equal stages of childhood, youth, adulthood, and old age. There is a natural contour of a life shaped by definite temporal boundaries. The psychological connections between our memories and intentions that unify our past and future from the conscious present and make each life an integrated whole are influenced by these boundaries. Kass asserts that "the 'lived time' of our natural lives has a trajectory and a shape, it's meaning derived in part from the fact that we live as links in the chain of generations" (Kass 2003a: 13).[6] He worries that regenerative medicine, and thus decelerated aging, could lengthen the lifespan in a way that would disrupt this natural trajectory by causing a radical imbalance between the last stage of life and the preceding three.

But a life with a disproportionately long last stage would not be bad for all people. On the contrary, for those who could retain physical and mental vigor for many years, a much longer life would be better than a shorter one. It could significantly increase their total lifetime well-being. As David Gems puts it: "Depending partly on whether one retained the mental plasticity of youth as one aged and on whether one opted for an open-ended life plan, extending a life has the potential to improve it" (Gems 2003: 38).[7] Such a life might enable people to pursue a series of rewarding projects or careers that would not be available to them within a normal lifespan.

The concern raised by Kass about altering the contour of a life presupposes a conception of life viewed as a whole from the *outside*. Viewed from the *inside*, though, the idea of a disproportionately long last stage of life might have no effect on our subjective attitudes toward time and could enable us to have more fulfilling lives on the whole. By nature, we seem more inclined to have asymmetrical attitudes about different times of our lives than to be neutral about them. We care more about what we might experience in the future and less about what we have experienced in the past.[8] Not only do we care more about events that might harm us in the future than about events that have harmed us in the past. We also care more about events that may benefit us in the future than about events from which we have benefited in the past. Although a final period of life that was considerably longer than earlier stages might weaken the psychological connections between our youth and old age, the connections between earlier and later periods of a long last stage of life could be strong enough to sustain a robust sense of personal identity. This would include not only numerical identity, the idea of persisting as the same individual from earlier to later times. It would also include what Marya Schechtman has called "narrative identity," where the unified subjective values and interests of one's biographical life would remain fundamentally unchanged as one lived further into the future (Schechtman 1997: Chapter 5).[9] Again, provided that we retained our mental capacity and were able to continue initiating, pursuing, and completing a series of projects, a life with a disproportionately long last stage would not obviously have negative psychological effects for us but could have positive ones instead.

A much longer life could also provide the opportunity to make amends for regretful choices of the past. It could allow for insight and moral growth and

[6] See also Kass 2003b. Fukuyama makes similar claims in Chapters 6 and 8 of Fukuyama 2002.

[7] Gems 2003: 38. For a similar view, see Harris 2000: 59, 2007.

[8] Although he argues for an attitude of temporal neutrality toward the different stages of life, Derek Parfit insightfully discusses asymmetries in our attitudes toward time in Parfit 1984: Chapter 8.

[9] David DeGrazia expresses a similar view (DeGrazia 2005).

maturity that usually come only through years of experience and reflection. Consider the case of Tolstoy's Ivan Ilych. It is only when he is diagnosed with a terminal disease that he realizes that the choices he made in pursuing a superficially successful but profoundly empty career were based on an illusion. It is possible that, for someone like Ilych, the gift of a much longer life would allow him to come to the same realization and consequently alter his choices and actions for a more fulfilling and meaningful life.

On the other hand, a limited lifespan of 80 years forces us to make choices more thoughtfully and deliberatively. It inclines us to take more responsibility for our choices and to be more aware of their foreseeable consequences. We would be less likely to have this attitude if we could live for 150 years. John Hick expresses this basic idea in his comment on the difference between finite and infinite lives:

> It is the very finitude of our earthly life, its haunting brevity that gives it shape and value by making time precious and choice urgent. If we had before us an endless temporal vista, devoid of the pressure of an approaching end, our life would lose its present character as offering a continuum of choices, small and large, through which we participate in our own gradual creating. There is thus much to be said for the view that the formation of persons through their own freedom requires the boundaries of birth and death (Hick 1993: 189).

If one accepts Hick's view, then one might say that if Ivan Ilych had not been diagnosed with terminal cancer and had continued living for many more years, he would not have had the insight into the meaning of life that he experienced just before his death. A longer life for him might not have involved any self-transformation but only more of the same illusion. His life on the whole would not have been any different, apart from containing more years. Another reason for questioning the desirability of a longer life is that the psychological distress resulting from bad choices could be worse in such a life. We would have to face the consequences of our mistakes for a longer period.

Suppose that a longer life would be good for persons and better than a shorter but more limited life of 80 years. Would we reach a point beyond which we would cease being interested in undertaking new projects or completing existing ones? Would our lives become devoid of meaning and degenerate into a state of terminal boredom? This is the fate of Elina Makropulos, the 342-year-old character in Karel Capek's play, *The Makropulos Secret*, the philosophical implications of which have been discussed in a well-known chapter by Bernard Williams (1973: 82–100). The core of Williams' discussion is the distinction between *conditional* and *categorical* desires. Conditional desires are desires for things that are conditional upon being alive. These desires do not provide reasons for continuing to live and to have a longer life. Categorical desires are desires that are not conditional upon being alive but provide reasons for continuing to live. For example, if one expects to live for roughly ten years after retirement, then one may desire to do volunteer work to make the remaining period of life meaningful. But this desire would not provide a reason to stay alive and therefore would be a conditional desire. In contrast, if one is engaged in medical research and has an intense desire to find a cure for cancer, then this desire may give one a reason to stay alive. As such, it would be a categorical desire.

Desires to initiate, engage in, and complete a series of projects over an indefinite period of time could very well be categorical rather than conditional desires. Such desires would not merely be contingent on remaining alive. They might motivate one to genetically alter the normal process of aging so that one might live well beyond the current limit of the human lifespan. This critically assumes that one will always have categorical desires as long as one exists, and that these desires will sustain an indefinite series of meaningful projects. Yet the example of Elina in Capek's play suggests that categorical desires could weaken over time. Even if genetically engineered arrested or decelerated aging ensured continued physical and mental vigor, there is no way of knowing whether one would have categorical desires indefinitely. It is possible that, beyond a certain point, additional life years would have diminishing marginal value for a person. On this view, each additional year will have less value for a person the more years of life that person has already had. Life may be valuable for people up to a certain point, after which it might have diminishing value. This could mean that a very long life could have a net disvalue for a person. A longer life would not necessarily be a better life, especially if it included a long period of mental decline before death.

We may be biologically programmed to have categorical desires and reasons to remain alive for only so many years. There may be a limit to these desires that is beyond our conscious awareness and current scientific knowledge. Admittedly, this is speculative and thus an open question. The desire to live depends on positive factors such as meaningful activity, opportunity, and human relations, as well as negative factors such as pain and suffering. The experience of these factors can vary from one person to the next. Whether one opted for substantial life extension would depend on how one valued life in the light of these factors. It would also depend on one's attitude toward the potential benefits and risks involved in genetic manipulation of the mechanisms of aging. These points do not suggest that genetically engineered life extension should be entirely a matter of personal choice. Individual decisions to have these interventions may entail social costs and therefore cannot be separated from public policy considerations. These considerations may constrain individual choices for life extension.

Would a substantially longer life alter our conception of human nature?[10] The length of the human lifespan is not fixed but malleable. It has increased significantly over the past two centuries, yet our understanding of what it means to be human has not changed. A substantially extended lifespan would be unique in the sense that the last stage of life would be considerably longer than earlier stages. Initially, the most notable effects of arrested aging would occur in what we presently describe as late adulthood. It is possible that all the stages of life would be more equally extended after a few generations with longer life spans. Nevertheless, this phenomenon alone would not fundamentally alter our cognitive and emotional understanding of our humanity. There will not be universal agreement on the implications of these changes. But there will be enough general agreement to retain a

[10] Fukuyama and Kass would answer this question affirmatively, hence their worries about a 'post-human' future.

shared sense of what it means to be human. Our minds have the capacity to adapt to changing conditions and could accommodate a life with a long last stage within the existing concept of ourselves as persons or human beings. However, if we retained physical vigor for many years, only to experience a prolonged period of cognitive decline during a large part of these years, then this could alter our conception of human nature. But it would not be a function of the length of life as such, or with the fact that the last stage of life was longer than earlier stages.

10.5 Conclusion

Regenerative medicine could retard the aging process. Therapies derived from stem-cell research could benefit many people by controlling many aging-related degenerative diseases and by relieving the pain and suffering these diseases cause. These therapies could result in a moderate extension of the lifespan, which could further benefit people by enabling them to have more quality life years. Yet if neural regeneration could not keep pace with physical regeneration, then there may be a trade-off between sustained physical vigor and cognitive decline. This decline would be worse in a longer life. Moreover, a moderately longer lifespan could burden the next generation in different ways. But provided that the goal of regenerative medicine was to treat degenerative diseases for those already suffering from them, it would be justified.

Genetic manipulation of the aging process to substantially extend life for its own sake would be more difficult to justify. It could disrupt molecular mechanisms that ordinarily suppress growth factors and could lead to cancers and other diseases. It could also considerably burden the young if it meant that the elderly would be dependent on them for a prolonged period of care. Because it would be a form of enhancement rather than medically indicated therapy, and because it could burden younger generations, this type of intervention should not be publicly funded. Assuming that it would not entail social costs, individuals should be allowed to choose to have it and assume any risks. This would include paying for any untoward consequences of it.

Some argue that any claims about even moderate life extension should be made tentatively. The possible reemergence of deadly infectious diseases, and the emergence of new epidemics such as obesity, may preclude any extension of the lifespan for younger populations. Those who are now in or beyond the fifth decade of life may benefit from regenerative medicine. But the prospects of a longer life for younger people are not as good. S. Jay Olshansky and other biodemographers have analyzed the effect of obesity on longevity in the United States and have concluded that the "steady rise in life expectancy during the past two centuries may soon come to an end" (Olshansky et al. 2005: 1138). Further, they argue that "past gains in life expectancy have largely been a product of saving the young, and since future gains must result from extending life among the old, another quantum leap in life expectancy can occur only if the future is different from the past" (Olshansky et al. 2005:

1139). Epidemiological evidence suggests that the future will not be different from the present and recent past, at least not in any positive respects. With the incidence of obesity and endocrine and metabolic disorders such as diabetes increasing in developing and developed countries, the potential for any extension of the human lifespan is unlikely to be realized. But there is a more important point of these observations. They strongly recommend that, before we tinker with the molecular mechanisms of aging to extend life, we should address the causes of many diseases that threaten to prevent a significant number of people from completing what we now consider a normal lifespan.[11]

References

Brock D (2002) Priority to the Worst Off in Health Care Resource Prioritization. In: Rhodes R, Battin M, Silvers A (eds) Medicine and Social Justice: Essays on the Distribution of Health Care. Oxford University Press, New York: 362–372

Callahan D (1987) Setting Limits: Medical Goals in an Aging Society. Simon & Schuster, New York

Callahan D (1990) What Kind of Life: The Limits of Medical Progress. Simon & Schuster, New York

Callahan D (1993) The Troubled Dream of Life: Living with Mortality. Simon & Schuster, New York

DeGrazia D (2005) Human Identity and Bioethics. Cambridge University Press, New York

Fries J (1980) Aging, Natural Death and the Compression of Morbidity. New England Journal of Medicine 303: 130–136

Fukuyama F (2002) Our Posthuman Future: Consequences of the Biotechnology Revolution. Farrar, Straus & Giroux, New York

Gems D (2003) Is More Life Always Better? The New Biology of Aging and the Meaning of Life. Hastings Center Report 33 (July–August): 31–39

Greaves M (2007) Darwinian Medicine: A Case for Cancer. Nature Reviews Cancer 7: 213–221

Guarente L, Kenyon C (2000) Genetic Pathways that Regulate Aging in Model Organisms. Nature 408: 255–262

Harris J (2000) Intimations of Immortality. Science 288: 59

Harris J (2007) Enhancing Evolution. The Ethical Case for Making Better People. Princeton University Press, Princeton, NJ.

Hayflick L (1965) The Limited In Vitro Lifetime of Human Diploid Cell Strains. Experimental Cell Research 37: 614–636

Hayflick L (1977) The Cellular Basis for Biological Aging. In: Hayflick L, Finch C (eds) Handbook of the Biology of Aging. Van Nostrand, New York: 159–186

Hayflick L (2001) The Future of Aging. Nature 408: 267–269

Hayflick L (2001–2002) Anti-Aging-Medicine: Hype, Hope, and Reality. Generations: 20–26

Hayflick L, Moorhead P S (1961) The Serial Cultivation of Human Diploid Cell Strains. Experimental Cell Research 25: 585–621

Hekimi S, Guarente L (2003) Genetics and the Specificity of the Aging Process. Science 299: 1351–1354

---

[11] I am grateful to Teresa Yu for helpful discussion and to Bert Gordijn and Ruth Chadwick for many helpful comments and suggestions on an earlier draft.

Hick J (1993) Disputed Questions in Theology and the Philosophy of Religion. Yale University Press, New Haven

Jonsen A, Siegler M, Winslade W (2002) Clinical Ethics. 5th edition, McGraw-Hill, New York

Juengst E T et al. (2003) Biogerontology, 'Anti-Aging Medicine' and the Challenges of Human Enhancement. Hastings Center Report 33 (July–August): 21–30

Kass L (2003a) Ageless Bodies, Happy Souls: Biotechnology and the Pursuit of Perfection. The New Atlantis 1: 9–28

Kass L (2003b) Beyond Therapy: Biotechnology and the Pursuit of Happiness. Harper Collins, New York

Kirkland J (2002) The Biology of Senescence: Potential for Prevention of Disease. Clinical Geriatric Medicine 18: 383–405

Kirkwood T (2001) Time of Our Lives: The Science of Human Aging. Oxford University Press, Oxford

Kirkwood T (2008) A Systematic Look at an Old Problem. Nature 451: 644–647.

Lithgow G J, Kirkwood T B (1996) Mechanisms and Evolution of Aging. Science 273: 80

Mahowald M (2003) Reflections on the Human Embryonic Stem Cell Debate. Perspectives in Biology and Medicine 46: 131–141

McHugh P (2004) Zygote and 'Clonote'—The Ethical Use of Embryonic Stem Cells. New England Journal of Medicine 351: 209–211

McKerlie D (2001) Justice Between the Young and the Old. Philosophy & Public Affairs 30: 152–177

Nesse R, Williams G (1994) Why We Get Sick: The New Science of Darwinian Medicine. Times Books, New York

Olshansky S J, Carnes B A (2001) The Quest for Immortality: Science at the Frontiers of Aging. W. W. Norton, New York

Olshansky S J et al. (2005) A Potential Decline in Life Expectancy in the United States in the 21st Century. New England Journal of Medicine 352: 1138–1145

Parfit D (1984) Reasons and Persons. Clarendon, Oxford

Sandel M (2004) Embryonic Ethics —The Moral Logic of Stem-Cell Research. New England Journal of Medicine 351: 207–209

Schechtman M (1997) The Constitution of Selves. Cornell University Press, Ithaca, NY

Williams B (1973) Problems of the Self. Cambridge University Press, Cambridge

Williams G (1957) Pleiotropy, Natural Selection and the Evolution of Senescence. Evolution 11: 398–411

Chapter 11
Germline Genetic Modification

Rebecca Dresser

11.1 Introduction

For several decades, scientists and ethicists have considered the possibility of altering genes at the beginning of human life. Human germline genetic modification began to attract widespread attention as early as the 1960s (Evans 2002: 55–57). At that time, scientists and scholars began examining the benefits and harms that could come from attempting to alter genes at the earliest stage of human development.

Genetic changes made in gametes or the fertilized egg would be maintained through subsequent development, including development of germ (sperm and egg) cells. This form of genetic alteration would affect children developing from modified embryos; the alterations could also be passed to the children's descendants. Accordingly, the benefits of any positive changes would be magnified; but any negative effects would be magnified, as well. The potential long-term effects complicate the effort to predict whether germline interventions would produce more benefit than harm.

Germline interventions could also be performed with different aims in mind. Germline modification could be attempted to remove or reduce the impact of genes linked to illness. Alternatively, the modifications could be designed with the goal of "adding or augmenting characteristics or traits not related to disease, such as muscle mass or height" (Genetics and Public Policy Center 2005: 13). A third mixed approach would be to make "preventive" modifications intended to increase a person's disease resistance (Genetics and Public Policy Center 2005).

The difficulties in predicting future effects led most scientists, as well as the general public, to support a ban or moratorium on germline genetic interventions in humans. By the late 1990s, however, certain scientists and other commentators were challenging this position. Their challenge brought germline interventions back into the spotlight. At the beginning of the 21st century, there was a resurgence of scholarship and public discussion about germline interventions (Genetics and Public Policy Center 2005).

This chapter describes the general arguments for and against human germline modification, but it analyzes germline genetic modifications from a vantage point that differs from most ethics and policy discussions. Writers addressing the topic often limit their discussions to the benefits and harms that could materialize if germline

B. Gordijn, R. Chadwick (eds.) *Medical Enhancement and Posthumanity*,

modifications were widely available. In this chapter, however, I consider the technology as it stands today. The question for contemporary society is not whether it would be a good or a bad thing if germline modifications were performed in humans. Instead, today's ethical inquiry should focus on whether to pursue human germline genetic intervention as a research goal. For us, the relevant questions are the following: What is the potential value of research aimed at human germline genetic modification and what price would be paid in attempting to develop the technology?

Examining germline modification from a research perspective expands the ethical inquiry beyond the usual analysis. Although it is important to examine the consequences and concerns that could exist if a speculative technology like germline modification were clinically available, it is also important to consider the ethical implications of embarking on research to develop the technology. Biomedical research is performed with a variety of goals in mind, but not all of those goals have equal moral and social value. Not all research objectives should be pursued with equal vigor, and some might not be worth pursuing at all.

Evaluating the merits and drawbacks of a research program also enriches the policy analysis of human germline modification. Policy conversations about potential future technologies tend to focus on whether they should be banned or regulated. But such conversations should also consider the matter of financial support. Resource allocation choices can influence technology development in ways similar to more formal policy measures. Policy analysts adopting a research perspective will consider how actively public and private entities should promote development of germline genetic modification in the face of competing demands on research resources.

Different types of interventions can have germline effects. For example, certain studies aimed at altering genes in the somatic cells of living individuals (so-called gene therapy) carry a remote possibility of producing changes in a research subject's germ cells, as well (Frankel & Chapman 2000). This possibility merits attention, but it raises different ethical and policy issues than those raised by a concerted attempt to develop interventions to alter the human germline. This chapter focuses on interventions that are aimed at and have a high probability of altering the genes humans pass to offspring. Such interventions would involve genetic modification of the early embryo, or of gametes used to create the embryo. I use the term preimplantation genetic modification (PGM) to refer to such interventions, because alterations would occur before researchers transferred the embryo to a woman's uterus for gestation.

11.2 Human Germline Modification: Early Ethical Analysis

Much commentary in the scientific and bioethics literature presents arguments for and against germline genetic alteration. To date, writers have considered the potential impact of the intervention's widespread use. They have focused on whether germline alterations would be good or bad for parent-child relationships, social justice, and the future of humanity (Harris 1992; Parens 1995; Walters & Palmer 1997; Resnik et al. 1999; Shanks 2005; Genetics and Public Policy Center 2005).

The primary concern about effects on the family is based on the possibility that germline genetic modification would allow parents to "design" their children to have certain desirable attributes. If this happened, adults could begin to think of children as objects to be manipulated, rather than as persons to be loved no matter what their talents and appearance. This could threaten the unconditional love that parents ideally have for their children. Children who failed to measure up to genetic specifications might be rejected by disappointed mothers and fathers.

The ability to improve children genetically could also influence general social expectations about parenthood. Pressures could develop for parents to use genetic modification despite their personal reluctance to do so. Adults having children with disabilities could be deemed "bad parents." Disabled children themselves could experience even more disadvantages than they do today. Because there would be fewer disabled people, the political power of disability groups would diminish, along with their ability to lobby for benefits. Critics also worry that germline modifications, particularly those aimed at enhancement, would be available solely to the better-off segments of society.

Worries about effects on future generations center on the possibility that modifications seen as beneficial at one point could later become harmful, due to a deterioration in the altered genes' functional capacities or the emergence of new diseases or other environmental threats. A related set of objections emphasizes the damage that humans have done in other attempts to control or change natural organisms.

Writers supporting germline modification believe that these concerns are overstated and do not warrant restrictions on a technology that offers the possibility of creating healthier and happier individuals now and in the future. They expect that future applications of science and medicine, as well as appropriate regulation, will be sufficient to manage any problems that could arise.

11.3 Renewed Enthusiasm for Germline Modification

Until recently, scientists and scholars portrayed human germline genetic alterations as a distant prospect. In turn, the debate over ethical implications was abstract and speculative. In the late 1990s, however, this situation changed. Certain scientists, ethicists, and other commentators began to speak of PGM in more concrete terms.

Three factors contributed to this shift. The first was knowledge generated by the Human Genome Project and related research. Scientists anticipated that this work would yield significant gains in understanding the links between genes and human traits, including disease susceptibility, physical characteristics, and behavioral attributes. Second was progress in modifying the genes of nonhuman animals. Improvements in transgenic techniques had made genetic alteration of laboratory animal embryos a routine part of molecular biology. Third was the accumulation of disappointing results in human trials of somatic cell genetic modification. The lack of clear success, together with the significant harm imposed on a few trial participants, brought home the impediments to achieving safe and effective post-birth genetic alterations. After more than a decade of human studies, no one could ignore the problems with using viral vectors and other conventional methods to deliver properly functioning genes to living individuals (Stock & Campbell 2000a; Kimmelman 2005).

A collection of researchers and others responded to these developments by calling for more serious consideration of human germline modification. These individuals contend that modifying genes early in development offers the best opportunity to deliver functional genes to mammals, including humans. For example, geneticist Mario Capecchi believes that "many of the technical hurdles encountered in human somatic gene therapy are obviated in the apparently more radical human germline gene therapy" and that "plausible scenarios can already be envisioned for methodologies by which human germline gene therapy could now be accomplished" (2000: 41). Molecular biologist Leroy Hood predicts, "fifty years from now we will be doing everything through the germline rather than in somatic tissues" (2000: 83).

Other scientists portray germline modifications as attainable and well worth pursuing. Biologist Lee Silver argues, "there is every reason to believe that genetic engineering could become feasible on human embryos in the near future" (2000: 68). To James Watson, co-discoverer of DNA's structure:

> It seems obvious that germline therapy will be much more successful thansomatic. If we wait for the success of somatic therapy, we'll wait until the sun burns out. We might as well do what we can to take the threat of Alzheimer's away from a family or breast cancer away from a family (Stock & Campbell 2000b: 79).

And Daniel Koshland, a former editor of *Science*, predicts that children produced through "germline engineering will compete very well with [children] conceived the natural way." Koshland goes further to suggest that "the genetically engineered child may have a good edge over the child conceived the ordinary way" (2000: 26).

Similar statements come from experts in other fields. A group of European scholars describes genetic modification of human embryos as "no longer a science fiction scenario" and "expected to be safe and effective in the foreseeable future if current research efforts are continued" (Waters 2002). Commentators Gregory Stock and John Campbell believe such modification is also inevitable. For them, "the real question about germline engineering is not whether the technique will be feasible, but when and how it will" (2000a: 5).

How should we evaluate these assertions? Should we share this optimism about the technology and join these commentators in endorsing research aimed at human germline genetic modification in human embryos? Or would caution and reflection be more defensible responses to the prospects for human PGM? What would be the value of pursuing this research and what would be the price of doing so?

11.4 What Are the Chances of Success?

Biomedical research projects should be evaluated according to their ability not simply to advance knowledge, but to generate health benefits. The value of biomedical research depends on the magnitude of its potential benefits and the prospects for achieving those benefits. Given that research resources and scientific talents are limited, research sponsors and policymakers should consider which research aims are more and less worth pursuing. Proposals for research to develop human germline genetic modification should be considered in this framework.

One factor to consider in evaluating research aims is the probability that scientists will succeed in achieving those aims. To evaluate the possibilities for successful modification of the human germline, we must review the state of the relevant science.

Laboratory researchers injecting foreign genes into the fertilized eggs of mice, rats, and other species have created genetically altered (transgenic) animals capable of passing genes to descendants. Through modifying genes in animal embryos with disorder-producing mutations, researchers have also produced multiple generations of animals free of the relevant disorder (Frankel & Chapman 2000). Scientists have reported success in modifying genes linked to behavior, too. A highly publicized example was the creation of transgenic mice who performed unusually well in standard learning tests (Wade 1999).

Yet these achievements by no means signal that germline modifications will soon be ready for human trials. Even the strongest supporters concede that methods used to alter genes in the laboratory are too dangerous and inefficient for human application. The most common techniques for creating transgenic animals can produce new mutations and other serious damage. As a result, few genetically altered embryos survive to become healthy animals. Moreover, few of the healthy animals carry and express the foreign genes to the desired degree. The ones that do must be bred with each other to produce animals with the desired genotype and phenotype. Animals born with health problems or without the desired modification are discarded (Frankel & Chapman 2000; Friedmann 2003).

Existing methods of creating transgenic animals involve adding foreign genes to early embryos. The risks and variable expression levels associated with gene addition lead many scientists to believe that human applications would require techniques to repair or replace unwanted genes (Blaese 2003; Evans 2003). Preliminary investigations are being conducted on such techniques, but none has progressed beyond the early stage of exploration (Taubes 2002; Culver 2003).

Scientists have begun using embryonic stem cells and one gene replacement technique called targeted homologous recombination to create transgenic animals. Researchers grow the stem cells in culture, then attempt to modify genes in the cells. Homologous recombination produces the desired genetic change in a very low percentage of stem cells. Researchers isolate the cells in which the desired alteration occurred and inject them into mouse blastocysts, which are then transferred for gestation.

This technique raises at least two concerns that could prevent it from being appropriate for human application. The longer stem cells are maintained in culture, the greater the likelihood that they will undergo chromosomal and other changes that could produce health problems in a later-born organism. Second, the resulting animals are chimeras, with alterations in just some of their cells. Researchers have been unable to direct the level of foreign gene expression in these animals.

Consequently, further breeding is required to obtain transgenic animals with the proper genotype and phenotype (Blaese 2003; Friedmann 2003).

Another approach to creating transgenic animals involves nuclear transfer technology, popularly known as cloning. In this approach, a genetically altered cell is placed in an enucleated oocyte and the resulting embryos implanted for gestation (Capecchi 2000; Friedmann 2003). Whether this would be possible in humans is unknown; whether it could be done with the requisite level of safety and efficacy is even more uncertain (National Academy of Sciences 2002).

In 2000, investigators reported success in producing transgenic animals using artificial chromosomes. Researchers hope that this method will enable them to introduce both new genes and the regulatory DNA sequences that would promote proper gene functioning. On the other hand, adding large amounts of DNA could be difficult and might produce undue damage. Thus, it is not yet known whether this method will produce modified animals more efficiently and effectively than standard transgenic techniques. Again, much more research would be required to determine whether human applications should be considered (Resnik et al. 1999; Friedmann 2003). Also possible are approaches that would alter genes in the sperm or eggs used to create a genetically modified embryo. A variety of methods are being explored in the laboratory, but the inquiry is just beginning. At this point, it is unclear whether any of the above methods will prove safe and effective enough to apply to humans (Genetics and Public Policy Center 2005: 13–21).

Besides the problems in developing safe and effective genetic modification techniques, efforts to perform human PGM could be hampered by the complexity of many human traits. For numerous conditions and characteristics, the relationship between genotype and phenotype is poorly understood (Couzin 2005). Many traits portrayed as candidates for genetic modification are polygenic, which means that they are influenced by two or more different genes. Environmental conditions also affect how genetic traits are manifested in individuals. In addressing the possibilities for enhancing children through genetic modification of embryos, cognitive scientist Steven Pinker has observed that "there is an enormous role for chance in the development of a human being" and that "even if a gene had some consistent effect, whether the effect was desirable would depend on what the other tens of thousands of genes are doing" (2003). The number of variables influencing the impact of many genes could make it impossible to control characteristics commonly associated with enhancement, such as intelligence (Gordon 1999).

In sum, the obstacles to successful human PGM are formidable, possibly insurmountable. At this point, it would be "foolish and irresponsible to try to alter or manipulate a complex system we barely understand" (Resnik 2002: 169). At minimum, dramatic advances in knowledge, as well as the emergence of novel techniques for genetic alteration, would be prerequisites to human applications of germline modification. Even with these advances, modifying complex traits might never succeed, or might succeed so rarely that the objective could reasonably be deemed unattainable.

On the other hand, one should never say "never" in science. Because future scientific developments cannot be predicted with certainty, it would be inappropriate to label this research aim an impossible goal. Because unexpected discoveries in later decades or centuries could lay the foundation for safe and effective PGM, we cannot defensibly conclude that successful human germline modification would be impossible. But based on the state of the current research, predictions that it could come in the foreseeable future seem more science fiction than science fact.

11.5 A Worthwhile Objective?

Another factor to consider in evaluating a research objective is whether that objective is sufficiently valuable to merit the effort. This depends not only on the value of the objective; it also depends on what it could cost to achieve the objective.

Even opponents concede that many people would value the fruits of successful human germline genetic modification; indeed, many of the ethical concerns about parent-child relationships, social justice, and effects on future generations rest on the assumption that genetic modifications to prevent disease and achieve various physical and mental enhancements would be in great demand among would-be parents. If scientists were able to devise safe and effective PGM methods that prevented disease and enhanced physical and mental abilities in later-born children, many children could have better lives. Modifications could improve the lives of their descendants, too, if genes promoting health and enhancing desirable traits were passed to offspring. Families could benefit, and society might be better off as well, for some modifications could serve to reduce health care costs or advance other economic and social interests. These judgments are based on prediction, but prediction is a necessary element of assigning value to any research goal.

In the real world, though, judgments about the moral and social value of a research aim should not be made in isolation. Instead, the evaluation must also consider potential losses that could accompany pursuit of that aim. According to this approach, a research objective might be attainable and of material value, but achieving it would impose unacceptable burdens and costs.

A germline modification research program would expose human subjects to serious risks and consume resources that could be used to support other valuable research projects. Moreover, in most cases, the benefits that could be gained from this form of genetic modification could also be gained through less risky and costly alternative measures.

11.5.1 Risks to Human Subjects

Germline modification research would present unavoidable risks to human subjects. Genetic modifications affecting early embryos could have a significant impact on later-born individuals. Risks to subjects would be especially great in the first phase of human trials. Laboratory studies would enable researchers to reduce risks, but preliminary work could never eliminate the uncertainty that always exists when interventions are initially tried on humans.

Although genetic modification techniques could be refined thorough animal research, species differences would complicate efforts to ascertain how a specific genetic modification would affect human subjects (Pennisi 2005). Many genes are believed to be pleiotropic, which means that they influence a number of different traits. Moreover, certain pleiotropic genes deemed undesirable, such as those that increase susceptibility to a disease, may also have positive effects, such as decreasing susceptibility to another disease (Burke 2003; Evans 2003). The genetic alteration in the mice that exhibited enhanced learning abilities may have had pleiotropic effects, for those mice also exhibited an unusual sensitivity to pain (Weiss 2001).

Altering a gene with pleiotropic effects would have multiple consequences to a developing human. Unexpected harms could materialize; such harms could be experienced by children developing from modified embryos and by descendants of those children. Exposing children, and possibly future generations, to this level of risk would require strong justification in the form of significant potential benefit to others (Dresser 2004a, b). Studies aimed at enhancement benefits would provoke the greatest controversy, for they would impose risks on offspring for reasons other than improved health. There could be wide disagreement over whether enhancement goals would justify exposing children and their descendants to potential harm in this form of human research (Dresser 2004b).

11.5.2 Consumption of Research Resources

A research program aimed at human PGM would also consume significant resources. At this point, it is far from certain that PGM would be safe and effective for human application. Resolving this uncertainty would demand the attention of a multitude of researchers, and their work would require substantial funding. Would PGM be a worthy use of our research resources and scientific talent?

Answering this question requires us to consider priority setting in biomedical research. The funds available to support research are limited. The clearest limits apply to government funds, but nonprofit organizations and industry sponsors also face decisions about how best to allocate their available research dollars. Like government research agencies in other nations, the U.S. National Institutes of Health (NIH) devotes its resources to biomedical research aimed at improving human health. Public health priorities are established using specific criteria, such as the number of people with a health problem, its effect on life expectancy, the level of disability it causes, and its financial and social costs. Proposals for both basic and applied research are evaluated in light of their potential effect on important health problems (NIH 1997, Institute of Medicine 1998).

As I discuss below, alternatives to PGM will offer the vast majority of prospective parents an opportunity to avoid having children with serious genetic diseases. In the future, alternatives to genetic modification aimed at avoiding polygenic disorders and enhancing socially valued traits could be available, too. The availability of alternatives lessens the justification for devoting limited research funds to studies aimed at developing human PGM.

Priority setting in biomedical research raises complex and difficult issues (Dresser 2001; Callahan 2003), but any ethically defensible set of criteria would assign human germline modification a low score in the competition for research dollars. Many competing research areas have a greater probability of providing more significant benefits. In NIH terms, PGM research would be high risk, low reward – the probability of failure would be substantial and the benefits of success small, given that many PGM aims could be achieved through alternative means. In light of the relatively low magnitude of PGM's distinct benefit and the scientific impediments to securing that benefit, PGM would be a debatable use of biomedical research resources (Chapman 2003).

In contrast to government funding agencies, commercial research sponsors put the potential for profit at the forefront in resource allocation decisions. Some observers think that the private sector will find PGM an inviting target for research and development, particularly PGM aimed at enhancement (Silver 2000; Stock 2002). But investing in PGM seems unwarranted in this context, as well. Less risky and costly alternatives will probably become available to people hoping to improve the health and lives of their children. Though safe and effective germline genetic enhancements could be great moneymakers, the possibility of developing such enhancements appears remote at this time. As a practical matter, it seems unlikely that sensible entrepreneurs will want to make large investments in a technology where returns are so distant and doubtful. Thus, even those adopting a market approach have reasons to classify PGM as a low-priority research aim.

Furthermore, I would argue that both public and private research sponsors ought to consider the social value of research aims in allocating their limited funds. Setting priorities according to criteria resembling those used by the NIH would be consistent with corporate good citizenship. Responsible philanthropists should also consider the public good when they distribute resources for research. In light of immense unmet domestic and worldwide research needs, research on human germline genetic modification ought to be ranked among the least compelling candidates for funding by any organization.

Commentators addressing the risks and costs of PGM research sometimes suggest that studies aimed at other objectives will inevitably generate the knowledge necessary to perform germline modification in humans. Thus, for example, laboratory work aimed at creating transgenic animals will lead to safer and more effective gene alteration methods. Research aimed at assisting infertile people, such as work on methods of oocyte freezing, will make it easier to develop human PGM (Silver 2000; Stock 2002). It is likely that scientific discoveries in other areas will be relevant to human PGM. But forecasts such as these oversimplify what it would take to bring human PGM to the clinic. Advances in other fields could never obviate the need for research tailored to specific PGM applications. At minimum, extensive human trials would be required before any particular genetic modification could be made available as a medical intervention. Safe and effective PGM will not magically appear as a result of animal and infertility research; instead, developing human PGM would demand substantial investment and expose children to potential harm in the research process.

Besides risks to human subjects and forgone opportunities to advance arguably more important biomedical research, PGM research could contribute to broader social harms, such as objectification of children or greater health disparities between the rich and poor. Such results are possible and should be considered, but they are also more speculative than the human subjects and research funding consequences. The latter risks are sufficient, in my view, to make PGM a questionable research aim.

11.5.3 PGM Alternatives

The existence of alternatives strengthens the basis for questioning the value of a research program aimed at human germline modification. Supporters of germline modification contemplate two kinds of benefits that would justify its application: avoidance of genetic diseases and enhancement of normal human characteristics. In many cases, however, there would be less risky and expensive ways to obtain those benefits.

Today, prospective parents seeking to avoid having children with serious genetic disorders may achieve this goal through prenatal genetic testing. In the future, the option of preimplantation genetic diagnosis (PGD) is expected to offer most couples a way to have children unaffected by such disorders (Robertson 2003). The PGD alternative will be most helpful to couples at risk for having children affected by monogenic disorders, but if researchers locate single genes that substantially contribute to certain polygenic disorders, PGD could also help couples seeking to avoid having children affected by those disorders. Indeed, if researchers discover single genes that are highly correlated with certain physical and behavioral traits, PGD could even offer prospective parents a limited number of enhancements:

> Although PGD involves a diagnostic test, as opposed to the genetic manipulation or genetic "engineering" of the embryo, the information it reveals could conceivably allow a parent to select an embryo based on many factors other than the absence of a disease-causing gene mutation. Over time, these factors could grow as science uncovers the links between individual traits that play a role in intelligence, appearance, and complex behaviors (Genetics and Public Policy Center 2004: 6).

In these situations, there would be no reason to resort to the higher-risk, higher-cost PGM procedure.

Prenatal diagnosis and PGD offer ways for couples to have healthy children and in the future, PGD will probably offer prospective parents additional ways to enhance the health and welfare of their children. A negative feature of these methods is that they often result in the destruction of embryos and fetuses. Human PGM is sometimes praised as a means to avoid embryo discard or pregnancy termination (Walters & Palmer 1997), but this praise is misplaced. Even PGM proponents expect that efforts to alter the genes of early embryos could produce new damage or otherwise go awry. Thus, PGM would require embryo and fetal testing, and prospective parents would still face decisions about embryo destruction and abortion (Resnik et al. 1999; Frankel & Chapman 2000).

Admittedly, certain PGM objectives could not be achieved through other means. When someone has two copies of a gene for a dominant trait, or both members of a couple have two copies of a gene for a recessive trait, all of the embryos they produce will have the unwanted genes. PGM could offer individuals in these relatively unusual situations an opportunity to have genetically related children unaffected by the undesired trait (Danks 1994). On the other hand, such individuals could also have children through adoption or donated gametes, or have an affected child and seek treatment for that child. During the time it would take to develop PGM, there would presumably be other advances that could make the latter alternative more desirable (Evans 2003).

By the time PGM became available, couples seeking enhancements might also be able to select less risky and expensive interventions, such as drugs and even somatic cell genetic interventions, to meet their enhancement objectives. For example, researchers could develop improved drugs to deliver human growth hormone to increase the adult height of children genetically predisposed to be short. And as one researcher has pointed out, "the very technological advances that would facilitate the development of [germline modification] could well be those that would make somatic cell gene therapy so safe, efficient, and inexpensive as to obviate the need for germline manipulation in many instances" (Evans 2003: 96–97). (Of course, it would also be important to evaluate the ethics of providing such interventions.)

PGM's distinct contribution would be to supply children with selected genes that were absent in biological parents. These might be genes that some humans have naturally, or genes not found naturally in humans (Resnik et al. 1999; Stock 2002). As noted earlier, there is good reason to believe that interventions aimed at altering polygenic traits could never achieve the safety and efficacy levels that would support human use. The obstacles to safe and effective modification of monogenic traits are less daunting, but success is far from assured. Some speculate that single-gene alterations in embryos could produce resistance to diseases, such as HIV (Silver 2000). It is possible to imagine a situation in which this would be an effective approach, but the question is whether to channel limited research resources to studying germline modification as a means to fight infectious disease, given the likely cost and limited abilities to deliver this form of treatment to a human population.

11.6 Decisions About Germline Modification Research: The Social Dimensions

Accurate communication about biomedical research could supply a foundation for public deliberation over whether human germline genetic modifications are worth pursuing. All too often, however, the public receives distorted messages about high-profile research areas. The popular media, together with some scientists and other commentators, exaggerate the likelihood that effective clinical interventions will emerge. These sources typically downplay the actual state of the science and the number of advances that would be necessary before safe and effective therapies could be offered. They also fail to mention the risks that investigational interventions could present to human subjects and the alternative research avenues that could be explored if different investment decisions were made.

Public discussions of human germline genetic modification exhibit many of these shortcomings. Commentators make unrealistic predictions about the future availability of PGM and the time frame for technology development. They also fail to acknowledge the opportunity costs of attempting to develop this form of genetic modification. Instead, the possibility of creating designer babies is usually described without reference to the potential losses that could accompany the research necessary to explore that possibility.

Experts and journalists should give public audiences a less rosy, more qualified picture of what PGM could offer prospective parents. Questions such as, "if you could do so safely, would you use an artificial chromosome to extend the life span of your child?" (Stock & Campbell 2000c: 101) should not be the only ones put to the public. Questions like the following should also be posed:

> Would you opt for a traumatic and expensive procedure that might give you a slightly happier and more talented child, or might give you a less happy, less talented child, or might give you a deformed child, and probably would make no difference? (Pinker 2003: D1).

If human PGM were developed, prospective parents would be as likely to face the second question as they would the first. Public discussions of designer babies should acknowledge this possibility.

A fair process for determining research priorities is also needed. The challenge is to develop better mechanisms for deciding which research goals are most – and least – worth pursuing. An open and transparent evaluation of research aims is easiest to justify for publicly funded research. Taxpayers supplying the support for government-funded research have legitimate claims to information access and representation in decision-making about the agency's research goals. Nonprofit and private-sector research supporters should consider being more open in their research priority setting, too. It would be good ethical practice for philanthropic organizations and industry sponsors to consult outside experts and members of the public when determining which research programs to pursue (Genetics and Public Policy Center 2005).

11.7 Conclusion

The gap appears to be widening between the health system's ability to generate new biomedical knowledge and its ability to translate that knowledge into actual health benefits (Lenfant 2003; Zerhouni 2003). Even cutting-edge basic scientists are among those disturbed by this situation. At the 2003 annual meeting of the American Advancement of Science, President Floyd Bloom, a neurobiologist, urged colleagues and government officials to reconsider the current emphasis on molecular biology research (AAAS 2003; Tuma 2003). Bloom observed that this research is unlikely to produce concrete medical benefits in the short term. In today's health care crisis, he argued, policy reforms and social science research are more promising avenues to health promotion and disease prevention.

We should challenge the call for an active research program targeted at human PGM. There are formidable obstacles to developing safe and effective germline genetic modifications. Embarking on this course would put human subjects at risk to develop a technology with limited justification. Given the alternative approaches that allow parents to avoid having children with genetic diseases and the likelihood that most enhancements would be too difficult to achieve, the risks presented by human germline modification research outweigh its potential benefits. Moreover, we ought to channel our limited resources elsewhere. Public and private resources are needed to investigate a huge array of research questions that could have a major impact on important health problems. In the context of human health needs, PGM is a low-priority scientific objective.

Research Supported by the National Institutes of Health, National Human Genome Research Institute.

References

American Association for the Advancement of Science, AAAS (2003) AAAS President Calls to Restore American Health System. http://www.eurekalert.org/pub_releases/2003–02/aaft-apc020303.php Accessed February 19, 2003

Blaese R M (2003) Germ line modification in clinical medicine: is there a case for intentional or unintended germ line changes? In: Chapman A R, Frankel M S (eds) Designing Our Descendants: The Promises and Perils of Genetic Modifications. Johns Hopkins University Press, Baltimore, MD

Burke W (2003) Genomics as a probe for disease biology. New England Journal of Medicine 349: 969–974

Callahan D (2003) What Price Better Health? Hazards of the Research Imperative. University of California Press, Berkeley, CA/Los Angeles, CA

Capecchi M (2000) Human germline gene therapy: how and why. In: Stock G, Campbell J (eds) Engineering the Human Germline. Oxford University Press, New York

Chapman A (2003) The implications of inheritable genetic modifications for justice. In: Chapman A R, Frankel M S (eds) Designing Our Descendants: The Promises and Perils of Genetic Modifications. Johns Hopkins University Press, Baltimore, MD

Couzin J (2005) To what extent are genetic variation and personal health linked? Science 309: 81

Culver K W (2003) Gene repair, genomics, and human germ line modification. In: Chapman A R, Frankel M S (eds) Designing Our Descendants: The Promises and Perils of Genetic Modifications. Johns Hopkins University Press, Baltimore, MD

Danks D (1994) Germ-line gene therapy: no place in treatment of genetic disease. Human Gene Therapy 5: 151–152

Dresser R (2001) When Science Offers Salvation: Patient Advocacy and Research Ethics. Oxford University Press, New York

Dresser R (2004a) Genetic modification of preimplantation embryos: toward adequate human research policies. Milbank Quarterly 82: 195–214

Dresser R (2004b) Designing babies: human research issues. IRB: Ethics & Human Research 26(5): 1–8

Evans C H (2003) Germ line gene therapy: can we do it, do we need it, where do we start, and where might it lead? In: Chapman A R, Frankel M S (eds) Designing Our Descendants: The Promises and Perils of Genetic Modifications. Johns Hopkins University Press, Baltimore, MD

Evans J (2002) Playing God? Human Genetic Engineering and the Rationalization of the Public Bioethical Debate. University of Chicago Press, Chicago, IL

Frankel M S, Chapman A R (2000) Human Inheritable Genetic Modifications: Assessing Scientific, Ethical, Religious, and Policy Issues. Available at http://www.aaas.org/spp/dspp/sfrl/germline/main.htm Accessed April 24, 2003

Friedmann T (2003) Approaches to gene transfer to the mammalian germ line. In: Chapman A R, Frankel M S (eds) Designing Our Descendants: The Promise and Perils of Genetic Modification. Johns Hopkins, Baltimore, MD

Genetics and Public Policy Center (2004) Preimplantation Genetic Diagnosis: A Discussion of Challenges, Concerns, and Preliminary Policy Options Related to the Genetic Testing of Human Embryos. Available at http://www.DNApolicy.org Accessed April 25, 2006

Genetics and Public Policy Center (2005) Human Germline Genetic Modification: Issues and Options for Policymakers. Available at http://www.DNApolicy.org Accessed August 25, 2005

Gordon J (1999) Genetic enhancement in humans. Science 283: 2023–2024

Harris J (1992) Wonderwoman and Superman: The Ethics of Human Biotechnology. Oxford University Press, Oxford

Hood L (2000) The human genome project–launch pad for human genetic engineering. In: Stock G, Campbell J (eds) Engineering the Human Germline. Oxford University Press, New York

Institute of Medicine (1998) Scientific Opportunities and Public Needs: Improving Priority Setting and Public Input at the National Institutes of Health. National Academy Press, Washington, DC

Kimmelman J (2005) Recent developments in gene transfer: risk and ethics. BMJ 330: 79–82

Koshland D (2000) Ethics and safety. In: Stock G, Campbell J (eds) Engineering the Human Germline. Oxford University Press, New York

Lenfant P (2003) Clinical research to clinical practice – lost in translation? New England Journal of Medicine 349: 868–874

National Academy of Sciences (2002) Scientific and Medical Aspects of Human Reproductive Cloning. National Academy Press, Washington, DC

National Institutes of Health (1997) Setting Research Priorities at the National Institutes of Health. NIH Publication, Bethesda MD: 97–4265

Parens E (1995) Should we hold the (human) germline? Journal of Law, Medicine & Ethics 23: 173–176

Pennisi E (2005) Why do humans have so few genes? Science 309: 80

Pinker S (1 June 2003) Better babies? Why genetic enhancement is too unlikely to worry about. Boston Globe: D1

Resnik D B (2002) Bioethics of gene therapy. In: Encyclopedia of Life Sciences. Nature/MacMillan, London

Resnik D B, Steinkraus H B, Langer P J (1999) Human Germline Gene Therapy: Scientific, Moral and Political Issues. R. G. Landes, Austin, TX

Robertson J A (2003) Extending preimplantation genetic diagnosis: the ethical debate. Human Reproduction 18: 465–471

Silver L (2000) Reprogenetics: how reproductive and genetic technologies will be combined to provide new opportunities for people to reach their reproductive goals. In: Stock G, Campbell J (eds) Engineering the Human Germline. Oxford University Press, New York

Shanks P (2005) Human Genetic Engineering: A Guide for Activists, Skeptics, and the Very Perplexed. Nation Books/Avalon, New York

Stock G (2002) Redesigning Humans: Our Inevitable Genetic Future. Houghton Mifflin, New York
Stock G, Campbell J (2000a) Introduction: an evolutionary perspective. In: Stock G, Campbell J (eds) Engineering the Human Germline. Oxford University Press, New York
Stock G, Campbell J (2000b) The road ahead: a panel discussion In: Stock G, Campbell J (eds) Engineering the Human Germline. Oxford University Press, New York
Stock G, Campbell J (2000c) Other voices. In: Stock G, Campbell J (eds) Engineering the Human Germline. Oxford University Press, New York
Taubes G (2002) The strange case of chimeraplasty. Science 298: 2116–2120
Tuma R S (2003) AAAS President's Surprise Plea for Low-Tech Research. BioMedNet News. Available at http://news.bmn.com/news/story?day=030214&story=2-gm Accessed February 13, 2003
Wade N (2 September 1999) Scientists create a smarter mouse. New York Times: A1
Walters L, Palmer J G (1997) The Ethics of Human Gene Therapy. Oxford University Press, New York
Waters B (2002) European Scholars Support Development of Germ Line Modification. Available at http://www.eurekalert.org/pub_releases/2002–12/sari-ess121302.php Accessed April 4, 2003
Weiss R (29 January 2001) Study: rodents' higher IQ may come at painful price. Washington Post: A2
Zerhouni E (2003) The NIH roadmap. Science 302: 63–64, 72

Chapter 12
Bioelectronics and Implanted Devices

Ellen M. McGee

12.1 Introduction

The future may well involve the emergence of humans who are fundamentally coupled with bioelectronic devices, science fiction's "cyborgs." Revolutions in semiconductor devices, cognitive science, bioelectronics, nanotechnology and applied neural control technologies are facilitating breakthroughs in hybrids of humans and machines. The interactions of increased computing power, advances in prosthetic devices, artificial implants, and systems that blend electronic and biological components, are facilitating the merging of man with machines. Increasing numbers of body parts are being replaced with bio-electronic and mechanical items, acclimatizing us to the melding of the organic and non-organic. Used as curative devices for patients with sensory, motor or cognitive deficits, active medical implantable devices evoke little dispute, allowing those who are blind, or paralyzed, or without a limb, to surmount those conditions. Significant ethical concerns are, however, raised by the potential for using these technologies to enhance and augment human capabilities, and by the possibility that humankind, as we know it, may eventually be phased out, or become just a step in evolution. Endowing humans with night vision, X-ray vision and long-range zoom capacities, or the ability to sniff out mercury and carbon monoxide, appreciably changes human abilities. Of even more significance, is the radical enhancement possible through approaching brain-machine interfaces. Brain machine interfaces may enhance, augment or replace those most prized of human capacities, the ability to reason and remember. These interfaces will enable humans to be constantly logged onto the internet, to cyberthink and to instantaneously retrieve encyclopedic stores of information. Building in these interfaces, surgically implanting them in the brain, will allow for greater energy, and efficiency, and will enable humans to operate without radios, or TVs, printed newspapers, cameras, GPS units, credit cards, computer workstations, ATM machines, wireless, corded or mobile phones, and other separate devices (Maguire 1999) Brain-computer interfaces involve technologies which take information from the brain and externalize it as well as those which provide individuals with access to information from outside. The interaction of these technologies to allow for input-output interactions raises ethical issues of privacy and autonomy,

B. Gordijn, R. Chadwick (eds.) *Medical Enhancement and Posthumanity*,

justice, and even the meaning of being human. In the future, if it becomes possible both to clone an individual and to implant a chip with the uploaded memories, emotions, and knowledge of the clone's source, a type of immortality could be achieved. Alternatively, the uploaded self could be stored in a computer. Uploaded minds would not age; such humans could travel at the speed of light and communicate directly from mind to mind. In the future, each individual, and mankind, in general, may be faced with decisions about what kind of entity he/she chooses to be: (1) a natural, (2) an immortal with a body or (3) an entity that exists in virtual reality. Because of the vast probability that these technologies will transform humanity, global ethical and legal guidelines ought to be formulated and enforced.

While the scientific community, national governments, and international forums, have devoted considerable consideration to genetic technologies, and to a lesser extent, drug enhancements, human and electronic interfaces have received little public, social or ethical scrutiny. Neither of these future enhancements – genetic or pharmaceutical – will alter future humanity, as will bioelectronic systems that mix electronic and biological components. Genetic enhancements are restricted by the limitations of biology; hybrids of human and machine are not so restricted. Drugs to increase memory merely undertake an improvement of normal memory, not the abilities of a computer-enhanced mind to share information at a distance and to access encyclopedic data. Altering genes can only achieve an optimum of the biologically based human. Inserting genes from another biological system, for example, inserting the gene that enables the superior smelling capacity of dogs would certainly improve on human abilities, but since human intelligence is already superior to animals, improvements here would only reach to the highest level of genetically based intelligence. Bioelectronic implants can transform the human, bestowing benefits beyond the biological.

Although bioelectronic systems research is initially aimed at increasing the therapeutic options for patients with sensory, motor or cognitive defects, the uses of these developments for enhancement will be an extension subsequent to their development for therapeutic purposes. This trajectory of technology introduction is a familiar pattern in drug usage, and it is easy to foresee that bioelectronic devices which are initially devised to aid in restoring species typical functioning (Daniels 1985) will be used to provide the unimpaired with new sensory perceptions, and greater intelligence.

My purpose in this paper is to provide a picture of the state of the art in the development of brain-machine interfaces – by examining, first, sensory and motor devices, second, brain devices, third, the implications of nanotechnology for this field and finally, the possibilities inherent in brain chips, cloning and artificial intelligence. These sections incorporate an assessment of the ethical and social challenges arising in this area. Since raising ethical concerns without some hint of a means to address their challenges is inadequate, I end with a suggested principle for adoption, standards for implementation of the technology and an initial plan for a regulatory framework. The possible benefits of future technologies are incalculable; their possible harms are weighty. Both banning and total freedom are impractical, regulation is imperative.

12.2 Current Sensory and Motor Devices

Active medical implantable devices for functional electrical stimulation to replace neural capacities comprise a variety of sensory and motor devices, including, cardiac pacemakers, fabricated heart valves, implantable pumps that assist pulmonary function or circulation of the blood (among them the Left Ventricular Assisted Device, LVAD), and biochemical pumps that supply insulin or pain medications. Since 1957 over 60,000 cochlear implants, which directly stimulate the auditory nerve and enable totally deaf people to hear, have been implanted; an alternative auditory prosthesis is implanted directly into the cochlear nucleus in the brainstem. Various other technologies for ameliorating sensory or motor deficits are in early research. The *Abicor* is an artificial heart, in early testing, with several patients living with a plastic heart and an internal motor and electronics package. Cardiac pacemakers and defibrillators operate using wireless transfer of medical data, through the internet, to the physician. An artificial lung is in development at the University of Pittsburgh and clinical trials of this device will begin soon (Rossi 2006). It is anticipated that the artificial lung will initially serve as a bridge until a lung transplant becomes available, or to keep patients with serious lung infections alive until their lungs heal. An artificial vision system, announced in January 2000, enables the blind, using a cortical implant, to navigate independently, to "read" letters, and through a special electronic interface to "watch" television, use a computer, and access the Internet.[1] This cortical implant has been undergoing experimentation outside the United States (in order to circumvent Institutional Review Board and Food and Drug Administration approval) and is now assisting the blind to drive and navigate around spaces. Other optoelectronic implants are in development to treat visual diseases using retinal microchips, either positioned on the surface of the retina or implanted behind the retina.[2] Systems for functional neuromuscular stimulation are being used experimentally in cases of spinal cord severage,[3] and have proved effective in restoring motor functions to paralyzed limbs, allowing for upright mobility and restoration of bladder and bowel function.[4]

---

[1] Artificial vision system for the blind announced by the Dobelle Institute. Press Release. *Science Daily*. Available at: http://www.sciencedaily.com/releases20000100118065202.htm. Accessed January 15, 2001; Dobelle W, Antunes J, Coiteiro D, Girvin J. The first artificial vision systems in commercial distribution. Available at: http://www.dobelle.com/news.html. Accessed January 31, 2005.

[2] Optoelectronic implants to treat visual diseases. *OpticsReport*. Available at: http://www.opticsreport.com/content/article.php?article_id=1007. Accessed January 20, 2006.

[3] Study of an implantable functional neuromuscular stimulation system for patients with spinal cord injuries. ClinicalTrials.gov. Available at: http://www.clinicaltrials.gov/ct/show/NCT00004445. Accessed January 29, 2005.

[4] Implantable FES system for upright mobility and bladder and bowel function for individuals with spinal cord injury. *Spinal Cord (2005) 43:713–723*. Available at: http://www.nature.com/sc/journal/v43/n12/abs/3101797a.html. Accessed January 30, 2006.

Robotic arms, using electro active polymers, are pioneering efforts in the artificial-muscle search. Artificial knees, and smart legs, utilize embedded microprocessors for control, and are manufactured as "bionic" joints called the Rheo Knee, or the C-leg, which combine computer chip technology with hydraulics to do the walking for amputees. The Department of Veterans Affairs is supporting research on the "biohybrid" limb which will function using brain and nerve signals.[5] This prosthesis merges man-made components with human muscles, bones and the neurological system in order to create a system for movement similar to that which allows paralyzed individuals to move a cursor with their minds.

12.3 Brain Devices

Over 30, 000 people are now living with implants for Deep Brain Stimulation (DBS; Lozano 2006). Presently, pacemaker-like brain implants, with the ability to download upgraded software directly from outside to the implant, help Parkinson's patients and those with essential tremors (Ditlea 2004). Vagus nerve stimulators, made by Cyberonics, although controversial, have shown effectiveness in clinical trials for treating depression.[6] So, too, has deep brain stimulation (DBS) in which electrodes are implanted in the lobes at the midline of the brain, at Area 25, so that low voltage can be steadily streamed from a pacemaker (Dobbs 2005).

Initial work on linking the brain directly with both local and remote manipulators has been demonstrated by neuroscientists at Duke University who trained a monkey to control a mechanical arm just by thinking (Lemonick 2003). In March of 1998, a "locked in" victim of a brain-stem stroke became the first recipient of a brain to a computer interface, enabling him to communicate on a computer by thinking about moving the cursor (Headlam 2000); these bionic brain implants, developed by researchers at Emory University allow a computer interface to be operated by the power of thought. In November of 2003, a US company announced plans to request an investigational device exemption from the Food and Drug Administration to test a device that would allow the paralyzed to control a computer through a neural interface. The device, Braingate, has been tested in animals, and the company subsequently initiated human trials on severely paralyzed patients in 2004.[7] The first subject, a quadriplegic 25 year old, was successfully implanted with a brain chip which enables him to check e-mail, play computer games, control a television, and

---

[5] Wendy Y. Lawton. Research group exploring limb loss hopes biohybrid will bridge gap between human and machine. *George Street Journal, December 10, 2004*. Available at: http://www.brown.edu/Administration/George_Street_Journal/vol29/29GSJ06e.html. Accessed February 1, 2006.

[6] Harris G. Device won approval though F.D.A. staff objected, *The New York Times, February 17, 2006*.

[7] Cyberkinetics. Available at: http://www.cyberkineticsinc.com/content/index.jsp. Accessed May 29, 2005.

turn lights on and off by thought alone.[8] The goals of the NASA *Extension of the Human Senses Group* are to develop brain-computer interface technologies for augmentation purposes.[9] The Defense Advanced Research Projects Agency (DARPA) of the US Department of Defense has allotted $24 million to support research into the proposals of six different labs for brain-machine systems (Zimmer 2004). The objective of these projects is to control robots and airplanes through thought alone, and ultimately anticipates a future of soldier-controlled killer robots (Martin 2005).

Efforts to decode the information processing system that is the brain were jump-started by the discovery of Miguel Nicolelis and John Chapin that electrodes with flexible tips did not damage the brain and that enough information to recognize commands could be produced by decoding only a small number of the neurons in a brain (see Zimmer 2004). Recently, in a risky procedure aimed at restoring hearing for two deaf women a penetrating device was inserted directly into the brain stem (Graham-Rowe 2004a). A team, led by Ted Berger of the University of Southern California, is working on replacing the functions of the hippocampus which serves to "encode" experiences and store new memories before they are laid down elsewhere as long-term memories (Graham-Rowe 2003). The group has copied the *behavior* of the hippocampus, rather than waiting to *understand its intricacies*. This shift, from trying to map detailed neural function to exploiting the user's ability to learn, is expected to increase the pace of development.

Researchers at Washington University, using an implanted brain grid, have found that patients can imagine moving and thus control a cursor with thought alone; their goal is to create a brain-machine interface for long-term use.[10] Other scientists, at Caltech, have recently succeeded in using implanted electrodes to detect activity in monkeys' "parietal reach region," where higher-level thoughts such as "get the key and use it" are generated (Graham-Rowe 2004b). Decoding these higher levels cognitive activities, including accessing the degree of enthusiasm of the monkeys, represents an important step for brain implant technology. These results are promising for the development of neural prostheses that would enable users to move mechanical devices with thoughts, and monitor "not only patients' goals, what they want to reach for, but also their mood and motivation" (Begley 2004).

12.4 Nanotechnology

The field of nanotechnology, which involves the "recently developed ability to measure, manipulate and organize matter on the nanoscale – 1 to 100 billionths of a meter" (Roco & Bainbridge 2001) promises a transformation in the ability to

[8] Hooper S. Brain chip offers hope for paralyzed. Available at: http://www.cnn.com/2004/TECH/10/20/explorers.braingate. Accessed January 4, 2005.

[9] Extension of the human senses group. Available at: http://ic.arc.nasa.gov/projects/ne/ehs.html. Accessed February 10, 2004.

[10] Implanted brain grid reads minds. 6/10/2004. Available at: www.betterhumans.com/News/news.aspx?articleID-2004-06-10-2. Accessed August 21, 2004.

rebuild our bodies and brains. “The definition most frequently used by government and industry involves structures, devices, and systems having novel properties and functions due to the arrangement of their atoms on the 1 to 100 nanometer scale.”[11] Nanotechnology builds from the molecular level up, using engineered devices, rather than by using bulk materials. Presently nanotechnology is used to produce stain resistant clothes, clear sunscreen and skin care products, golf drivers, tennis balls that bounce longer, dental adhesives, rain repellents for windshields joint and muscle creams and smart drugs. Dramatic claims are made for nanotechnology’s future use in medicine: (1) as medical nanosensors which will be used diagnostically to search for a specific piece of disease related DNA, or radiation levels, (2) as monitors of hormone levels and to signal release of insulin, (3) as smart drugs to target specific organs or cells, (4) as miniature robots to ferry materials to cells, and (5) to repair damaged genes. Through nanotechnology techniques, robots, called nanobots, will work within our bodies to clean fatty deposits from the bloodstream, to destroy viruses, bacteria and cancer cells, to deliver drugs, and to assist in diagnosis. Robert Freitas has proposed the creation of artificial red blood cells, “respirocytes”, spherical nanorobots about the size of a bacterium, for use in transfusions, as treatment for anemia, in sports, and to augment functioning.[12] This medical nanomachine will have an onboard nanocomputer and sensors and be remotely reprogrammable by physicians. The Defense Advanced Research Projects Agency (Darpa) is engaged in producing biologically based devices for the detection of chemical and biological warfare agents. It is projected that by the 2020s it will be possible to send multitudes of nanobots through the capillaries of the working brain for noninvasive scanning that will enable us to model and simulate the entire brain (Kurzweil 2005). Futurist Ray Kurzweil projects that due to miniaturization and cost-reduction, nanobot technology will, within 25 years, result in the ability to scan and reverse engineer the human brain (see Kurzweil 2005).

12.5 Enhancement

As researchers succeed in the goals of developing sensory replacements, artificial lungs, hearts, limbs, and brain interfaces, the prospect of utilizing their work to facilitate the enhancement of humans through bioelectronics arises. A distinction, the therapy/enhancement distinction (Parens 1998), is commonly made between interventions which are therapeutic in their intent, used to treat disease or disability, and interventions which either (1) augment or improve on normal species function, or (2) bestow entirely new capacities. Enhancements of the first type are exemplified

[11] Foresight Nanotech Institute. About nanotechnology. Available at: http://www.foresight.org/nano/whatisnano.html. Accessed February 2005.

[12] Nanomedicine and the future of healthcare 2002-11-06. *Plausible Futures Newsletter*. Available at: http://www.plausiblefutures.com/index.php?id=54173. Accessed June 23, 2005.

by adapting methods used to restore auditory and visual capabilities in order to provide non-disabled individuals with access to a wider spectrum of vision and hearing. These extra-senses will include those for sonar and polarized light, electromagnetic senses, internal organ monitoring and the ability to adjust the intensity of the senses, or even to shut them off. As regards brain chip implants, it seems apparent that there are real distinctions between using the technology for therapy and enhancement. Enabling those who are paralyzed or naturally less cognitively endowed to achieve on a more equitable level is therapeutic, and brings a capacity that was below species typical functioning up to the norm. Bioelectronic systems research will pave the way for augmenting human motor abilities, allowing for "supernaturally" fast running or out of the ordinary muscle power. The Olympic motto, *Faster*, *Higher*, *Stronger* could be achieved in an unexpected manner; "with Freitas's respirocytes (robotic red blood cells; Freitas 1998) runner could do an Olympic sprint for 15 minutes without taking a breath" (see Kurzweil 2005: 254). These capacities would benefit soldiers or anyone needing to flee an attacker, and nurses, who would be better able to lift patients. Human/machine interfaces will come, for the possibility of these technologies to improve the capacities of humans is predictable, as is the impetus to implement. Humans with the capacity for cyber thought, total recall, and supra intelligence will have entirely new capacities. This step in the evolution of humans will bring a multitude of new problems, including possible interference with privacy and autonomy rights, but, hopefully, can be self-directed and guided. Thus, there is a need for thoughtful, worldwide discussions and meaningful regulation.

12.6 Ethical Concerns in Therapeutic Usage

When used for therapy, implanted chips and bioelectronics do not provoke acrimonious debate. Nevertheless, the concerns that do emerge with curative use of implanted chips – questions of safety, fairness, access, and the costs of implementing this technology – need to be addressed.

12.6.1 Safety

As with all devices, there are both short and long term risks. Short-term risks include those associated with surgery: bleeding, infections, and adverse reactions to anesthesia. Long term risks are more challenging to evaluate, but certainly may included immune reactions to foreign substances; it may be difficult to develop nontoxic materials, that do not cause an adverse reaction in the body. Related to these issues are those of warranty availability, liability responsibilities of manufacturers, industry wide standards for devices, methods of facilitating upgrades, and procedures for training users in implementation of the systems. Further, it will be necessary to collect data on the usefulness of implants and on whether some types of users benefit more than others. Some individuals, such as the developmentally delayed and those with dementia, may not be able to learn to use the system. Others will require counseling to help in reaching decisions about implantation.

12.6.2 Fairness, Access and Costs

It is not likely that a health system already straining to provide drug and surgical benefits to citizens will be able to include these advances in its care package either through insurance or government programs. Moreover, these concerns will be complicated by this, as other, technology's ability to initiate a constantly changing standard of normalcy. This will be made all the more difficult to restrain, as the derivative of change will be positive – thus providing strong feedback leading to increasingly greater expectations, and greater demands on an already overburdened health care system. Methods must be devised to limit the inequities in therapeutic availability arising from developments in this area. Certainly efforts should be made to avoid the type of situation which has resulted in the lack of HIV/AID drugs for a majority of the world's sufferers; perhaps in this area, too, a commitment should be made to tier pricing where developing countries pay the lowest possible price or get the technology for therapeutic purposes at cost.

12.7 Ethical Issues in Enhancement Applications

More knotty technical, ethical, and social questions are raised by this technology's potential for enhancement and even control of humans. Brain implants used to provide vision to the blind are highly desirable devices. Extending their use in order to provide night vision, X-ray vision, and long-range zoom capacities to the normally sighted raises considerably different issues. Enhancement in and of itself is not necessarily objectionable; vaccines, in vitro fertilization, breast enhancement surgery, are all instances of readily accepted and widely sought enhancement technologies. However, brain machine interfaces will put new forms of stress on privacy, autonomy, and justice, and more importantly, on what it means to be human. These interfaces can assist not only those with failing memory, but may even bestow fluency in a new language, enable "recognition" of previously unmet individuals, and provide for the sharing of sensory and cognitive data mind to mind. Projected users of these devices will fall into three groups.

First will be those with a disability for whom the devices will be therapeutic. Second stage users will come from the military, which will use implanted computing and communication devices to interface with weapons and information systems. Third stage users for implanted devices will be individuals involved in any type of information intensive businesses (Maguire & McGee 1999). Funding for these developments is supported by the Defense Advanced Research Projects Agency:

"DARPA is interested in creating new technologies for augmenting human performance through the ability to non-invasively access these codes in the brain in real time and integrate them into peripheral device or system operations."[13] Brain-computer interfaces promise to change the capacities of humans to such a degree that they become fundamentally different. Humanity itself, at least those (former?) members of Homo sapiens who have access to the technology will be substantially different.

Not all regard this prospect favorably. Both essentialists, including those who argue for bodily integrity, and creationists, argue against development of implantable chips.[14] Many, including Fukuyama, fear tampering with human nature as we know it; he argues that human nature, which provides continuity to our species and defines our values and politics, should not be altered (Fukuyama 2002). Leon Kass, former head of the President's Council on Bioethics, writes, "If there is a case to be made against these activities – for individuals – we sense that it may have something to do with what is natural" (Kass 2003). The notion that nature is somehow good and technology evil is common and erroneous, since the human has always been a fabricator of means to enhance his existence. Technology itself is not evil; the uses that men devise may be.

There are those who believe that modifying brain function to produce a superior human interferes with God's creation. This view logically includes positing restrictions on curing disease and disability and is contradicted by religious views that call for man to partner with God in creation (Berry 2000).

More realistic than these critiques, are the multitude of technical, ethical and social concerns that should be resolved before proceeding with implantable chips. The concerns include: apprehensions about safety, risk, and informed consent, issues of manufacturing and scientific responsibility, anxieties about the psychological impacts of enhancing human nature, worries about possible usage in children, concerns about increasing the divide between the rich and the poor, and most troublesome, issues of privacy and autonomy. As is the case in any technology assessment, it is unlikely that we can reliably predict all effects. Nevertheless, the potential for harm must be considered.[15]

12.7.1 Safety of Enhancement Devices

Safety concerns are paramount, and, as discussed previously within the context of therapeutic devices, both surgery and long-term use of implants may generate risks. The development of non-toxic materials is imperative, as is a consideration of warranties, quality oversight of software and hardware, liability responsibilities of manufacturers, and developing trouble-free methods for upgrades. Surely minimizing

[13] BAA 01–42, Addendum 1, Special focus area: brain machine interfaces. Available at: http://www.darpa.mil/baa/baa01-42mod1.htm. Accessed January 20, 2006.

[14] For a fuller discussion of these critiques see Maguire and McGee 1999 for debate.

[15] In this section I have drawn from McGee and Maguire 2001.

additional surgeries must be a priority. These matters will in all likelihood be resolved, in clinical therapeutic trials, before enhancement devices are implanted.

12.7.2 Informed Consent

Brain implants should be subject to principles of informed consent. Usage for children, prisoners, the military, and citizenry of despotic regimes is highly problematical. The question of free adaptation is rendered more complicated by the likelihood of social and economic pressures for improvement.

12.7.3 Psychological Questions

The psychological impact on the self needs to be a subject of research since the boundaries between self and others and even groups will be eroded, if not eliminated. The boundaries between real and virtual world will blur, and a self constantly wired to the collective will be transformed. The emergence of a Borg type collectivity or hive mind, where personal identity is lost and assimilation is the preeminent value is a real possibility.[16] Selves will have relationships and interact in highly realistic virtual reality environments, transforming the sense of both the individual and reality. Whether this will be a benefit or burden is unclear.

12.7.4 Justice Issues

Unless there is universal access to these technologies, inequalities will increase; the injustice involved in increasing the divide between humans in the developed and developing worlds, between genders and between enhanced and non-enhanced children is disquieting. Although it is possible that costs, as with many technologies, will rapidly decline, it is probable that there will be a division between different classes of people the "naturals" and the "enhanced." This would, in all likelihood, lead to strife and even greater power and economic imbalances.

12.7.5 Autonomy

Unquestionably, the most troubling aspect of this new technology is the potential for control of persons. Microchips could enable not only global tracking of individuals,

[16] Borg. *Wikipedia*. Available at: http://en.wikipedia.org/wiki/Borg. Accessed June 26, 2006.

but also be used to "see" and "hear" what an individual is experiencing. Brain implants (as demonstrated with robo-rat) could be used to change behavior and attitudes. Individual's thoughts and emotions, could be monitored, controlled or directed; it would be easy to ascertain where anyone is and with whom they are in touch. For those with "nothing to hide" it becomes easy to accept surveillance and even loss of autonomy. The larger question is whether it is a "good" for humanity. Uses for children, prisoners, the military and, eventually, ordinary citizens pose trenchant questions of autonomy and privacy. The development of cyber-soldiers could facilitate warfare, but forestall the liberty of personnel; tracking and monitoring of children could have beneficent aims, and still violate norms of privacy.

12.8 Brain Chips, Cloning, and Ethics

More critical problematical ethical uncertainties surface when we consider the possibility of both cloning a human and uploading memories to a chip,[17] and these uncertainties involve the question of the nature of man. For some, human identity is biological. Cloning involves the duplication of an organism; it is a later born identical twin. Insofar as the self is identified with a particular body, a clone to some extent duplicates that self.[18] Cloning the self would ensure a certain type of immortality. However, insofar as the self is other than the genetic body, fully replicating the self requires more than biological identity. Certainly a major facet of an individual's identity involves narrative identity. By 2040, it may be possible to store the data representing all of a human being's sensory experiences, all that we have encountered, read, and experienced, in a storage device implanted in the brain. This data could be collected by biological probes receiving electrical impulses, and would enable a user to recreate experiences, or even to transfer (transplant) memories from one brain to another. Another technique for achieving this goal is to implant a chip behind the eye in order to record all of a person's thoughts, sensations, and experiences. British Telecom's Artificial Life Team is working on this device, dubbed Soul Catcher 2025; since estimates are that it will be ready for use in 2025. Dr. Winter's claim is that "by combining this information with a record of the person's genes, we could recreate a person physically, emotionally and spiritually." (Archives Society of Alberta 1996; In actuality it would probably be necessary to implant multiple chips in order to capture all the sensory data which is sent to the brain.) A different approach is that of Gordon Bell from Microsoft's Media Presence Group who is recording a lifetime's worth of articles, books, cards, CDs, letters, memos, papers, photos, pictures, presentations, home movies, videotaped

---

[17] Parts of this section borrow significantly from my article, becoming Borg to become immortal. Forthcoming *Cambridge Quarterly of Healthcare Ethics*.

[18] As pointed out by the editor Bert Gordijn in a personal communication: "It is most likely that there would be genetic and epigenetic differences between two clones,...caused by mutations... or by different environments triggering different patterns of expression."

lectures, and voice recordings and storing them digitally, along with creating software to selectively replay this information.[19]

> Current technology can extend corporal life for a few decades. Both one-way and two-way immortality require part of a person to be converted to information (*Cyberized*), and stored in a more durable media. We believe that two-way immortality where one's experiences are digitally preserved, and which then take on a life of their own will be possible within this century.[20]

It is an open question whether brain machine interface technology will, in the near future, enable uploading our memories to a chip. Some researchers argue that as we develop capacities to scan the brain, research that is ongoing, we will learn to do so in order to download it, thus not even needing to store the raw data as it is generated. It is theoretically possible that we will map the locations and interconnections of neurons and synapses, and eventually be able to transfer an analog of the brain and its memory to a digital-analog computer (Kurzweil 2002). Indeed Ray Kurzweil claims that "By the end of this century, I don't think there will be a clear distinction between human and machine" (McCullag & Kurzweil 2000). Futurologist, Ian Pearson of BT posits that at some point it should be possible to make a "full duplex mind link between man and machine."[21] Thought transmission between humans could then be achievable, backup copies of our brains could be made, and a global network would be part of our consciousness. One result of uploading minds is that immortality could be assured since uploaded minds would not experience death. However, reformatting our mind files and storing them in another medium does not ensure immortality unless survival is ensured by continually upgrading to the latest hardware and software (see Kurzweil 2005: 329–330). Once mind is uploaded, these new beings could travel at the speed of light, have enhanced memory and knowledge capabilities, and communicate from mind to mind. Further ethical concerns arise from the possibility that memory storage would enable justice officials to have perfect knowledge of an individual's responsibility for, or lack of involvement in a crime; the right not to incriminate oneself could be abrogated. In addition, questions are raised about the dangers of total recall even for the individual, since forgetting seems to play a significant role in mental health.

Once mind is uploaded to a chip, psychological continuity of personal identity could be immortalized in a series of cloned selves, bestowing immortality, and raising anew philosophical questions regarding personal identity. If all that is

---

[19] Gemmel J, Bell G, Lueder R, Drucker S, Wong C. My life bits: fulfilling the memex vision. *Microsoft Research*. Available at: http://research.microsoft.com/ jgemmell/pubs/MyLifeBitsMM02.pdf. Accessed January 7, 2005.

[20] Bell, G, Gray J. Digital immortality. Available at: http://research.microsoft.com/research/pubs/view.aspx?msr_tr_id=MSR-TR-2000–101. Accessed February 9, 2006.

[21] Pearson I. The future of human evolution. Available at: www.bt.com/sphere/insights/pearson/human_evolution.htm. Accessed January 28, 2005.

required for the persistence of personal identity is the sustaining of memory and physical continuity (Olson 2002), then the clone with a previous or ongoing individual's memories uploaded to a chip implanted and activated would be the same person ongoing in time. Arguments minimizing cloning's effects and claiming that cloning is unlikely to affect a person's sense of self or identity (Brock 2002) become irrelevant when the clone receives all the memories and experiences of a previous individual. In this case, concerns about the loss of an open future for the clone and the impacts upon autonomy and freedom are warranted. Certainly, the cloned person's individuality and uniqueness could be overwhelmed to such an extent that the new individual might simply be the ongoing previous individual now experiencing a new history; a clone's independent learning might even be suppressed to facilitate this. The extent to which the clone's identity would be impacted by the implant would depend upon the age of implantation, and the control exerted over the new memories of the host clone. In considering the question of whether such an implant would produce an extension of the same person or a duplicate, one disquieting question is: how many can exist at the same time? If only one, then it would be an extension, if more than one, duplication. It is, in some real sense, the same person, and not the same person, just as I am not the same today as I was yesterday, because things have happened in the meantime and this changes who I am. What the ability to transfer memories does is to enable this evolution of "self" across a much longer time than a single body might normally exist, possibly forever.

A multitude of other questions emerge when contemplating this eventuality. When would the chip be implanted? Or enabled? What would it be like to be an already aware individual with an ongoing history imprisoned in a child's body? Would the cloned, implanted entity feel like a unique person? Who would the clone be? Should this be allowed? Or promoted?

The question "what is man?" seems to have no definitive answer. Yet, mind is surely the most salient feature of Homo sapiens. Once memories can be transferred from one brain to another or perhaps even several others – even to a computer or other species- questions regarding personal identity, the nature of memory, and the meaning of memory will be even more insistent.

12.9 Artificial Intelligence

At the moment human intelligence is superior to that of machines, at least in terms of general intelligence. In some areas, of course, machines already exceed human intelligence: in pattern recognition, intelligent data mining, detecting fraud, doing calculations, and diagnosing medical conditions. As machines progress, they will successfully compete with humans, and given sufficient time, surpass humans. This will result after AI achieves human levels due to the "speed, memory, capacity, and knowledge sharing that nonbiological intelligence already exhibits" (see Kurzweil 2005: 407). Several researchers in a variety of articles and books have projected the coming superiority of artificial intelligence.[22] Intelligent machines could then supersede mere humans.

> We are re-evolving artificial minds at ten million times the original speed of human evolution, exponentially growing robot complexity....Within three decades, fourth-generation universal robots ... will be able to abstract and generalize – perhaps replace us.[23]

Based on the speed with which computers are gaining processing power, already existent input/output technologies, and the research potential for understanding the principles of operation of the human brain and copying its workings (either through computational neuroscience or emulating "the scanned brain on a computer by running a fine-grained simulation of its neural network),"[24] artificial intelligence and super-smart robots may well be developed within a few decades.

If an individual's brain is completely scanned and "recreated in a neurocomputer of sufficient capacity, we'll have an entity that acts very much like" that individual (Kurzweil 1999a). Our minds could be copied to another medium, even a robot. Several futurists and transhumanists have projected that this ability to capture and reinstantiate our minds would free mankind from the necessity of a biological substratum or body. We would then be nonbiological conscious entities. This post-carbon future would, according to both Moravec and Kurzwil, free us from the vulnerabilities of the body, and is a prospect they embrace (Moravec 1998; Kurzweil 1999b). These minds will exist in virtual environments, having experiences in virtual reality. The underlying assumption here is that the significant aspect of humans is mind, that we are not constituted by our bodies; the vision here elevates intelligence and rationality and disvalues the physical in the form of body.

Unless humanity embraces cyber technology, its hegemony may eventually yield to intelligent machines. If cybernetic technology is guided to allow the development, or evolution of humans that are not merely human, are cyborgs, the supremacy of humans could be ensured, at least until the time when the machines evolve the next generation without our assistance (Kurzweil 2005). As humans transform their bodies, replacing parts with nonbiological systems with improved function, and enhanced human brains become one with nonbiological portions of intelligence, the nature of man will be radically altered. If cloning is combined with cyborg technology one possible evolutionary path will be defined. Other possibilities, however, include that of humanity being destroyed by its future self-creating technology. Nanotechnology raises specific concerns, including the possibility that self-replicating entities could escape our control, and that the software directing nanobots could be compromised. The possibility that self-replicating nanobots, stronger, faster and more intelligent than humans will be malevolent has led for

---

[22] Bostrom N. When machines outsmart humans. *Futures. Vol. 35–37:759–764.* Available at: http://www.nickbostrom.com/2050/outsmart.html. Accessed April 16, 2005; Kurzweil 1990.

[23] Moravec R. Robots, re-evolving minds. *Kurzweil AI net.* Available at: http://www.kurzweilai.net/meme/frame.html?main=/articles/art0145.html. Accessed April17, 2005.

[24] Bostrom N. When machines outsmart humans. *Futures. Vol. 35(7):759–564.* Available at:_www.nickbostrom.com/2050/outsmart.html. Accessed April 17, 2005.

calls to bring to a halt the development of these technologies before humanity is destroyed. A preventive ethic needs to be universally adopted to deal with the dangers of these future technologies. The Foresight Institute has proposed that nanotechnologists relinquish the development of physical entities that can self-replicate in a natural environment.

> Any use of self-replicating systems is avoided except in approved and controlled circumstances. Any developers who design or build self-replicating machines adopt systematic security measures to avoid unplanned distribution of their designs and technical capabilities. Both potential benefits and risks of alternative technologies are explored actively, in a balanced and rigorous manner.[25]

These restrictions are indispensable since nanotechnology will enable and be used to fulfill the promise of bioelectronic devices and implanted chips, since reducing size will enhance efficacy. But, greater than these concerns is the need for dialogue about the wisdom of promoting these developments. What kind of existence will make for a meaningful future for humanity? Humanity needs to reflect on its relation to body, and on whether virtual reality would be a satisfactory substitute for experience. If body is important in our self-constitution then existence as Intelligences needs to be precluded. Nevertheless, some, who value being embodied, may be desirous of augmentation or enhancing of mental function using implanted brain chips. Many countries of the world have already banned reproductive cloning which would impact on the option of combining cloning and implanted uploaded chips. For many, the thought of becoming a "brain in a vat," intelligence within virtual reality, will be rejected. The prospect of being a mind in a robot, likewise, may not be humanly desired. Not every scientific possibility need be accepted. Regulation is possible, as with nuclear materials, environmental controls, research on humans, and uses of active infectious agents. Nations and world societies need to assess the risks to society as a whole, and to the nature of humanity and its self-evolution from the development of these technologies.[26] International dialogue leading to policy positions about the kinds of evolution desired for human kind must be organized and reasonable regulations implemented. Development and implementation of technology is not inevitable; reflection and restriction is possible. Since implanted bioelectronic chips are a likely future technology, policies and regulations should be devised to mitigate their possible deleterious effects. These policies should entail self-regulation by the involved scientific communities, and extend to include national and international regulation. Regulation, which is preferable to prohibition, should proceed from the standpoint of preventive ethics. The precautionary principle should guide scientific research in this field, and guide policy formation since the risks of harm are uncertain.

---

[25] Jacobstein N, Reynolds G. *Foresight Guidelines on Molecular Nanotechnology*, Foresight Institute and IMM. Available at: http://www.foresight.org/guidelines/current.html#Preamble. Accessed January, 2006.

[26] For a fuller discussion of needed regulations see: McGee E. Becoming Borg to become immortal. Forthcoming *Cambridge Quarterly of Healthcare Ethics*.

12.10 Suggestions for Action

Public forums need to be created where scientists could elucidate the forthcoming developments and citizens could openly debate cybernetic technologies' future. Where public funds are invested, public accountability should be secured. "Deliberative Polling" represents a promising avenue for this type of forum (Fishkin 2006). Decision makers must be held responsible for developing regulations for these enhancement technologies.

Most nations have medical device regulating bodies. The International Standards Organization (ISO) has introduced international standards for the world community. In the United States before a medical device can be marketed it must be approved by the Food and Drug Administration (FDA). In the United States implantable brain chips and other bioelectronic devices would be listed as Class III devices inasmuch as they are implanted and could present a health risk. The development of such technologies is, then, already subject to governmental regulation. However, this type of analysis, which is only concerned with safety and efficacy, is inadequate to consider the social and policy questions of these enhancement devices. Therefore a new system, parallel to the existing human subjects review process, should be instituted for enhancement technologies. The complexity of the issues surrounding enhancement techniques makes providing policy difficult, and requires new regulatory bodies both nationally and internationally.

The implications of these devices on the evolution of human nature necessitate both national and international consideration. Nations and world societies are stakeholders in assessing the costs to mankind from these technologies. Many international authorities and structures already exist ranging from those that govern economic, environmental, and intellectual property law, to those that govern international public health law through the World Health organization. Since these bioelectronics will be developed internationally, marketed globally and affect human nature universally their regulation needs to extend from the self-regulation of scientists to the national and international levels. Self-regulation by those involved in brain implant technology should be pursued, in order to recommend and establish standards of safety, efficacy, privacy, autonomy, consent and justice. I suggest that a new principle be adopted for enhancement technologies: the risk/benefit ratio applied in evaluating safety and effectiveness should be higher than that required for therapeutic interventions. In view of the complexity of issues and the magnitude of the transformations possible, there is increased risk for unforeseen problems, and a greater need for preventive ethics.

Further, requirements must be made for (1) reversibility in the event of adverse events, (2) informed consent, and (3) limited access for initial studies. Reversibility would preclude permanency of problems; informed consent would restrict usage to competent adults (although if it is shown that the implants, studied in a therapeutic trial, help the demented or retarded, surrogate decision-making should be allowed); limiting studies would secure time for evaluation before widespread implementation. Effective regulation of the scenario described, where a clone is created and implanted with a brain chip containing all of a previous individual's thoughts and memories could be effectively banned by national and international prohibitions on human reproductive cloning.

12.11 Conclusion

It should be evident from the material and discussion presented here that the development of brain-machine interfaces is a looming reality. My presentation of the innumerable sensory, motor and brain devices, and of developments in nanotechnology and artificial intelligence should be sufficient to make the case for forthcoming developments that will change humanity as we know it. Inasmuch as the ethical and social challenges that arise in this area are unaddressed and unregulated, and are not only different in degree, but possibly in kind, from other enhancement techniques (since they truly involve the creation of "supra humans") there is an urgent need for world-wide dialogue and action. The principle I have recommended and the standards suggested should serve as an impetus to the development of policy and regulatory organizations worldwide. Great benefits can be expected from bioelectronics and implanted devices; possible harms need to be examined and precluded. Scientific, national and international action should commence.

References

Archives Society of Alberta (1996) September, vol 16, no 2. Available at: www.archivesalberta.org/vol16_2/brain.htm. Accessed January 7, 2005

Begley S (2004) Prosthetics operated by brain activity move closer to reality. The Wall Street Journal Science Journal, July 9, 2004: B1

Berry J (2000) The Care of Creation. Inter-Varsity Press, Leicester, UK

Brock D W (2002) Human cloning and our sense of self. Science, April 12, vol 296: 314–317

Daniels N (1985) Just Health Care. Cambridge University Press, New York

Ditlea S (2004) Cyborgs of New York. The Daily News, June 8, The Front Page

Dobbs D (2005) A depression switch. The New York Times Magazine, April 2: 50–55

Fishkin J (2006) The nation in a room. Boston Review, March/April

Freitas R (1998) Exploratory design in medical nanotechnology: a mechanical artificial red cell. Artif Cells Blood Substit Immobil Biotechnol, July 26 vol 4: 411–430

Fukuyama F (2002) Our Posthuman Future. Farrar, Straus & Giroux, New York

Graham-Rowe D (2003) World's first brain prosthesis revealed. New Scientist, March 12, 2003. Available at: http://www.newscientist.com/article.ns?id=dn3488. Accessed June, 2003

Graham-Rowe D (2004a) First brainstem implants aim to tackle deafness. New Scientist, January 19. Available at: http://www.newscientist.com/article.ns?id=dn4540. Accessed May, 2004

Graham-Rowe D (2004b) Brain implants 'read' monkey minds. New Scientist, July 8, 2004. Available at: http://www.newscientist.com/article.ns?id=dn6127. Accessed August 10, 2004

Headlam B (2000) The mind that moves objects. The New York Times Magazine, June 11: 63–64

Kass L (2003) Ageless bodies, happy souls: biotechnology and the pursuit of perfection. The New Atlantis, no 1 (Spring): 9–28

Kurzweil R (1990) The Age of Intelligent Machines. MIT Press, Boston, MA

Kurzweil R (1999a) Spiritual Machines, September 13, 1999. Available at: http://www.pbs.org/newshour/gergen/september99/gergen_9–13.html. Accessed February, 2000

Kurzweil R (1999b) Spiritual Machines: When Computers Exceed Human Intelligence. Viking, New York

Kurzweil R (2002) The coming merging of mind and machine. In: Fritz S (ed) Understanding Artificial Intelligence: 90–99

Kurzweil R (2005) The Singularity Is Near. Viking, New York

Lemonick M (2003) Robo-monkey's reward. Time, October 27: 45–44

Lozano A (2006) Functional neurosurgery and deep brain stimulation: opportunities and challenges. Available at: http://www.loc.gov/today/cyberlc/feature_wdesc.php?rec=3715. Accessed February 16, 2006

Maguire G Q (1999) Transforming humanity: toward the implantable walkstation. Available at: http://web.it.kth.se/ maguire/Talks/LIU-990824.pdf. Accessed June 5, 2000

Maguire G Q, McGee E M (1999) Implantable Brain Chips? Time for Debate. Hastings Center Report 29, no 1: 7–13

Martin R (2005) Mind Control Wired Magazine Issue 13.03, March 2005. Available at http://www.wired.com/wired/archive/13.03/brain.html. Accessed January 30, 2006

McCullag D, Kurzweil R (2000) Rooting for the machine. Wired News, November 3. Available at: http://www.wired.com/news/technology/0,1282,39967,00.html. Accessed January 31, 2005

McGee E M, Maguire G Q (2001) Implantable brain chips: ethical and policy issues. Lahey Clinic Medical Ethics Journal, Winter

Moravec H (1998) Mind Children: The Future of Robot and Human Intelligence. Harvard University Press, Cambridge

Olson Eric T (2002) Personal Identity. The Stanford Encyclopedia of Philosophy (Fall Edition). In: Zalta E N (ed) Available at: http://plato.stanford.edu/archives/fall2002/entries/identity-personal. Accessed April 17, 2005

Parens E (1998) Is Better Always Good? The Enhancement Project. In: Parens E (ed) Enhancing Human Traits: Ethical and Social Implications. Georgetown University Press, Washington, DC: 1–28

Roco M C, Bainbridge W S (2001) (eds) Societal Implications of Nanoscience and Nanotechnology. NSSET Workshop Report, March, 2001. Arlington, VA. Available at: http://www.wtec.org/loyola/nano/NSET.Societal.Implications/nanosi.pdf. Accessed, June 22, 2005

Rossi L (2006) Artificial Lung on the Horizon. Reports University of Pittsburgh Researcher. Available from: http://www.discover.pitt.edu/media/pcc010514/fakelung.html. Accessed January 30, 2006

Zimmer C (2004) Mind over machine. Popular Science, February. Available at: http://www.popsci.com/popsci/medicine/article/0,20967,576464-1,00.html. Accessed January 31, 2005

Chapter 13
Converging NBIC Technologies for Improving Human Performance

A Critical Assessment of the Novelty and the Prospects of the Project[1]

Bert Gordijn

13.1 Introduction

In recent times, optimistic views have been advanced about the convergence of nanotechnology, biotechnology, information technology and cognitive science and the way in which this so-called NBIC convergence could and should be used to enhance human performance (Roco & Bainbridge 2003a, b; Roco & Montemagno 2004a; Roco 2004). These ideas have been elaborately developed and presented in several 'NBIC workshops' in the USA.[2] This contribution focuses on two claims made by the proponents of the NBIC convergence. Firstly, it is argued that the project of "Converging Technologies for Improving Human Performance" represents something genuinely new and quite unique.[3] Secondly, it is maintained that

[1] Reprinted by permission of the American Society of Law, Medicine & Ethics, copyright 2006.

[2] The first of these NBIC workshops was entitled "Converging Technologies for Improving Human Performance". Organized by the National Science Foundation (NSF) and the Department of Commerce (DOC) it was held in December 3–4, 2001 at the NSF in Virginia. The contributions made at this workshop were published in a report with the same title (Roco & Bainbridge 2003c). The second NBIC workshop was held in February 5–7, 2003 in Los Angeles. A selection of this workshop's papers appeared in a second volume (Roco & Montemagno 2004b). Finally, two further NBIC workshops were held in New York City in February 25–27, 2004 and in Kailua-Kona (Hawai) in February 23–25, 2005. As a result further edited volumes focusing on NBIC convergence are to be expected. Quickly after the publication of the first report, the idea of improving human performance by means of NBIC convergence triggered a considerable variety of international critical reactions. In the USA, however, the idea that NBIC convergence should be furthered and used for improving human performance seems to have attained broad acceptance as an inspiring regulative idea within large parts of the nanotechnology community.

[3] For example, the authors claim that "we stand at the threshold of a new renaissance in science and technology" (Roco & Bainbridge 2003b: 1). Moreover, "the sciences have reached a watershed" (Roco & Bainbridge 2003b: 2). There are "paradigm changes" (Roco 2004: 12) and we can expect to see "revolutionary changes in technology, economy, and society, as well as human potential" (Roco 2004: 12). In addition, it is stated that "at this unique moment in the history of technical achievement, *improvement of human performance* becomes possible" (Roco & Bainbridge 2003b: 3). Finally, it is argued that converging technologies will bring about a "turning point in the evolution of human society" (Roco & Bainbridge 2003a: x).

B. Gordijn, R. Chadwick (eds.) *Medical Enhancement and Posthumanity*,

the future prospects of this project are extraordinarily positive.[4] In order to critically assess these two claims I will first focus on the question of whether there is indeed anything genuinely new about the project of improving human performance by means of converging NBIC technologies. Next I will analyze whether the project warrants that we be optimistic about its future prospects.

13.2 Is There Anything New Under the Sun?

What, if anything, is truly new about the project of improving human performance by means of converging NBIC technologies? The notion of improving human performance is itself certainly not a new idea. It has been around since time immemorial.[5] The desire to realize this notion seems to be more or less innate. If it is not the idea of improvement of human performance *per se* that is new, what about the idea of using *science and technology* to improve our performance?

13.2.1 Using Science and Technology for the Improvement of Human Performance

The idea that science and technology can and should be used to enhance human performance was firstly developed in an elaborated manner in the 17th century. Prior to this, science and technology played only a minor role in theorizing about improving human performance, if at all.[6] In the 17th century this situation changed under the influence of rapid developments in the natural sciences and technology. As achievements mounted the idea of using scientific and technological means to enhance human performance gradually emerged. A good example illustrating this new outlook is Francis Bacon's utopian tale *New Atlantis* (1627) where the author unfolds his design for an ideal future society, in which science would assume the position he believed it rightly deserved. In the style of a travel account, Bacon describes how a sea captain discovers an island on which a well-organized scientific

[4] After all, NBIC convergence will enable us to deal with all manner of future challenges by "substantially enhancing human mental, physical, and social abilities" (Roco & Bainbridge 2003b: 3). Moreover, converging technologies will not only initiate "a new renaissance" (Roco & Bainbridge 2003b: 13) but also determine "a tremendous improvement in human abilities, societal outcomes, the nation's productivity, and the quality of life." (Roco 2004: 2). Finally, converging technologies will bring about "world peace, universal prosperity and an evolution to a higher level of compassion and accomplishment" (Roco & Bainbridge 2003b: 6).

[5] Ancient man, for example, operated with the regulative idea of 'becoming like God' (*homoiosis theoi*). This regulative idea originated in the teachings of the Orphic religion.

[6] The Franciscan monk Roger Bacon (1214–1294) was a notable exception. As early as the 13th century he fantasized about ships without oarsmen, wagons that could move by themselves and machines which could fly through the air.

research center of the type necessary for science to progress satisfactorily – according to Bacon's theory of science in *Novum Organum* (1620) – constitutes the central institution. This utopian research community had already mastered many technical instruments for the enhancement of human performance which, at the time of Bacon's Europe, people could only dream about: microscopes, modern weapons, telephones, microphones, steam engines and airships, to name but a few.

In the 18th century, physics, chemistry and biology flourished. Discoveries, new theories and technical inventions were copious. In the course of these developments, optimism regarding the future prospects of using science and technology for the improvement of human performance grew substantially. An interesting representative of this Enlightenment optimism is Marquis de Condorcet. In his work *Esquisse d'un tableau historique des progrès de l'esprit humain* (1795) he describes the benefits and seemingly endless possibilities of enhancement which mankind could hope to reap from scientific progress, especially in the medical field.

Condorcet anticipated current views on the possibilities of using medical knowledge and technology to improve human performance. Presently, these ideas seem to abound. What has drastically changed, however, is the circumstance that they are now linked to real and substantial medical developments and progress. Whereas in the 17th and 18th century, enthusiasm was reserved for theoretical considerations and hypothetical mind games, present euphoria is chiefly directed at real-life research fields.[7] Thus, a true distinction can be made between the hypothetical context of Condorcet and the real possibility of achieving radical improvements of human performance in a 21st century medical technological context. This does not automatically imply that the project of improving human performance by means of converging NBIC technologies has any inherent aspects of novelty or uniqueness. However, this historically new medical technological setting, in which the project is embedded, is certainly relevant when it comes to assessing its possible future impact.

13.2.2 NBIC Convergence

Against the background of the aforementioned historical precedents, neither the notion of improving human performance *per se* nor the idea of using science and technology to improve human performance can be regarded as innovative. The next candidate to lay a claim to novelty is NBIC convergence itself. However, in order to assess this claim caution is appropriate. After all, the *verbatim* expression 'NBIC convergence' may be new, but this does not imply that the idea it refers to is innovative as well. In order to assess the latter claim, it should first be clear what the slogan 'NBIC convergence' exactly means. Unfortunately, the analysis of the concept of NBIC convergence – as presented by its advocates – demonstrates that this notion still lacks sufficient clarity.

[7] See for example Fossel 1996, Kaku 1997, Kurzweil 1999, Schwartz 1998, Silver 1997.

First, it is not clear whether NBIC convergence is primarily regarded in a descriptive manner or whether it is first and foremost viewed from a normative perspective as something desirable that should be actively furthered and promoted.

A second question concerns the specific aspects of the four NBIC provinces of science and technology that are converging or should be converged. Does NBIC convergence – as conceptualized by its advocates – primarily involve: (1) academic research scenes, (2) vocabularies and discourses, (3) epistemological objects of different strands of research, (4) research methods, (5) scientific media (journals, newsletters etc.), (6) aims of different strands of research, (7) theories, or (8) any other aspect of the NBIC provinces of science and technology? As there are many possible answers, it is theoretically conceivable that certain features of the NBIC provinces of science and technology are converging while others are diverging. Moreover, from a normative point of view it might be the case that we should converge only particular characteristics of the NBIC sciences whereas other aspects should be left alone. Yet, the advocates of NBIC convergence fail to make clear what specific kind of convergence they have in mind.

A third question has to do with convincing evidence (be it empirical or theoretical) that might substantiate statements about NBIC convergence. Corroboration of any kind seems to be fundamentally lacking. Sometimes, for example, the proponents of NBIC convergence seem to focus on convergence in the sense of a reduction of theories.[8] However, concrete examples of a reduction of one NBIC theory to another are absent. Also empirical evidence of any kind, for example concerning convergence of research scenes or scientific media, is lacking.

Given these open questions, the concept of NBIC convergence - as thus far presented by its advocates – is still quite nebulous. Therefore, it is difficult to assess the groundbreaking character of this concept.

13.2.3 Cross-Fertilization and Synergism

If the proponents of NBIC convergence wish to hold on to the concept of convergence, a more elaborated and better substantiated version of this concept might mitigate the above-mentioned problems. Alternatively, they might also skip the troublesome concept of convergence and instead focus on 'cross-fertilization' and 'synergism'. These less intricate concepts might be used synonymously in the sense that results in one scientific or technological discipline can reinforce developments in another and vice versa. Unquestionably, the idea of NBIC cross-fertilization or NBIC synergism is more understandable and acceptable than the idea of NBIC

[8] See for example Roco and Bainbridge 2003b: 2, 13. Another proponent of NBIC convergence in the same volume, however, seems to use the word 'convergence' as something that is the direct opposite of reductionism (Canton 2003: 72).

convergence, at least from a descriptive point of view. After all, it is undisputed that scientists from different NBIC disciplines benefit from another's research.[9]

Supposing that 'NBIC convergence' does indeed boil down to cross-fertilization and synergism, the main idea – with both its descriptive and normative dimension – would then be that the existing cross-fertilization and synergism between NBIC disciplines should be further stimulated in order to enhance human performance. However, if this were indeed a sound interpretation of the ideas of the proponents of NBIC convergence, neither the phenomenon of 'NBIC convergence' nor the idea could be regarded as genuinely groundbreaking. After all, throughout history there have been many periods of cross-fertilization and synergism between different technological or scientific disciplines. In addition, the general idea that cross-fertilization and synergism between different domains of human activity – be they primarily scientific, technological, political, cultural or commercial – should be stimulated to maximize results is quite commonplace. Accordingly, several authors have argued that improved human performance might be achieved by means of cross-fertilization or synergism of different scientific or technological fields.[10]

13.2.4 Technological Transformation of Human Beings

Although the concepts of improving human performance (*per se* or by means of science and technology) and synergism of the four component technologies are not of themselves truly innovative, this does not mean that the NBIC project has no novel dimension whatsoever. Rather the aspect of novelty appears to be hidden in the way proponents of NBIC convergence intend to achieve improved human performance, i.e. by technologically reshaping ourselves.

Up to now we have been improving our performance through education, study and exercise. Furthermore, we developed houses, clothes and of all manner of technological instruments like telephones, telescopes, cars and computers, thus technologically transforming our natural surroundings to serve the improvement of our performance.

In addition to these traditional ways of improving performance the proponents of NBIC convergence now advocate that we start improving our performance by technologically transforming our own blueprint. Of course, we have already taken

---

[9] There are several well-known examples of cross-fertilization or synergism between NBIC disciplines. For example, progress in computing has enabled the rapid sequencing of the human genome as well as the swift development of new neuroimaging technologies. Vice versa, progress in genetics and neuroscience is stimulating computer science by furthering the development of DNA computers and artificial neural networks.

[10] Lee Silver, for example, coined the word 'reprogenetics', a discipline based upon the cross-fertilization and synergism between the traditional fields of reproduction medicine and genetics. He assumes that in the nearby future reprogenetics will enable many new options (for example by means of germ line interventions) for the enhancement of human performance (Silver 1997). Apart from that, the specific idea of NBIC synergy seems to have been clearly anticipated in Antón et al. 2001.

first cautious steps to technologically reshape ourselves, for example by means of cosmetic surgery and dentistry, smart drugs, mood enhancers, sports doping and growth hormones. Yet, the outlook of the proponents of NBIC convergence fundamentally diverges from past practice and experience. In the dominant view of the current medical establishment, enhancement by means of technological transformation is still seen as relatively peripheral and highly ambivalent. In the NBIC convergence program, on the other hand, it is esteemed as something pivotal and highly positive. Moreover, the kind of medico-technological auto transformation that is advocated by the proponents of NBIC convergence has a more drastic dimension. It involves radically transforming ourselves in order to improve our sensory, motorial and cognitive skills and abilities.

After all, they propose the use of brain-to-brain interaction and brain-machine interfaces (using direct connections to our neural system). Furthermore, we are to have new organs, new skills and new genes (Roco & Bainbridge 2003b: 7). With an information-gulping sixth sense, for example, we might be able to instantaneously gulp down the information of an entire book making it a structural part of our wetware "ready for inferencing, reference, etc., with some residual sense of the whole, as part of the gulp experience" (Spohrer 2003: 110). If these future prospects of 'NBIC convergence' come true, we will be entering a genuinely new Age which will bear witness to pervasive use of NBIC sciences and technologies to transform our biological design for the purpose of enhancing performance.

13.3 Should We Be Optimistic?

At this early stage it is not easy to say just where the project of improving human performance by means of NBIC technologies will lead. However, let us suppose – for the sake of the discussion – that future developments in NBIC sciences and technologies will indeed enable us to reshape our biological design, just as the advocates of NBIC convergence envision.

It is incontestable that some enhancements of our design might turn out to have genuinely valuable effects. At first sight, it is not difficult to imagine a plethora of positive aspects attached to having better sensory, motorial and cognitive skills and abilities. Yet, it seems likely that there may be also negative consequences that emerge in proportion to the magnitude of the adjustments and modifications that are introduced through NBIC.

13.3.1 Changing Attitudes Towards the Body

Widespread use of NBIC enabled enhancement technologies will result in an increasingly close association of the body with technology, which could trigger a negative change in attitudes towards the body. Firstly, the body and its functions will more and more become a product of technology. In the future, for example, complete warehouses of NBIC manufactured biohybrid replacement cells; tissue and organs (possibly even better than the originals) could perhaps be set up. Hence, those who could afford them could purchase replacement body parts whenever they needed anything. Furthermore, bioelectronic systems to improve normal sensory, motorial and cognitive properties and skills will become increasingly common practice. Widespread and invasive use of such bioelectronic systems that will enhance central bodily functions will make it increasingly difficult to distinguish between our body's own functions and technology's functions.

Secondly, the body will progressively become a part of technological systems and networks. For instance, the body and its functions might constantly be checked and monitored with the help of nanosensors registering all manner of emerging health threats. These detecting gadgets might be linked with computer systems enabling automatic responses for a broad variety of common disorders and ailments (for instance by activating certain nanometric drug release systems).

Both developments will contribute to a more technologically inspired image of the body as something very similar to a machine. The body will increasingly be regarded as a whole, made up of many different components that might be fixed, enhanced or replaced if necessary. Development, functions and appearance of the body will be seeming less and less fixed by nature and to be accepted without change, and more and more controllable by technology. Instead of feeling in charge to see after our own health we might increasingly trust technology to take over this responsibility. In the process however, the body will be treated almost like the inanimate material of a machine. Hence, the body might become increasingly de-hallowed and de-mystified.

13.3.2 Privacy and Autonomy

NBIC enabled technological enhancement of the human body and its functions might seriously infringe autonomy and privacy. Standard use of neuro-implants to improve cognitive ability in human beings might further intensify their links to computers, especially when contact to diverse databases would no longer be made via the fingers on a computer keyboard, but directly via the brain, which would be permanently connected to selected databases. In addition, neuro-implants might also facilitate intensive links to other human beings by establishing brain-to-brain interfaces. Communication with geographically remote people would then be permanently given via a direct link from brain to brain.[11] The proponents of NBIC

---

[11] Direct links from brain to brain would depend upon a greatly improved understanding of how thoughts are formulated in the brain. Otherwise every interface would be through the senses (i.e. one might see scrolling in front of their eyes, a download of information, but this would need to be read as with any other visual data).

convergence even speculate about humanity becoming "like a single, distributed and interconnected brain" by the end of this century (Roco & Bainbridge 2003b: 6). They expect that this will mean "an enhancement to the productivity and independence of individuals" (Roco & Bainbridge 2003b: 6).

However, various side effects are conceivable in conjunction with these applications which would facilitate easy access to the privacy of other human beings. The digital fragments left over every time a computer is used could help to retrace and register the exact movements and actions of any individual. Furthermore, the excessive networking of human brains would enable their visual impressions to be registered, their thoughts to be recorded and so on. At any one time a selected individual could thus be localized and registered in a broad variety of respects – including his "inner life". Easy access to all areas of human privacy, even the most intimate, would then pave the way to subtle manipulating and control. For example, direct networking of human brains would mean that human beings could receive – and subconsciously be influenced by – all manner of subliminal information. Thus, excessive networking of human brains might facilitate mass deceptions by a central agent. This would not only infringe upon people's privacy, but also upon their autonomy.

13.3.3 Medicalization

Widespread NBIC interventions to enhance sensory, motorial and cognitive ability as well as our physical appearance could be accompanied by the problem of medicalization. It is quite probable that once a certain number of people have undergone enhancing interventions, others would feel themselves under increasing pressure to do likewise. Without such interventions they might fear not being able to keep up with the growing number of enhanced individuals around them. In time, the attitude could become ingrained that in order to be successful in life one has to submit one's body to all manner of enhancing interventions available. As a result, attitudes towards conventional human abilities could change quite negatively. Average abilities could become almost akin to defects, in need of elimination. People could become afraid that their bodies and skills are fundamentally inadequate. As a result, enhancement interventions could trigger a process of medicalization of thus far absolutely ordinary functioning human abilities and normal physical appearances.

13.3.4 Personal Identity

When a human being thinks about his own person, he particularly examines issues such as: What am I good at? How do I perform? Do I act responsibly? What is my particular character? What makes me unique? What can I remember? What is my life history? If a human being were regularly subjected to new NBIC-enabled technological interventions to improve his sensory, motorial or cognitive abilities, it could become increasingly difficult to answer such questions. Improving the cognitive abilities of an individual, for example, could mean that certain of his own mental efforts almost cease, becoming extremely dependent on high-performance implants. As a result, that individual human being might find it increasingly difficult to say which of his thoughts and actions still constitute a *personal* achievement. Thus, it is difficult to foretell whether our satisfaction with our NBIC-enabled higher achievements will be increased, or whether our expectations will merely shift to the right.

If not only cognitive, but also emotional enhancement systems were to become available for implantation, it might become increasingly difficult to determine the characteristics specific to an individual. If, in addition, many different people were to share the possibility of being permanently connected to databases, the exclusiveness of possessing particular information would become relative, which in turn would reduce the uniqueness of those people.

Implantation of brain-to-brain communication systems – which would 'wire up' different individuals to enable them to instantaneously exchange their conscious thoughts and experiences – could blur the borderline between the self and the cyberthink community. In the face of such mental wiring, how are one's own thoughts and experiences and life history to be kept separate from those of others? And the borders between the real world and the virtual world would become increasingly blurred. As a result, it would become more and more difficult to determine one's own personal identity.

13.3.5 Blurred Self-Perception as a Human Being

Widespread and frequent use of NBIC technologies to enhance our biological design will make the symbiosis between man and technology increasingly narrower. We would not only become more and more embedded in all manner of technological systems and networks. Our bodies themselves would increasingly become a product of technology. This process can be referred to as 'artifactualization' of human beings.

This process of artifactualization will most probably be accompanied by a second process that is likely to be stimulated by future NBIC progress: technological systems will increasingly be developed along the lines of organic systems. This is already happening in the fields of artificial intelligence, artificial life, robotics and neural computing networks, to name just a few examples. In the long term it is hoped that certain technological systems will be able to imitate various human traits or skills. This process can be termed an 'anthropomorphization' of technology.

The combination of these two processes, the artifactualization of human beings and the anthropomorphization of technology, could in the long term lead to the following problem: pairs of opposites which have been around for hundreds of years, like 'nature – culture', 'organic – inorganic', 'conscious – unconscious' and 'living – non living' could become fundamentally nebulous. And yet for a very long time such pairs of opposites have represented essential elements within human self-perception. Their growing fuzziness or even disappearance would necessitate fundamental changes in human self-perception to fit the new situation. All in all, the increasing confusion and the fundamental changes in connection with human self-perception might give rise to feelings of uneasiness, creeping disorientation and even existential panic. The very foundations of our image of mankind are shaken.

13.4 Outlook

Genuinely groundbreaking in the project of improving human performance by means of converging NBIC technologies is the way its proponents intend to achieve improved human performance, i.e. by technologically reshaping ourselves. If the NBIC program were to be carried out to its extreme, it might in time come up with highly sophisticated and drastic enhancement technologies that could change man so radically that we could no longer speak of human beings in the conventional sense. In recent times, the prospect of mankind transforming into a posthuman race has increasingly led to widespread enthusiasm. Various movements propagating a complete surmounting of human nature already exist. Quite obviously, the mere idea of some kind of radical transformation from a human to a posthuman existence is enough to inspire huge enthusiasm.

Enthusiasm alone is not a guarantee of ethical desirability, however. This contribution's analysis has demonstrated that transforming and enhancing our biological design has seriously troublesome features. Therefore, a profound ethical debate seems advisable. Only a continued prospective painting of existing NBIC research trends, followed by an ethical analysis of their various aspects and consequences, can facilitate advance regulative intervention – in accordance with the ethical insights gained. In addition, anticipative ethical analysis appears to be especially indicated when – as is the case with the development and application of NBIC technologies to enhance human performance – further developments could have far-reaching consequences for mankind. Especially in cases such as these, ethical reflection should not wait until research is completed and findings are clearly revealed in practice.

References

Antón P S, Siberglitt R, Schneider J (2001) The Global Technology Revolution. Bio/Nano/Materials Trends and Their Synergies with Information Technology by 2015. RAND, Santa Monica, CA/Arlington, VA. Available at http://www.rand.org

Canton J (2003) The Impact of Convergent Technologies and the Future of Business and the Economy. In: Roco M C, Bainbridge W S (eds) NBIC Convergence for Improving Human Performance. Nanotechnology, Biotechnology, Information Technology and Cognitive Science. Kluwer, Dordrecht, The Netherlands/Boston, MA/London: 71–78

Fossel M (1996) Reversing Human Aging. William Morrow, New York
Kaku M (1997) Visions. How Science Will Revolutionize the 21st Century. Anchor Books/ Doubleday, New York
Kurzweil R (1999) The Age of Spiritual Machines. When Computers Exceed Human Intelligence. Viking, New York
Roco M C (2004) Science and Technology Integration for Increased Human Potential and Societal Outcomes. In: Roco M C, Montemagno C D (eds) The Coevolution of Human Potential and Converging Technologies. Annals of the New York Academy of Sciences, vol 1013. New York Academy of Sciences, New York. Availabe at: http://www.annalsnyas.org: 1–16
Roco M C, Bainbridge W S (2003a) Executive Summary. In: Roco M C, Bainbridge W S (eds) NBIC Convergence for Improving Human Performance. Nanotechnology, Biotechnology, Information Technology and Cognitive Science. Kluwer, Dordrecht, The Netherlands/Boston, MA/London: ix–xiii
Roco M C, Bainbridge W S (2003b) Overview. Converging Technologies for Improving Human Performance. Nanotechnology, Biotechnology, Information Technology and Cognitive Science (NBIC). In: Roco M C, Bainbridge W S (eds) NBIC Convergence for Improving Human Performance. Nanotechnology, Biotechnology, Information Technology and Cognitive Science. Kluwer, Dordrecht, The Netherlands/Boston, MA/London: 1–27
Roco M C, Bainbridge W S (2003c) (eds) NBIC Convergence for Improving Human Performance. Nanotechnology, Biotechnology, Information Technology and Cognitive Science. Kluwer, Dordrecht, The Netherlands/Boston, MA/London
Roco M C, Montemagno C D (2004a) Preface. In: Roco M C, Montemagno C D (eds) The Coevolution of Human Potential and Converging Technologies. Annals of the New York Academy of Sciences, vol 1013. New York Academy of Sciences, New York. Available at: http://www.annalsnyas.org: vii–viii
Roco M C, Montemagno C D (2004b) (eds) The Coevolution of Human Potential and Converging Technologies. Annals of the New York Academy of Sciences, vol 1013. New York Academy of Sciences, New York. Available at: http://www.annalsnyas.org
Schwartz W B (1998) Life Without Disease. The Pursuit of Medical Utopia. University of California Press, Berkeley, CA/Los Angeles, CA/London
Silver L M (1997) Remaking Eden. Cloning and Beyond in a Brave New World. Avon Books, New York
Spohrer J (2003) NBICS (Nano-Bio-Info-Cogno-Socio) Convergence to Improve Human Performance: Opportunities and Challenges. In: Roco M C, Bainbridge W S (eds) NBIC Convergence for Improving Human Performance. Nanotechnology, Biotechnology, Information Technology and Cognitive Science. Kluwer, Dordrecht, The Netherlands/Boston, MA/London: 101–117

Afterword
Advancing Posthuman Enhancement Dialogue[1]

Michael J. Selgelid

The preceding chapters shed light on the history of human enhancement and human strivings toward transcendence; the conceptual meanings of human enhancement, posthumanity, human nature, identity, and so on; and reasons for thinking that human enhancement and/or posthumanity are, ethically speaking, things we should pursue or avoid. The collection as a whole furthermore highlights important *interconnections between* the history, meaning, and ethics of human enhancement and the pursuit of posthumanity. Human enhancement and strivings towards posthumanity are not altogether new, but their meanings and methods have changed with time and technology – sometimes in radical ways. Ethical conclusions about "enhancement" or "posthumanity" should importantly depend on both the *meanings* of such things and the *methods* used in their pursuit. The lessons of history should, finally, inform normative judgments and policy decisions that need to be made both now and in the future. We should not underestimate the value of further examining the interconnections between historical, conceptual, and ethical issues revealed in this book. These relationships are complex, so we here have our work cut out for us.

The social consequences of a future consisting of "posthumans" that are different species (i.e., that cannot reproduce with human beings), for example, could be quite different from one where "posthumans" merely have (one or more) powers that surpass those of current humans; and social consequences will also depend on whether or not the posthuman powers we are talking about are made available (or actually provided) to everyone. We must be clear about what we are talking about before we can say whether or not provision of "posthuman" powers would be good or permissible. Otherwise, parties to the debate risk talking past one another. To transhumanists arguing that one kind of posthumanity could be a good thing, a response to the effect that another kind of posthumanity would be a bad thing misses its mark – if the aim was to refute the transhumanist vision being responded to. Though it may not be sufficient to resolve posthuman enhancement debates on its own, the (conceptual) clarity of analytic philosophy is essential for rational dialogue.

[1] The author thanks the Brocher Foundation in Hermance, and the Institute for Biomedical Ethics at the University of Geneva, in Switzerland, for hosting him as a visiting scholar and supporting his research on this topic during the first half of 2007.

B. Gordijn, R. Chadwick (eds.) *Medical Enhancement and Posthumanity*,

Further debate about posthuman enhancement, however, requires more than conceptual clarity and historically informed thinking. The papers in this volume reveal that the meaning, consequences, and ethics of enhancement largely (though not entirely) turn on key empirical questions. Is it likely that any given enhancement technology will actually be safe and effective? What will the actual benefits and costs (including opportunity costs) of particular technological advancements be? To what extent could such technologies extend our capacities? In what ways, if any, will posthumans themselves be limited? How would social relations actually be affected under different scenarios where lifespans are extended by different amounts (in different ways)? If super intelligent rational posthumans were or were not to become different species, then how would they treat the merely human? How confused would posthuman cyborgs' identities be – and how much would that bother them? What are the magnitudes of gains and losses of utility, equality, and liberty to be expected under various enhancement policy scenarios? How efficient/effective would various forms of regulation be? Whether or not a particular path of enhancement will actually be a good thing – and whether or not it should be forbidden, permitted, or required – will often depend on answers to questions like these.

Though the answers to such questions about the future will inevitably remain uncertain, we should address them as best as we can. Progress will here require more empirical study. In addition to science and history, other social science disciplines such as psychology, sociology, anthropology, politics and economics must play a larger role. A better division of intellectual labour is needed. Philosophers should more explicitly identify the empirical questions that the ethical questions turn on; and, when they lack special expertise for answering such questions themselves, they should seek more input from other disciplines. Philosophy may then come back in to provide ethical analysis of empirical findings. The central inclusion of historical analysis in the organization of this volume is a step in the right direction; this general kind of approach should be expanded in the future. In one respect, then, debates about enhancement and posthumanity will advance when philosophy attempts to do less, and when other disciplines do more, of the work required for ethical analysis and policymaking.

In other respects philosophy itself needs to do more – and I here point to the need for theoretical work of the deepest kind. The main political philosophy frameworks currently on the table may not be up to the job of resolving the policy questions raised in this volume even if we had more solid answers to the empirical questions at stake. I refer to the problem of conflicting values and the lack of a well developed theory for striking a balance between them. It is not altogether implausible, for example, that the path to enhancement would in fact (perhaps severely) promote inequality. Let's assume that a well-informed empirical analysis indicates that this will likely be the case. The big question then, from a policy standpoint, is how the goal to promote liberty should be balanced against the goal to promote equality. On the one hand, one might think that individuals should have liberty to benefit themselves and their children; but, on the other hand, equality and utility matter too.

I would guess that most philosophers, policy makers, and citizens would deny that liberty, equality, or utility should always take priority over the others, regardless of the extent to which the others are threatened. Citizens of modern democratic countries generally accept that tradeoffs should be made between such things,[2] but the elephant in the room that no one mentions is the lack of a well developed philosophical framework for making such tradeoffs in practice. How much equality, for example, should we be willing to sacrifice for a given amount of liberty, or vice versa? Each of the three main strands of political philosophy – libertarianism, (Rawlsian) egalitarianism, and utilitarianism – places extreme weight on the specific value it emphasizes. It is plausible to think that (and I would guess that most philosophers, policy makers and citizens would upon reflection agree that)[3] that each of these theoretical perspectives is partly accurate – because the things they emphasize (i.e. liberty, equality, and utility) matter. But it is also quite plausible to think that (and I would guess that most would upon reflection agree that) each of these views is partly wrong – because they place too much weight on the values they emphasize.[4] If this is correct, then we need a fourth – more moderate and pluralistic – theoretical framework that provides a principled wa y to strike a balance between liberty, equality, and utility.[5] Philosophically speaking, this is much to ask for – especially in light of the apparent incommensurabilities involved. Be that as it may, progress in debates over posthuman enhancement will require philosophical advancement in this direction.

As others have recently noted, the enhancement debate also indicates the importance of further research on questions about "quality of life" or well-being (Savulescu 2006). If enhancement involves making lives better, the question of what constitutes improvement is paramount. Is quality of life ultimately constituted by happiness (conceived as pleasure), preference satisfaction, or autonomy; or some combination of these, and perhaps also other, things (see Brock 1993; Kitcher 1996)? Insofar as social policy should be influenced by utilitarian considerations (i.e. measures of aggregate and/or average well-being), whose conception of well being should come into play? Again, these are philosophically challenging questions.

Debate about enhancement has grown steadily and gathered much momentum since the beginning of the millennium; and it is safe to say that the literature has now (at the time of this writing in 2007) reached a critical mass. The papers in this volume reveal that much progress has been made. Further advancement of posthuman enhancement dialogue requires both more empirical input from other disciplines and major developments in philosophical theory.

---

[2] Liberal democracies, for example, generally employ progressive taxation – which involves tradeoffs between equality and (negative) liberty.

[3] This kind of claim of course itself warrants empirical study.

[4] The suggestion that each of the three frameworks is partly flawed goes a long way towards explaining why there is debate (between libertarians, egalitarians, and utilitarians) to begin with – and why it has lasted so long. There are powerful counterexamples to each of the three main theories.

[5] For more on moderate pluralism see Selgelid (2002). Also see Sen (1999).

References

Brock D (1993) Quality of Life Measures in Health Care and Medical Ethics. In: Brock D, Life and Death. Cambridge University Press, New York
Kitcher P (1996) The Lives to Come. Simon & Schuster, New York
Savulescu J (2006) What Is an Enhancement and When Should We Enhance People? Enhancing Human Capacities: Ethics, Regulation, and European Policy, Conference held in association with the 8th World Congress of the International Association of Bioethics, 5 August, Beijing
Selgelid M J (2002) Societal Decision Making and the New Eugenics. Grey Series of the European Academy (Europaische Akademie) for the Study of Consequences of Scientific and Technological Advance, Bad Neuenahr-Ahrweiler GmbH, Germany 30. Available at: http://www.ea-aw.de/fileadmin/downloads/Graue_Reihe/GR_30_Eugenics_042002.pdf
Sen A (1999) Development as Freedom. Anchor Books, New York

Kolibri 360 GmbH
Ferdinand-Jühlke-Straße 7
99095 Erfurt, Deutschland
produktsicherheit@kolibri360.de